Pediatric Procedural Sedation and Analgesia

Edited by

Baruch Krauss, MD, EdM, FAAP
Instructor in Pediatrics
Harvard Medical School
Division of Emergency Medicine
Children's Hospital
Boston, Massachusetts

Associate Editor

Robert M. Brustowicz, MD, FACMQ
Assistant Professor of Anaesthesia
Harvard Medical School
Medical Director of the Autotransfusion Service and
Senior Associate in Anesthesia
Children's Hospital
Boston, Massachusetts

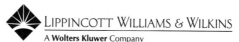

LIPPINCOTT WILLIAMS & WILKINS
A **Wolters Kluwer** Company
Philadelphia · Baltimore · New York · London
Buenos Aires · Hong Kong · Sydney · Tokyo

Editor: Elizabeth Greenspan
Managing Editor: Tanya Lazar
Marketing Manager: Katie Rubin
Project Editor: Paula C. Williams

Copyright © 1999 Lippincott Williams & Wilkins

351 West Camden Street
Baltimore, Maryland 21201-2436 USA

227 East Washington Square
Philadelphia, PA 19106

Printed in the United States of America

Library of Congress Cataloging-in-Publication Data

Pediatric procedural sedation and analgesia / edited by Baruch Krauss;
   associate editor, Robert M. Brustowicz.
         p.   cm.
   Includes bibliographical references and index.
   ISBN 0-683-30558-1
   1. Pediatric anesthesia.   I. Krauss, Baruch.   II. Brustowicz,
Robert M.
   [DNLM: 1. Conscious Sedation—in infancy & childhood.
   2. Analgesia—in infancy & childhood.   3. Analgesics—pharmacology.
   4. Hypnotics and Sedatives—pharmacology.   5. Surgical Procedures,
   Minor—in infancy & childhood. WO 440 P3714 1999]
   RD139.P435   1999
   617.9′6′083—dc21
   DNLM/DLC
   for Library of Congress   99-10331
                                                                      CIP

To purchase additional copies of this book, call our customer service department at **(800) 638–3030** or fax orders to **(301) 824–7390**. International customers should call **(301) 714–2324**.

99 00 01 02 03
1 2 3 4 5 6 7 8 9 10

For Dana, Benjamin, and Jeremy

(BK)

To my wife Barbara,

and my children,

Alex, Katherine,

Caroline, and Allison

(RMB)

Foreword

As a rule, a great book should never put anyone to sleep, but this text is an exception. If you follow the guidelines provided by the authors and you have the appropriate skills and equipment, you will be able to perform potentially painful procedures on patients who, while not under general anesthesia, will not be fully awake. Even more importantly, you will understand the physiology and pharmacology of the process in detail.

Drs. Krauss and Brustowicz have assembled a superb group of physicians, drawn primarily from both emergency medicine and anesthesiology, to provide a practical but scientifically grounded approach to procedural sedation in pediatrics. While they are not the first to address the topic of pediatric sedation, we believe they have made a unique contribution. Earlier works have often either been limited to offering a few simple pharmacological formulas or have been oriented to the milieu of the surgical amphitheater. In this text, Drs. Krauss and Brustowicz expand upon an appropriately detailed scientific foundation to build a practical approach to procedural sedation for any specialist, geared specifically for multipurpose environments that differ dramatically from the operating suite. Physicians in every discipline, whether novices or experienced practitioners, will benefit from their wisdom. On the one hand, emergency physicians, pediatricians, and family physicians should find a wealth of previously unexplored knowledge about physiology and pharmacology, which will enable them to expand their armamentarium and deliver sedatives in the safest possible fashion. On the other hand, many anesthesiologists will enjoy a fuller understanding of the demands of and the available options for sedation of acutely ill and injured patients in diverse settings.

We congratulate Drs. Krauss and Brustowicz for their timing and their foresight. For many reasons, the turn of the millennium calls for a book on pediatric procedural sedation. Consumer demand and growing expertise among many specialists have increased the frequency with which procedural sedation is administered and will continue to drive this trend. Yet the quality of the practice has not always kept pace with the rapid advances in the science, creating an opportunity for this book to fill the void. Additionally, we think Drs. Krauss and Brustowicz have shown great foresight in drawing upon the talent available in anesthesiology, pediatric emergency medicine, emergency medicine, and pediatrics. As is usually the case when individuals from diverse backgrounds join together, the whole is greater than the sum of the parts.

Gary R. Fleisher, MD, FACEP, FAAP
Professor of Pediatrics
Harvard Medical School
Chief, Division of Emergency Medicine
Children's Hospital
Boston, Massachusetts

Paul R. Hickey, MD
Professor of Anaesthesia
Harvard Medical School
Chairman, Department of Anaesthesia
Children's Hospital
Boston, Massachusetts

Preface

Baruch Krauss, MD, Robert M. Brustowicz, MD*
Boston, Massachusetts

The specialties of anesthesiology and emergency medicine have played a major role in the development of the field of pediatric procedural sedation.* Neonatal pain research by anesthesiologists in the mid 1980s establishing that neonates have the neurophysiologic apparatus to experience pain created an ethical imperative to recognize and treat pain in infants and children. At the same time, emergency physicians were beginning to perform nonelective procedures aided by anesthesia technology newly available in the outpatient setting.

Since that time, pediatric procedural sedation has developed into a unique discipline practiced in multiple outpatient settings by a variety of specialists. These include anesthesiologists providing pediatric procedural sedation outside of the traditional operative setting; adult and pediatric emergency physicians and nurses practicing in community hospitals and tertiary-care centers; general pediatricians and family practitioners in office or clinic practice; orthopedic, general, and plastic surgeons whose patients frequently require pediatric procedural sedation; radiologists in hospitals or free-standing imaging centers; gastroenterologists in endoscopy suites; and dentists in hospital and office-based practice.

In spite of the strong interest in and practice of pediatric procedural sedation, there has been no single text focused exclusively on this topic. Our goal was to produce a concise, practically oriented reference with individualized sedation recommendations and management guidelines for all nonelective procedures. This book is intended to be used by physicians as a quick reference guide for urgent patient care as well as a resource containing all the practical information relevant to pedi-

---

*"A technique of administering sedatives or dissociative agents with or without analgesics to induce a state that allows the patient to tolerate unpleasant procedures while maintaining cardiorespiratory function. Procedural sedation and analgesia is intended to result in a depressed level of consciousness but one that allows the patient to maintain airway control independently and continuously. Specifically, the drugs, doses, and techniques used are not likely to produce a loss of protective airway reflexes." (American College of Emergency Physicians. Clinical policy for procedural sedation and analgesia in the emergency department. Ann Emerg Med 1998;31:663–677.)

ix

atric procedural sedation. We used an evidence-based approach for each topic, reviewing the existing literature, starting with the original studies, especially in areas of controversy where differing recommendations existed. The final product represents our interpretation of the science found in the medical literature. As our knowledge base grows, undoubtedly some of the recommendations will change.

This book represents the first interdisciplinary effort in the field of pediatric procedural sedation between the specialties of anesthesiology and emergency medicine. Both specialties share a common foundation of skills in resuscitation, airway management, vascular access, and pharmacology. It is our belief that there is much to be gained from an exchange of ideas and information between our two specialties in the field of pediatric procedural sedation.

The book is divided into three parts. Part I provides a focused review of the physiology and pharmacology of pediatric procedural sedation, an in-depth discussion of individual agents used in pediatric procedural sedation, and guidelines for monitoring sedated patients. Part II describes the principles and management strategies for pediatric procedural sedation as applied to selected outpatient settings and for specific patient populations and includes guidelines for preparation, management, and discharge of sedated patients. Part III addresses the practical aspects of providing pediatric procedural sedation for nonelective procedures with individualized management guidelines for each procedure.

The principles that define our approach to pediatric procedural sedation, especially in regard to Part III, are listed below.

- If the risks of pharmacologic management outweigh the benefits in a given situation, then other means to control the patient (e.g., immobilization, general anesthesia in the operating room, or postponing the procedure if it is not emergent) should be used.
- All procedures should be done with the lowest level of sedation/analgesia possible.
- Multiple sedation/analgesia options are presented for each procedure to take into account the wide variation in approaches to pharmacologic management. There are a complex set of variables in children (discussed in detail in Part III) that must be assessed before each sedation so that the pharmacologic management is patient and procedure specific.
- When multiple sedation/analgesia options exist for a given procedure, the routes of administration are listed in the figures/tables in order of increasing levels of sedation (beginning with the noninvasive routes and ending with invasive routes capable of producing profound sedation/analgesia) and *are not listed in order of preference*. Therefore, an intravenous option may be the most appropriate choice but will still be listed last by design.

Space constraints in this edition limited our ability to sufficiently cover the following topics: rectal, transmucosal, and subcutaneous routes of administration;

nonpharmacologic interventions for acute anxiety and pain; analgesia for the patients with an acute surgical abdomen; rapid tranquilization; analgesia in the prehospital setting; and the combination agent Demerol/Phenergan/Thorazine.

We would also like to suggest another use for this text. Many anesthesiologists will be responsible for working with other departments within their institutions in establishing uniform standards for sedating patients and credentialing practitioners. This book can be used as a guide for the practitioner who may not have significant experience in these areas.

We hope that this text will enhance the overall safety of pediatric procedural sedation for all pediatric patients and serve to strengthen the ongoing collaboration between anesthesiologists and emergency physicians in pediatric procedural sedation.

Acknowledgments

We would like to thank our mentors
Gary Fleisher, Paul Hickey, and Mark Rockoff
for support and guidance and
Cindy Chow and Andrea Stephenson
for their invaluable secretarial help.

Contributors

Richard Bachur, MD, FAAP
Instructor in Pediatrics
Harvard Medical School
Division of Emergency Medicine
Children's Hospital
Boston, Massachusetts

Brian Bates, MD, FAAP
Clinical Assistant Professor of
    Pediatrics
University of Texas Health Science
Director of Children's Emergency
    Center
Methodist Women's and Children's
    Hospital
San Antonio, Texas

Kathleen Brown, MD
Assistant Professor of Emergency
    Medicine and Pediatrics
State University of New York at
    Syracuse
Syracuse, New York

Robert Brustowicz, MD, FACMQ
Assistant Professor of Anaesthesia
Harvard Medical School
Medical Director of the
    Autotransfusion Service and
Senior Associate in Anesthesia
Children's Hospital
Boston, Massachusetts

John Burton, MD, FACEP
Assistant Residency Director
Department of Emergency
    Medicine
Maine Medical Center
Portland, Maine

Carl Chudnofsky, MD, FACEP
Assistant Professor
University of Michigan
Ann Arbor, Michigan
Chairman, Department of
    Emergency Medicine
Hurley Medical Center
Flint, Michigan

Fran Damian, RN, MS
Director of Nursing and Patient
    Services
Division of Emergency
    Medicine
Children's Hospital
Boston, Massachusetts

Alan Doctor, MD, FACEP
Clinical Fellow in Anaesthesia
Harvard Medical School
Fellow in Critical Care
Children's Hospital
Boston, Massachusetts

Joel Fein, MD, FAAP
Associate Professor of Pediatrics
University of Pennsylvania School of
  Medicine
Division of Emergency Medicine
Children's Hospital
Philadelphia, Pennsylvania

**Michael Gerardi, MD, FACEP,
  FAAP**
Clinical Assistant Professor of Medicine
University of Medicine and Dentistry
  of New Jersey
Director of Pediatric Emergency
  Medicine
Children's Medical Center
Atlantic Health System
Livingston, New Jersey

Steven Green, MD, FACEP
Professor of Emergency Medicine
Loma Linda University School of
  Medicine
Director of the Emergency Medicine
  Residency Program
Loma Linda University Medical Center
Loma Linda, California

David Greenes, MD, FAAP
Instructor in Pediatrics
Harvard Medical School
Division of Emergency Medicine
Children's Hospital
Boston, Massachusetts

Kristine Henderson, MD
President, Bayou Anesthesia
  Associates
Fort Walton Beach Medical Center
Fort Walton, Florida

Constance Houck, MD
Instructor of Pediatric Anaesthesia
Harvard Medical School
Associate in Anesthesia
Children's Hospital
Boston, Massachusetts

Grant Innes, MD
Clinical Assistant Professor of
  Emergency Medicine
University of British Columbia
Department of Emergency
St. Paul Hospital
Vancouver, British Columbia

David Jaffe, MD, FAAP
Associate Professor of Pediatrics
Washington University School of
  Medicine
Chief, Division of Emergency
  Medicine
St. Louis Children's Hospital
St. Louis, Missouri

Mark Joffe, MD, FAAP
Associate Professor of Pediatrics
University of Pennsylvania School of
  Medicine
Division of Emergency Medicine
Children's Hospital
Philadelphia, Pennsylvania

Robert Kennedy, MD, FAAP
Associate Professor of Pediatrics
Washington University School of
  Medicine
Division of Emergency Medicine
Children's Hospital
St. Louis, Missouri

Babu Koka, MD
Assistant Professor of Anaesthesia
Harvard Medical School
Clinical Director of Anesthesia and
  Senior Associate in Anesthesia
Children's Hospital
Boston, Massachusetts

Baruch Krauss, MD, EdM, FAAP
Instructor in Pediatrics
Harvard Medical School
Division of Emergency Medicine
Children's Hospital
Boston, Massachusetts

William Levin, MD, FACEP
Assistant Professor of Medicine
New Medical College
Attending Physician Otolaryngology,
  Head and Neck Surgery
New York Eye and Ear Infirmary
New York, New York

Ronald Litman, DO
Associate Professor of Anesthesiology
  and Pediatrics
University of Rochester School of
  Medicine and Dentistry
Strong Memorial Hospital
Rochester, New York

Tamiko Long, MD
Auxillary Faculty
University of Utah
Primary Children's Medical Center
Salt Lake City, Utah

Shobha Malviya, MD
Assistant Professor of
  Anesthesiology
Director, Pediatric Pain Service
University of Michigan Health
  Systems
Ann Arbor, Michigan

Keira Mason, MD
Instructor of Anesthesia
Harvard Medical School
Director of Radiology Anesthesia
Children's Hospital
Boston, Massachusetts

Alejandro Mondolfi, MD
Department of Pediatrics
Centro Medico Docente La Trinidad
Caracas, Venezuela

Howard Needleman, DMD
Clinical Professor in Pediatric
  Dentistry
Harvard Dental Medical School
Associate Dentist-in-Chief
Children's Hospital
Boston, Massachusetts

Douglas Nelson, MD, FAAP
Associate Professor of Pediatrics
University of Utah
Section of Emergency Medicine
Primary Children Medical Center
Salt Lake City, Utah

Leila Mei Pang, MD
Associate Professor of Pediatrics
Division of Pediatric
  Anesthesia and Intensive Care
College of Physicians and Surgeons
  of Columbia University
Babies Hospital
New York, New York

Holly Perry, MD
Assistant Professor of Pediatrics
University of Connecticut Medical
  School
Hartford, Connecticut
Division of Emergency Medicine
Connecticut Children's Hospital
Hartford, Connecticut

Annie Pham-Cheng, DMD
Instructor in Pediatric Dentistry
Harvard Dental School
Assistant in Dentistry
Children's Hospital
Boston, Massachusetts

Alfred Sacchetti, MD, FACEP
Assistant Clinical Professor of
  Emergency Medicine
Thomas Jefferson University
Philadelphia, Pennsylvania
Research Director
Our Lady Lourdes Medical Center
Camden, New Jersey

Richard Saladino, MD
Assistant Professor of Pediatrics
Harvard Medical School
Division of Emergency Medicine
Children's Hospital
Boston, Massachusetts

Steven Selbst, MD, FAAP
Professor of Pediatrics
Thomas Jefferson University
Philadelphia, Pennsylvania
Vice Chairman, Department of
    Pediatrics
DuPont Hospital for Children
Wilmington, Delaware

Navil Sethna, MB, ChB
Assistant Professor in Anaesthesia
Harvard Medical School
Associate Director of Pain Treatment
    Service and
Senior Associate in Anesthesia
Children's Hospital
Boston, Massachusetts

**Michael Shannon, MD, MPH,
    FAAP, FACEP**
Associate Professor of Pediatrics
Harvard Medical School
Associate Director, Division of
    Emergency Medicine
Children's Hospital
Boston, Massachusetts

Mary Fallon Smith, RN, MS
Clinical Nurse Specialist
Division of Emergency Medicine
Children's Hospital
Boston, Massachusetts

Stephen Teach, MD, MPH
Assistant Professor of Pediatrics
George Washington University School
    of Medicine
Department of Emergency Medicine
Children's National Medical Center
Washington, DC

Thomas Terndrup, MD, FACEP
Professor of Pediatrics and Physiology
State University of New York Health
    Sciences Center at Syracuse
Syracuse, New York
Chairman, Department of Emergency
    Medicine

State University of New York at
    Syracuse
Syracuse, New York

Cheryl Vance, MD, FAAP
Assistant Professor of Emergency
    Medicine
University of California
Sacramento, California

Edward Walkley, MD, FACEP
Clinical Professor of Pediatrics
University of Washington
Director of Pediatric Services
Mary Bridge Children's Hospital
Tacoma, Washington

Mehernoor Watcha, MD
Associate Professor of Anesthesia and
    Director, Clinical Anesthesia Research
University of Pennsylvania School
    of Medicine
Children's Hospital of Philadelphia
Philadelphia, Pennsylvania

William Womack, MD, PhD
Staff Anesthesiologist
White-Wilson Medical Center
Fort Walton Beach, Florida

George Woodward, MD, FAAP
Assistant Professor of Pediatrics
University of Pennsylvania School of
    Medicine
Division of Emergency Transport
    Service
Children's Hospital
Philadelphia, Pennsylvania

William Zempsky, MD, FAAP
Assistant Professor of Pediatrics and
    Emergency Medicine
University of Connecticut School of
    Medicine
Division of Emergency Medicine
Connecticut Children's Medical
    Center
Hartford, Connecticut

Contents

PART ONE: SCIENTIFIC FOUNDATIONS

Section I: Physiology of Analgesia and Sedation

Section II: Monitoring

Section III: Pharmacology of Sedation

Section III: Approach to Procedural Sedation in Selected Settings

Section IV: Approach to Procedural Sedation for Selected Patient Populations

PART THREE: Nonelective Procedures

Section I: Introduction

Section II: Head, Ears, Eyes, Nose, and Throat

Part One

Scientific Foundations

Section I: Physiology of Analgesia and Sedation

Chapter 1
Airway and Respiratory Control

Alan Doctor

Alterations in airway reflexes, breathing control, pulmonary mechanics, and ventilation dynamics may accompany the levels of sedation commonly used in the outpatient setting. An understanding of the principles underlying normal pediatric pulmonary physiology will aid in managing both the planned and sometimes unplanned changes in pulmonary function that may accompany procedural sedation.

RESPIRATORY MECHANICS

Ventilation and maintenance of pulmonary architecture that optimizes efficient gas exchange are influenced and, in part, determined by the mechanical properties of the lung and chest wall.

COMPLIANCE

Compliance is an expression of the elastic properties of the lung and chest wall, which represents the change in lung volume for a given change in pressure, and primarily determines the ease of ventilation and lung volume maintenance. Lung compliance in the child is less than that in the adult and poorest in the newborn. Compliance is adversely affected by extremes in lung volume, with restrictions to thoraco-abdominal expansion and with increased pulmonary blood volume. Compliance is also determined in part by ventilatory history and the status of the surfactant system. Most relevant to sedation in the outpatient setting is the fact that compliance is also affected by posture, being highest in the erect position followed by prone and supine positions. Obviously, restrictive binding as a means of immobilization may adversely affect compliance.

AIRWAY RESISTANCE

Airway resistance can be thought of most easily as the main determinant of airflow velocity for a given pressure change between the mouth and alveolus. Resistance is directly proportional to the length of the airway and inversely proportional to the radius of the airway to the fourth power. Therefore, the relatively smaller airways of the child cause significantly greater resistance than is found in adults. The primary site of airway resistance in children is the upper airway (60%) and the large central bronchi (30%). Airway tone and caliber are often adversely affected during periods of sedation, significantly increasing the work of breathing in the child. Careful positioning and attentive clearing of accumulated secretions will minimize limitations to airflow in the sedated child. Lower airway resistance is rarely a factor during sedation for brief procedures in the outpatient setting.

LUNG VOLUMES

Basic Definitions

Before discussing ventilation dynamics, it is helpful to define landmark points in the respiratory cycle. Lung volumes are best discussed with the aid of a spirometer (Fig. 1.1). The beginning of the tracing in Figure 1.1 displays normal chest excursion during quiet breathing and defines tidal volume. A maximum inspiration and expiration follow, defining vital capacity and residual volume respectively. A

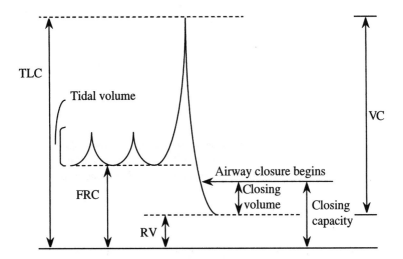

Figure 1.1. Stylized spirogram to illustrate the various lung volumes. The example illustrates a child with a closing capacity less than functional residual capacity. *TLC,* total lung capacity; *FRC,* functional residual capacity; *RV,* residual volume; *VC,* vital capacity.

critical point to note on the tracing is functional residual capacity (FRC), representing lung volume following normal expiration. FRC is the starting point in any given respiratory cycle and, as such, defines the mechanics of the ensuing ventilatory cycle. In addition, a lung that is over or under inflated at FRC will affect both the area available for gas exchange and the regional distribution of blood flow within the lung, possibly causing increased dead-space ventilation, $\dot{V}/\dot{Q}$ mismatch, or intrapulmonary shunting.

Factors Affecting FRC

During equilibrium in the static state, the balance of elastic forces acting within lung (towards collapse) and from the chest wall (towards expansion) determine lung volume at FRC. Other forces influencing static FRC include diaphragmatic tone, abdominal volume and pressure, posture, and lung disease. The factors affecting compliance mentioned above modulate lung volumes such as FRC. Likewise, restrictive binding, poor posture and positioning, and increased abdominal pressure will all act against FRC maintenance.

FRC in Relation to Closing Capacity

As lung volume approaches residual volume, there is a point, known as the closing capacity, at which small airways begin to close (Fig. 1.1). For a variety of reasons, both in the elderly and in young children, closing capacity is often greater than functional residual capacity. When the tidal range is partly within closing capacity, a portion of pulmonary blood flow will be distributed to alveoli with either little or no ventilation leading either to $\dot{V}/\dot{Q}$ derangement or to intrapulmonary shunting and hypoxia. It should be noted that although closing capacity is a relatively independent feature of pulmonary mechanics, any factor reducing FRC, such as those mentioned above, may bring the tidal range within closing capacity, impairing the efficiency of gas exchange.

FRC in Children

Because of chest wall mechanics in the child, static FRC is small (approximately 10% of total lung capacity [TLC]) relative to FRC in the adult (40 to 50% of TLC). An FRC of 10% TLC would be functionally insufficient, causing atelectasis with intrapulmonary shunting. Children overcome this mechanical disadvantage by never allowing their lungs to reach static FRC. When FRC is measured in the dynamic state in children, it approaches the expected 40% of TLC. Lung volume is maintained at dynamic FRC through tachypnea, increased intercostal muscle tone, and laryngeal braking. If expiratory time is limited such that inflation occurs before the cessation of expiratory flow, then the lung is dynamically prevented from reaching what would be its static FRC. Tachypnea limits the absolute expiratory time in each respiratory cycle and thus contributes to FRC maintenance. Children increase intercostal muscle tone during exhalation, thus stabilizing the chest wall, increasing its elastic recoil, and thereby augmenting lung volume. Laryngeal braking is active laryngeal closure during exhalation, generating a back pressure thereby aiding in FRC maintenance.

These adaptations to the child's mechanical disadvantage allow maintenance of FRC in the dynamic state. Because these mechanisms are active and may be attenuated during periods of sedation, they act as one of the physiologic limits to the depth of sedation that can be achieved without mechanical assistance.

GAS EXCHANGE

Following is a brief summary of the factors influencing gas exchange with reference to the potential adverse effects of sedation.

Carbon Dioxide

The partial pressure of CO_2 increases as it is added to alveolar gas from pulmonary blood and diminishes as the result of alveolar ventilation; the partial pressure is always related to the ratio of these two processes and is roughly expressed in the equation below:

Alveolar CO_2 concentration $(P_A CO_2)$ = carbon dioxide output/alveolar ventilation

For practical purposes, we can consider that CO_2 production will remain constant over the brief periods required for sedation during outpatient procedures. Alveolar ventilation, however, can vary dramatically over brief periods and radically affect $P_A CO_2$. Alveolar ventilation is the product of respiratory frequency and the tidal volume (less the volume of the physiologic dead-space, or the fraction of tidal volume not exposed to perfused alveoli). Except during extreme hypoventilation, the relationship between alveolar ventilation and alveolar CO_2 concentration is nearly linear, e.g., if alveolar ventilation is halved, CO_2 concentration will double.

Oxygen

The formula above is also the basis of the universal alveolar gas equation that describes both the changes in O_2 and CO_2 that occur with changes in ventilation:

Alveolar O_2 concentration = inspired O_2 concentration −
(O_2 uptake/alveolar ventilation)

$$P_A O_2 = P_I O_2 - (P_A CO_2 / R)$$

$P_A CO_2$ is used as a measure of alveolar ventilation:

R = respiratory quotient and is usually 0.8 (CO_2 production/O_2 consumption)

One can see that a balance of two processes also determines O_2 tension in the alveolus: the removal of O_2 by pulmonary capillary blood, and the replenishment by alveolar ventilation. The rate of removal is determined by O_2 consumption and is relatively fixed over the short term; therefore, one can see that P_AO_2 will also vary with alveolar ventilation. It is extremely important to note, however, that the hypoxia that develops from hypoventilation (unlike that from shunt, diffusion impairment, or $\dot{V}/\dot{Q}$ mismatch) is easy to correct simply by increasing the inspired oxygen concentration. For example, using the alveolar gas equation above we can calculate the following (we will use rough partial pressure of O_2 at sea level):

Alert baby	$P_AO_2 = 150-(40/0.8) = 100$
Hypoventilating baby	$P_AO_2 = 150-(80/0.8) = 50$

If we increase the inspired O_2 concentration merely to 28% (with a partial pressure of 200 torr), then

$$P_AO_2 = 200-(80/0.8) = 100$$

This principle illustrates the ease of correcting hypoxia resulting from hypoventilation during sedation and the method of preoxygenating the patient whenever hypoventilation is anticipated during sedation (Fig. 1.2). It should be noted that for all the reasons listed in the discussions on respiratory mechanics, and because of children's relatively high oxygen consumption (6 to 8 mL/kg/min relative to 3 to 4 mL/kg/min in the adult), children do not tolerate periods of hypoventilation as well as adults; therefore, it is critical to monitor oxygenation continuously during sedation and anticipate a need for the prompt administration of supplemental oxygen.

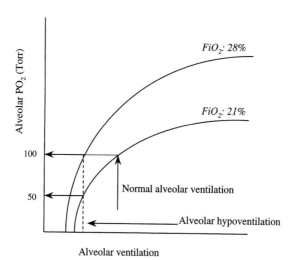

Figure 1.2. The effect of hypoventilation on alveolar PO_2. Also illustrated is correction of alveolar PO_2 by increasing the inspired oxygen concentration from 21 to 28%.

CONTROL OF BREATHING

The apneustic center in the pons and the respiratory center in the medulla are responsible for the control of breathing and act as the final integration station for the respiratory system. These two centers' outputs are modulated by input from both central and peripheral chemoreceptors and pulmonary proprioceptors, as well as other central neural centers, and are commonly affected by agents used for sedation. Although the chemical control of ventilation is primarily geared towards maintaining pH and CO_2 in the normal range, the response is amplified in the presence of hypoxia. One should remember that the control of breathing is relatively tenuous in patients with chronic hypercapnia who rely primarily on a hypoxic signal to maintain ventilation. Special care must be taken to maintain ventilatory drive in these patients when the combination of sedative agents and supplemental oxygen is deemed necessary.

PEDIATRIC AIRWAY

Airway Anatomy

The pediatric airway differs from the adult airway in both its anatomy and physiology in several ways with important clinical consequences. The relative size of the pediatric airway is much smaller than that of the adult, making the pediatric airway relatively susceptible to significant dynamic and fixed obstruction. The tongue is large in relation to the mouth, and if muscular tone is diminished, the tongue is prone to posterior displacement and airway obstruction. Such airway obstruction may be relieved by adjusting head position or with a jaw thrust maneuver. Infants are obligate nasal breathers, making nasal obstruction poorly tolerated until approximately 3 to 5 months. The tonsils and adenoids, although small in the neonate, may grow dramatically in childhood, achieving maximal size by 4 to 7 years; in some children the tonsils and adenoids are large enough to produce airway obstruction during sleep or during sedation.

The lumen of the lower pediatric airway is conical, rather than cylindrical in the adult, with the narrowest portion being the cricoid cartilage. The importance of this narrowing is apparent because the resistance to airflow is proportional to the fourth power of the radius. Note that 1 mm of edema or accumulated secretions will reduce the cross-sectional area of a 4-mm airway by 75% and increase the resistance to airflow by a factor of 16, significantly increasing the work of breathing. The same restriction in airway caliber in an 8-mm adult airway will decrease the cross-sectional area by 44% and only increase resistance by a factor of 3.

The relatively large size of the infant head and occiput, and the relative redundancy of tissue in the upper airway can cause positional obstruction in the sleeping or sedated infant. A small rolled towel beneath the neck in the supine infant usually will prevent or attenuate any obstruction of this nature.

Airway Reflexes

Motor reflexes involving the upper airway are cough, laryngospasm, apnea, and swallowing. The fluid control of these reflexes in the conscious child allows the complex coordination of swallowing, speech, and breathing. Laryngospasm and apnea are the reflexes of primary concern when planning sedation in the outpatient setting. Partially sedated patients in whom the level of consciousness is not sufficient for reflex control are particularly susceptible to laryngospasm or apnea in response to airway stimulation by secretions, blood, or mechanical manipulation. In addition, the "fail-safe" mechanism triggered by hypoxia to relieve laryngospasm may fail in the presence of central nervous system (CNS) depression. Therefore, patients must be monitored with vigilance, especially during the initiation and emergence from sedation, and care must be taken to minimize stimulation of the airway during periods of sedation.

IMPLICATIONS OF AN UPPER RESPIRATORY INFECTION

The average child will have three to eight viral upper respiratory infections (URI) per year. Historically, it has been common anesthetic practice to cancel elective surgery in children suffering from or recently recovering from a URI. This is because of the belief that the risks of perioperative respiratory complications are increased in this population. Occasionally, a child with a URI will present with a problem requiring emergency management typically facilitated with sedation.

The relevant pathologic changes that occur in children with an active URI include increased small airway edema and increased closing capacity, increased upper and lower airway resistance caused by the accumulation of secretions and mucosal edema, and perhaps most concerning, increased upper and lower airway hyperreactivity (considered vagally mediated). The airway hyperreactivity may last up to 6 weeks after a URI.

Reports of patients with a URI developing pulmonary complications while undergoing surgery are mostly those patients undergoing general anesthesia with an endotracheal tube in place (a potent airway stimulant). Complications are much less common in patients undergoing minor procedures under general anesthesia without endotracheal intubation. This information must be extrapolated with caution to the sedated and nonintubated patient outside the operating room in whom the risk of laryngospasm may increase because of the differences in anesthetic depth and technique.

Experience has shown that a recent or active URI is a risk factor for pulmonary complications, although most of the evidence is in children requiring intubation, a potent stimulus for precipitating bronchospasm. In addition, this risk is considered amplified in the child with underlying reactive airway disease. No published experience exists regarding pulmonary complications in the nonintubated sedated patient with an active or recent URI outside the operating room.

The decision to proceed with sedation in the child who has an active or recent

URI as an aid to an emergency procedure should be made because of the known increased risk of pulmonary complications in the like environment of the operating room. If the decision is made to sedate a child who has an active or recent URI, the child should be premedicated with an anticholinergic, such as atropine or glycopyrrolate, to dry secretions and block vagal tone to attenuate irritant-induced airway hyperreactivity. In addition, humidified oxygen should be administered to prevent inspissation of secretions.

SUGGESTED READING

Bell C, Hughes CW, Oh TH, eds. The Pediatric Anesthesia Handbook. St. Louis: Mosby Year Book, 1991.

Motoyama EK, Davis PJ, eds. Smith's Anesthesia for Infants and Children. St. Louis: Mosby Year Book, 1996.

Nunn, JF. Nunn's Respiratory Physiology. Oxford: Butterworth-Heinemann, 1993.

West, JB. Respiratory Physiology—The Essentials. Baltimore: Williams & Wilkins, 1995.

Chapter 2
Physiologic Considerations

Leila Mei Pang

This chapter reviews the physiologic considerations and their clinical implications for procedural sedation and analgesia related to the cardiovascular, gastrointestinal, renal, and hepatic systems.

CARDIOVASCULAR SYSTEM

In the normal patient, as much as 80% of the systemic blood volume resides in the venous system. Baroreceptors in the carotid sinus, liver, and spleen sense pressure changes via the sympathetic nervous system, causing veins to constrict or dilate altering venous return to the heart. When exposed to opioids, veins become less elastic and passively dilate, and blood sequesters in the dilated veins, decreasing cardiac output. Children who are hypovolemic before being sedated become effectively more hypovolemic because of this passive venous dilation.

The duration of fasting can also affect the circulating blood volume and, hence, preload, especially if the agent used for sedation can potentially produce respiratory depression, depress myocardial contractility, or decrease peripheral vascular resistance (afterload). Thus, the patient's vascular volume should be assessed before proceeding with sedation, because a hypovolemic patient may not tolerate any decrease in vascular resistance.

Clinical Implications

The clinical implications are as follows:

- Intravenous barbaturates exert a negative inotropic effect and decrease stroke volume and can cause significant changes in blood pressure and cardiac output.
- Opioids decrease vascular resistance, increase total vascular capacity, and blunt the reflex response to hypovolemic hypotension. Hypotensive effects of phenothiazines may be exaggerated when used in combination with opioids.

- Intravenous propofol induction and continuous infusion can significantly decrease mean arterial pressure, oxygen saturation, and heart rate.
- Intravenous ketamine, in a normal patient, supports the circulation, producing no change in arterial blood gases, systemic or pulmonary artery pressure, heart rate, cardiac index, or pulmonary-to-systemic arteriolar resistance ratios. However, in the hypovolemic patient, ketamine can decrease cardiac output, heart rate, and vascular resistance.
- Benzodiazepines have a direct myocardial depressant at the cellular level, but in clinical concentration ranges, the cardiovascular effects are minimal.

GASTROINTESTINAL SYSTEM

The effect of orally administered drugs depends on multiple factors including the following:

- Rate and extent of absorption from the gastrointestinal (GI) tract
- Ablility of the drug to dissolve in physiologic solutions
- Physicochemical nature of the drug
- Composition of the membranes through which the drug must pass
- Nature of the GI juices
- Rate of gastric emptying
- Degree of gastric motility
- Intestinal blood flow

Most weakly acidic or basic lipid-soluble drugs, which are non-ionized at physiologic pH, when given orally are absorbed in the small intestine so that delayed gastric emptying delays drug absorption. Some medications affect gastric pH and the volume of gastric juice.

Drugs also can be administered rectally, especially in patients who have nausea, vomiting, or diseases of the upper gastrointestinal tract. Drugs readily cross the rectal mucosa, but because of the small surface area, absorption is often slow and erratic.

Determining the patient's volume status requires analysis of changes in heart rate, mean arterial pressure, capillary perfusion, moistness of mucous membranes, tears, skin turgor, and weight. Correction of fluid and electrolyte imbalances before sedation minimizes reflexes that maintain cardiovascular homeostasis. In emergent cases, full presedation correction of extracellular fluid deficits may not be possible before sedation is needed, but these deficits should be corrected as much as possible. Peritonitis, perforated viscous, intussusception, bowel obstruction, and major trauma are all characterized by continuing large fluid and protein shifts that require fluid resuscitation before sedation can be administered safely.

NPO Status

The duration of fasting, or NPO (nothing by mouth), should depend on the patient's age, size, and general medical condition (see chapters 13 and 17). The younger the child, the smaller the glycogen store, and the more likely that hypoglycemia can occur with prolonged fasting. Prolonged periods of fasting predispose children to irritability and thirst, which can increase gastric fluid volume and decrease gastric fluid pH, thus increasing the potential for aspiration of gastric content during sedation. Giving patients clear liquids 2 to 3 hours before sedation stimulates peristalsis but does not stimulate gastric acid secretion if no protein is given. Solids include milk; water or clear sweetened fluids, such as apple juice, Pedialyte, or soda, are considered clear liquids.

Despite attempts to reduce gastric volume a group of patients is still at an increased risk for regurgitation and aspiration of stomach contents. Table 2.1 lists conditions in which there should be a high index of suspicion for gastroesophageal reflux. In these children, presedation medication with agents designed to reduce gastric volume and pH should be considered. Table 2.2 lists drugs that can be considered for the patients at high risk for regurgitation; these drugs should be given 1 to 3 hours before the anticipated sedation. No functional differences exist between the child and adult that should affect gastrointestinal absorption.

RENAL SYSTEM

The ultimate route of elimination of most drugs or their metabolites is by way of the kidney. Because many drugs are simply filtered by the kidney, the glomerular filtration rate influences drug excretion and action. Renal disease can alter plasma and tissue proteins, thereby affecting protein binding, the amount of free versus bound drug in the circulation, and the rate of clearance by the liver.

In patients with renal failure, standard doses of sedative drugs may have exag-

Table 2.1. Conditions Associated with Gastroesophageal Reflux

Recurrent pneumonias
Cerebral palsy/mental retardation
Gross obesity
Tracheoesophageal fistula
Bronchopulmonary dysplasia
Esophageal dysmotility
Incompetent gastroesophageal sphincter
Delayed gastric emptying time
Pathology associated with ileus, vomiting, and electrolyte disorders
Increased intra-abdominal pressure

Table 2.2. Presedation Medication

Drugs	Dosage
Antacids	
Bicitra	30 mL
Prokinetic agents	
Metoclopramide	0.1 mg/kg
H_2-histaminergic receptor blockers	
Cimetidine	5–10 mg/kg
Ranitidine	2–2.5 mg/kg
Famotidine	0.3–0.4 mg/kg up to a maximum of 40 mg

gerated or prolonged effects because of the loss of renal mechanisms for drug elimination and biochemical abnormalities of uremia that alter drug availability.

Maintaining effective intravascular volume is the most definitive strategy to preserve renal perfusion and prevent renal impairment during procedural sedation. Ongoing fluid losses must be replaced. It is preferable to err on the side of overhydration, because the consequences of fluid overload can be more easily reversed than the highly lethal ischemic renal failure that can result from intravascular volume contraction and poor perfusion.

Chronic renal failure is usually associated with a chronic anemia. It must be noted that the reserve necessary to tolerate stress may be significantly decreased in these patients. Depending on the clinical problem, presedation transfusion may be needed.

Clinical Implications

Implications for procedural sedation in the patient with renal disease in the presence of normal electrolytes, normal growth and development, and normotension are minimal.

Benzodiazepines and barbiturates may produce excessive sedation because of relative hypoproteinemia, decreased protein binding, and impaired renal elimination of active metabolites. Similarly, opioid analgesics are associated with excessive sedation and respiratory depression because of impaired elimination of active metabolites. These three classes of drugs (benzodiazepines, barbiturates, opioids), however, can be administered safely if they are titrated in small incremental doses to the desired effect under direct observation and monitoring.

HEPATIC SYSTEM

Metabolism or excretion through the liver or kidney terminates or alters the activity of most drugs. Although all tissues have some ability to metabolize drugs, the liver is the principal organ of drug metabolism. The overall rate of metabolism depends on the size of the liver, the metabolizing ability of the appropriate microsomal enzyme system, and the amount of free drug available. Liver volume relative to body weight decreases from birth to adulthood, with the relative volume in the first year of life being twice that at age 14. The hepatic enzyme systems responsible for the metabolism of drugs are cytochrome P-450, cytochrome P-450 reductase, and nicotine adenine diphosphate hydrogenase (NADPH). Alpha 1-acid glycoprotein is the major binding protein for many of the alkaline drugs (specifically opioids and local anesthetics).

Hepatic clearance of drugs with high (e.g., propofol, ketamine) or intermediate (e.g., methohexital, midazolam) extraction ratios depends largely on hepatic blood flow. The elimination rate of drugs with low hepatic extraction ratios (e.g., diazepam, lorazepam) depends on enzymatic activity of the liver and is independent of hepatic blood flow. Factors that decrease hepatic blood flow include hypocapnia, congestive heart failure, volume depletion, circulatory collapse, beta-adrenergic blockage, and norepinephrine administration. In addition, liver disease can influence pharmacokinetics in several ways. It can alter protein content, thereby changing the degree of protein binding. Alterations in hepatic blood flow will affect drug clearance. Moderate to severe liver disease will alter enzymatic activity, thereby affecting drug metabolism.

Increased plasma and extracellular fluid volume seen in patients with chronic liver disease may present as a decreased sensitivity to a drug because of the increase in the volume of distribution of the drug. Altered portal flow or portacaval shunting may increase bioavailability of an orally administered drug because of the reduced first-pass metabolism. However, drugs in patients with liver disease tend to produce a more profound and prolonged effect. Heightened sensitivity should be expected from centrally acting drugs.

Sodium abnormalities are common in patients with liver disease secondary to inappropriate antidiuretic hormone secretion. When the serum sodium falls below 120 mEq/L, altered mental states and seizure activity may occur. Secondary hyperaldosteronism can be associated with profound hypokalemia.

Clinical Implications

Benzodiazepines are highly bound to plasma albumin. Therefore, liver disease, which alters albumin concentration, protein binding, and tissue distribution, will prolong the elimination of this class of drugs. Benzodiazepines undergo oxidative metabolism in the liver to biologically active metabolites, which, in turn, undergo secondary biotransformation by conjugation with glucuronic acid to inactive metabolites. Oxidative metabolism can be impaired by a decrease in hepatic function and by the presence of metabolic inhibitor drugs such as cimetidine, resulting in a prolonged and more profound sedative effect. Conjugative processes are not affected by these factors. The effect of midazolam is enhanced by pretreatment with H_2-receptor antagonists such as cimetidine and ranitidine.

Patients with liver disease have alterations in metabolism and excretion of barbiturates and opioids. These patients have an increased sensitivity to barbiturates, opioids, and phenothiazines. In patients with decompensated liver disease, sedatives (e.g., diazepam, phenobarbital) and opioids (e.g., meperidine) can cause prolonged depression of consciousness if used in standard doses.

Promethazine is a histamine antagonist with antiemetic and sedative properties. It is extensively metabolized by the liver; therefore, its duration of action may be prolonged by severe liver disease. Phenergan is metabolized more rapidly in children than in adults.

Chlorpromazine may be used in patients with hepatic disease; however, caution is advised because metabolism may be delayed or modified. Chlorpromazine is metabolized by hepatic microsomal enzymes. The oxidized metabolite is biologically active. Children tend to metabolize this drug more rapidly than adults.

Opioids are metabolized by the liver. Thus, hepatic disease may increase bioavailability. The accumulation of the biologically active metabolite of meperidine or normeperidine may produce tremors and seizures. Respiratory depressant and sedative effects are prolonged by phenothiazines either by alterations in the rate of metabolic transformation or alterations in neurotransmitters involved in the action of opioids.

SUGGESTED READING

Morray JP, Lynn AM, Stamm SJ, et al. Hemodynamic effects of ketamine in children with congenital heart disease. Anesth Analg 1984;63:895–899.

Nakae Y, Kanaya N, Namiki A. The direct effects of diazepam and midazolam on myocardial depression in cultured rat ventricular myocytes. Anesth Analg 1997;85:729–733.

Chapter 3

Noninvasive Monitoring for Procedural Sedation

Kristine Henderson, William Womack

Outpatient sedation and analgesia, like any procedure performed in medicine, should be performed with care and forethought. Sedation and analgesia are frequently performed in different areas outside of the operating room, many of which were not designed with anesthetic needs in mind. Noninvasive monitoring of vital signs is essential (and ultimately mandated) to optimize the safety of sedation and analgesia in the outpatient setting. Required monitors, medications, and materials must be assembled and readily available before undertaking the sedation. In addition, the personnel must be adequately prepared and trained.

PERSONNEL

Practitioners from many specialties provide sedation and analgesia in the outpatient setting. When the primary caregiver is providing sedation to perform a procedure that will occupy his or her attention, a second person must be monitoring the patient to ensure patient safety. The primary caregiver must be a credentialed provider (M.D., D.O., or D.D.S.) and should have current training in advanced cardiac life support (ACLS) as well as basic life support (BLS). In addition, this individual must have completed specialized training in sedation/analgesia, either through residency training or via a hospital-sponsored course. The primary provider establishes the sedation/analgesia and may then perform the procedure for which the sedation was necessary. The primary provider is also responsible for managing any aberrations in vital signs and for ordering supplemental sedation as needed.

The secondary provider may be a monitoring technician or nurse. This individual is dedicated to monitoring the patient during the procedure and may only assist the primary provider with minor, easily interrupted tasks. He or she should notify the physician of significant changes in monitored parameters. This caregiver must be trained in BLS. In addition, some hospitals are requiring that monitoring technicians complete an examination, ensuring that they are aware of the range of normal vital signs and possible complications of sedation/analgesia.

EQUIPMENT

Because sedation/analgesia is performed for many reasons in many disparate settings, it is important for clinicians to carefully familiarize themselves with the surroundings before beginning the procedure. Equipment that is suitable for children must be available when sedating a pediatric patient. All items on the following list must be immediately available:

- Code Cart
    - -Including: defibrillator, airway equipment, emergency medications
    - -The contents of the cart must allow the patient to be supported until transported to a medical facility or other part of the hospital for further stabilization
    - -All equipment and medications should be checked and maintained on a scheduled basis
- Oxygen source
    - -A positive-pressure-oxygen-delivery system (wall or oxygen tank) capable of administering greater than 90% oxygen for at least 60 minutes
    - -Back-up source
- Self-inflating bag-valve-mask
    - -With oxygen tubing
- Suction source
    - -Wall: generates airflow of 300 L/min, vacuum of 300 mm Hg
    - -Portable: most units only generate 100 mm Hg suction and may be inadequate to handle a massive aspiration
    - -Tubing, Yankauer tip, and soft suction catheters
- Vascular access equipment
    - -Intravenous catheters, tourniquet, alcohol swabs, tape, and intravenous tubing and fluid
- Pharmacologic antagonists
    - -Naloxone or Nalmefene for reversal of opioids
    - -Flumazenil for reversal of benzodiazepines
- Pulse oximeter
    - -With alarms *on*
- Noninvasive blood pressure measuring device
    - -Manual or automatic

- Electrocardiogram (ECG) monitor and pads
    - -ECG on defibrillator may be used for three-lead monitoring
- Means of two-way communication
    - -Telephone, intercom, or "runner"
- Adequate lighting
    - -And a back-up flashlight
- Electrical outlets
    - -And emergency back-up outlets
- Adequate space
    - -For procedure and for resuscitation if needed
- Medical record of monitored parameters

Equipment for inhaled sedation must have the capability of delivering 25 to 100% oxygen at a flow rate appropriate for the size of the patient and a scavenger device for waste gases.

MONITORING

The physiologic parameters which must be monitored include the following:

- Level of consciousness
- Ventilation
- Oxygenation
- Hemodynamics

The minimum frequency for recording these parameters is as follows:

- Before the procedure
- After each dose of sedative
- Upon completion of the procedure
- At the beginning of the recovery period
- Before discharge from care

However, it is recommended that all monitored parameters be recorded at more frequent intervals depending on the particular procedure and the required level and depth of sedation.

Level of Consciousness

Patients should be capable of age-appropriate purposeful responses, either verbal or nonverbal (thumbs up, hand squeeze), throughout the procedure. This should be checked and recorded at frequent intervals. Mere withdrawal from painful stimulus is not considered a purposeful response and thus signals a deeper level of sedation. If a deeper level of sedation is required for the procedure, more stringent monitoring guidelines should be followed. The following guidelines are identical to the basic monitoring standards for general anesthesia:

- Oxygenation, ventilation, circulation (including ECG monitoring), and temperature should be continually evaluated.
- End-tidal CO_2 monitoring (capnography) is strongly encouraged.
- Vital signs should be assessed and recorded every 5 minutes throughout the procedure and recovery period.

Ventilation

The adequacy of ventilation, including respiratory rate and a quantitative assessment of airflow, must be monitored by at least one of the following methods:

- Observation of respiratory activity—"look, listen, and feel"
- Continuous auscultation of breath sounds—monaural precordial stethoscope or standard stethoscope
- Capnography

Capnography measures exhaled carbon dioxide via infrared absorption spectrometry. Although capnography has been the standard of care for monitoring patients in the operating room, its routine use in nonintubated patients is only now gaining acceptance in many nonoperative settings as technology has improved and cost has declined. Portable, handheld, lightweight monitors are now available as both single parameter capnograph units and as dual parameter capnograph and pulse oximeter units. Carbon dioxide monitoring can be applied to a face-mask or nasal cannula providing real-time, breath-by-breath measurement of respiratory rate, including display of the capnograph waveform. Analysis of the shape of the waveform can allow early detection of problems such as hypoventilation during sedation, impending upper airway obstruction, as well as response to beta agonist treatment (Fig. 3.1). The addition of capnography provides an earlier indication of respiratory depression than pulse oximetry and respiratory rate alone.

It should be noted that impedance plethysmography, available as a "respiratory rate" readout on many standard ECG monitors, is *not* an acceptable method for assessing ventilation. Impedance plethysmography measures changes in impedance across the chest wall; therefore, a patient with airway obstruction or laryngospasm who is making an effort to breathe will have a "respiratory rate" reading (despite zero air exchange) until all respiratory efforts cease.

Oxygenation

The adequacy of oxygenation and the need for supplemental oxygen is assessed using pulse oximetry. Pulse oximeters measure the percent of hemoglobin that is bound to oxygen via absorbance spectrometry of red and infrared light and are ac-

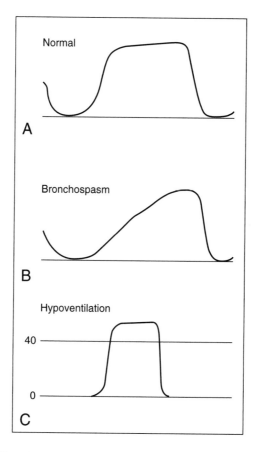

Figure 3.1. **A.** Normal capnogram shape. **B.** "Shark fin" shape of obstructive capnogram (bronchospasm). **C.** Hypoventilation.

curate down to approximately 75% SpO2. This is because in vivo calibration of pulse oximeters at low SpO2 is potentially dangerous, and animal data may not apply to human. Testing of pulse oximeters by several manufacturers has shown that at 75% SpO2 bias is scattered uniformly, with 7% underestimation and 7% overestimation of SpO2. Pulse oximetry is *not* a substitute for monitoring ventilation, because there is a variable lag time between the onset of hypoventilation or apnea and a change in oxygen saturation.

Pulse oximetry may be affected by numerous extrinsic factors, but a decline in oxygen saturation should always prompt an evaluation of respiratory rate, adequacy of ventilation, and adequacy of circulation. Once it is assured that the patient is doing well, the source of the pulse oximetry interference can be sought. Such factors may include the following:

- Bright external lighting: inadequate waveform
- Patient movement or shivering: inadequate waveform
- Dark nail polish: factitious low SpO2 reading
- Methemoglobinemia: oximetry reading will approach 85% regardless of true oxygenation level because of spectrophotoelectric absorption of methemoglobin
- Intravenous dyes: factitious low SpO2 reading
     -methylene blue, indocyanine green, indigo carmine
- Adhesive residue from reusable oximeter probes: factitious low SpO2

In addition to pulse oximetry, an oxygen analyzer is recommended during nitrous oxide administration to assure appropriate levels of oxygen delivery.

Circulation   The three circulatory parameters of interest include the heart rate, blood pressure, and, in some patients, the electrocardiogram. Pulse oximetry and ECG are ideal because they provide a continuous measure of pulse rate. Heart rate must be measured by at least one of the following methods:

- Palpation of the pulse
- Auscultation of heart sounds
- Oscillometric blood pressure machine
- Pulse oximetry monitor
- ECG monitor

Blood pressure may be measured noninvasively by several methods. Manual auscultation using Korotkoff sounds is the most widely available and least expensive method of measuring blood pressure, although automated noninvasive blood pressure (NIBP) machines are becoming more prevalent. Manual auscultation is useful in situations in which the automated monitors do not function well, such as when the patient is shivering, moving, or has an irregular heartbeat. The primary disadvantage is that it is time consuming and labor intensive, which distracts the monitoring provider from other tasks. As with all forms of noninvasive blood pressure measurement, the selection of an inappropriate cuff size will cause measurement error.

Automated NIBP monitors measure blood pressure based on oscillometry. The cuff pressure is raised above the systolic blood pressure, then gradually decreased while oscillations in cuff pressure from arterial pulsations are sensed. The pressure at which the peak amplitude of oscillation occurs is the mean blood pressure; the systolic and diastolic pressures are then calculated internally, based on manufacturer-specific formulas.

Pulse oximetry waveform analysis is a method of blood pressure assessment that involves inflating a cuff on the extremity with the pulse oximeter attached and noting the disappearance and reappearance of the pulsatile waveform. This technique is especially useful in sick neonates that do not have an arterial catheter in place.

Noninvasive blood pressure measurement may be a source of disturbance to the patient, particularly to the lightly sedated child undergoing a painless procedure such as a CT scan or EEG. In this setting, it may be appropriate to check blood pressures only before and after the procedure. A good waveform on the pulse oximeter demonstrates that peripheral perfusion is adequate. Although this may be adequate for healthy children, it may be inappropriate for the rare child with hypertension or significant cardiac disease, or for American Society of Anesthesiologists (ASA) class III and IV patients.

If pulse oximetry is providing an adequate waveform, the addition of continuous ECG monitoring is only necessary for patients with pre-existing cardiac disease, or during procedures associated with dysrhythmias (e.g., central line placement). If an ECG is used, a three-lead ECG is adequate for detection of dysrhythmias. Electrodes are placed on the right and left arms and the left leg and Lead II is selected. The p wave will usually be upright and easily seen. If the patient has cardiac disease, and monitoring for ischemia is necessary, electrodes are placed on all four extremities and a fifth lead (V_5) is placed on the anterior axillary line at the fifth intercostal space. ST segment analysis of leads II and V5 will detect 80 to 95% of all ECG-detectable ischemia.

Temperature

Continuous monitoring of temperature is not necessary for patients undergoing sedation/analgesia. However, it must be remembered that pediatric patients, especially infants, lose heat more rapidly because of their greater surface-to-volume ratio. Some of the places where a patient may undergo sedation may be kept at relatively low temperatures, such as in the radiology suite. In this setting, take precautions to prevent excessive radiant heat loss by covering the patient as much as possible, especially the head. Many practitioners consider temperature monitoring prudent during extended procedures in cool settings.

SUGGESTED READING

American Academy of Pediatrics, Committee on Drugs. Guidelines for monitoring and management of pediatric patients during and after sedation for diagnostic and therapeutic procedures. Pediatrics 1992;89:1110–1115.

American Society of Anesthesiologists Practice Guidelines for Sedation and Analgesia by Non-Anesthesiologists. Anesthesiology 1996;84:459–471.

Andrews JS. Conscious sedation in the pediatric emergency department. Curr Opin Pediatr 1995;7(3):309–413.

Bell C, Conte AH. Monitoring oxygenation and ventilation during magnetic resonance imaging: a pictorial essay. J Clin Monit 1996;12:71–74.

Block FE Jr. A carbon dioxide monitor that does not show the waveform is worthless. J Clin Monit 1988;4:213–214.

Cote CJ. Sedation for the pediatric patient. Pediatr Clin North Am 1994;41(1):31–58.

Cote CJ, Rolf N, Liu LMP, et al. A single-blind study of combined pulse oximetry and capnography in children. Anesthesiology 1991;74:980–987.

Egleston CV, Aslam HB, Lambert MA. Capnography for monitoring non-intubated spontaneously breathing patients in an emergency room setting. J Accid Emerg Med 1997;14:222–224.

Gilger MA, Jeiven SD, Barrish JO, et al. Oxygen desaturation and cardiac arrhythmias in children during esophagogastroduodenoscopy using conscious sedation. Gastrointest Endosc 1993;39 (3):392–395.

Guidelines for Nonoperating Room Anesthetizing Locations, and Standards for Basic Anesthetic Monitoring. American Society of Anesthesiologists (ASA) Standards, Guidelines, and Statements, Oct 1995.

Hart LS, Berns SD, Houch CS, et al. The value of end-tidal CO_2 monitoring when comparing three methods of conscious sedation for children undergoing painful procedures in the emergency department. Pediatr Emerg Care 1997;13 (3):189–193.

Langbaum M, Eyal FG. A practical and reliable method of measuring blood pressure in the neonate by pulse oximetry. J Pediatr 1994;125 (4):591–595.

Liu LMP, Liu PL. Monitoring in pediatric anesthesia. Semin Anesth XI 1992;(3):243–251.

London MJ, Hollenberg M, Wong MG, et al. Intraoperative myocardial ischemia: localization by continuous 12-lead electrocardiography. Anesthesiology 1988;69:232.

Maxwell LG, Yaster M. The myth of conscious sedation. Arch Pediatr Adolesc Med 1996;150:665–667.

Chapter 4
Benzodiazepines

Mehernoor Watcha

The experience of being in the presence of an apprehensive, crying, struggling child undergoing a procedure is distressful for all, including the parents, health care personnel, and the child. In such a situation, physicians are often asked to provide pharmacologic sedation to reduce patient struggling, permit the procedure to be completed, and consequently improve the overall experience. In this chapter, we will discuss the role of benzodiazepines, a group of drugs that has become popular in recent years for providing sedation in children. Benzodiazepines provide anxiolysis, sedation and amnesia, and help improve the overall experience of children undergoing procedures in the outpatient setting. Diazepam is the prototypical benzodiazepine, but midazolam has become more widely used in recent years. Midazolam has become the benzodiazepine of choice for procedural sedation. In European countries, triazolam had briefly gained some popularity. These drugs are discussed below with an emphasis on midazolam, because it is more widely used and more information is available about it in the pediatric population.

GENERAL INDICATIONS

Benzodiazepines have been used as sedative-hypnotic agents for 1) the management of procedural anxiety, 2) amnesia during procedures, and 3) the control of seizures. In adults, benzodiazepines have been used to treat alcohol withdrawal, panic disorders, and muscle spasms.

MECHANISM OF ACTION

Benzodiazepines are a group of drugs that have a benzene A ring fused to a 7-member diazepine B ring. All clinically active drugs in this group have a 5-aryl substitution C ring. Replacement of the C ring with a keto function at position 5 and a methyl substitution at position 4 results in the antagonist flumazenil. Second-generation benzodiazepines have been synthesized in the hope of separating out the sedative, anxiolytic, and muscle relaxant properties of this group; however, drugs with more selective action have not been identified.

Benzodiazepines act at the gamma-aminobutyric acid ($GABA_A$) receptor, a membrane chloride channel that mediates inhibitory neurotransmission. Benzodiazepine agonists increase the chloride current generated by $GABA_A$ receptor activation, potentiating the GABA effects of calming the patient, relaxing skeletal muscles, and, in high doses, producing sleep.

Although diazepam is considered the prototypical benzodiazepine, it has been replaced in clinical practice by midazolam. The advantages of midazolam relate to its shorter half-life and water-solubility. Triazolam has a more acceptable taste than midazolam, but a longer onset and duration of action.

PHARMACOKINETICS

Data on the pharmacokinetics of diazepam and triazolam in the pediatric patient population are sparse, but are available for midazolam.

Absorption

Absorption varies with the route of administration of midazolam. Mean bioavailability of intramuscular midazolam in children is 87%. Intranasal absorption is good, with a mean bioavailability of 55% and a peak plasma level of 72.2 ± 27.3 ng/mL reached in 10.2 ± 2 minutes after a dose of 0.1 mg/kg. Midazolam is also readily absorbed from the gut but undergoes first-pass hepatic metabolism, resulting in a bioavailability of 27% with an oral dose of 0.15 mg/kg, and 15% with an oral dose of 0.45 or 1 mg/kg. The rectal route has a bioavailability of 18% with peak serum concentrations achieved in 30 minutes.

Satisfactory sedation for gastrointestinal endoscopy has been achieved with blood levels of >200 ng/mL, but lower concentrations permit ease of separation from parents before induction of anesthesia. In anesthetized children, blood levels peaked at 182 ± 57 ng/mL within 12.6 ± 5.9 minutes after intranasal administration of 0.2 mg/kg midazolam, and 48 ± 16 ng/mL within 12.1 ± 6.4 minutes after rectal administration. Triazolam reaches a peak concentration of 8.5 ± 3.0 ng/mL 74 ± 25 minutes after oral intake, in keeping with clinical evidence of a slower onset of action than midazolam.

Distribution

Midazolam is widely distributed in the body, including the cerebrospinal fluid (CSF) and brain, and is highly protein bound. The volume of distribution of midazolam at a steady state has been variously reported as 1 to 1.9 L/kg after oral administration. The volume of distribution is twice as high after intranasal compared with the IV route.

Elimination

Midazolam is rapidly metabolized by hydroxylation. Approximate half-life for oral and intranasal administration are similar (2.2 hours). Elimination half-life is increased in neonates below 39 weeks gestation, in critically ill patients with cardiac failure, and in the obese. Triazolam has a long elimination half-life of 213 ± 144 minutes.

ROUTES OF ADMINISTRATION

Oral

Midazolam and diazepam have been administered by the oral, intranasal, rectal, intramuscular, and intravenous routes. The oral route is most commonly used, and satisfactory sedation can be achieved in 30 to 45 minutes with 0.5 mg/kg of oral midazolam, a dose that takes into consideration the first-pass hepatic effect. Higher doses of 0.75 to 1.0 mg/kg midazolam are associated with increased side effects such as dysphoria, blurred vision, and loss of balance and head control. Disguising the bitter taste of the drug is also a problem (see below). Triazolam has been suggested as an alternative to midazolam because the taste is considered more acceptable; however, it has a longer onset and duration of action, with sedative effects lasting as long as 180 minutes, leading to delayed discharge.

Although the oral route of administration is the most acceptable, convenient, and easiest method of delivery, a liquid oral formulation of midazolam is not currently available in the USA, hence, the oral administration of the injectable preparation. However, this preparation is bitter, and smaller children often either refuse to ingest it or promptly spit it out. The taste has been disguised by the addition of flavors including cherry or chocolate syrup, apple juice, Kool Aid, etc., and children are instructed to swallow all of it as quickly as possible. An oral formulation of midazolam with a more acceptable taste is currently undergoing clinical trials in the USA. Oral preparations of diazepam and triazolam are available.

Oral Transmucosal Midazolam

Midazolam reportedly has been administered via the sublingual route where transmucosal absorption results in rapid sedation. However, the bitter taste of the drug limits this route of administration. In a study of sublingual midazolam, many of the children who received it via this route did not comply with instructions and swallowed it. Thus, it is unclear if true transmucosal or oral absorption occurred.

Intranasal

The nasal route of administering midazolam was described a decade ago when concerns for residual gastric volume with oral drugs was higher than warranted. Intranasal application of benzodiazepines provides a more rapid onset of clinically effective sedation than the rectal or oral routes (7 to 10 minutes vs 25 to 40 minutes for midazolam). The usual intranasal dose of midazolam is 0.2 to 0.5 mg/kg, but the efficacy may vary if a diluent is administered or in the presence of an upper respiratory infection (URI). If midazolam is administered with saline, some of it may end up in the oropharynx and not undergo transmucosal absorption. In the presence of a URI, increased nasal secretions may decrease contact of the drug with nasal mucosa, but increased vascular congestion may increase absorption of that amount, which does come in contact with the mucosa. Although effective, intranasal midazolam is irritating to the nasal mucosa, increasing the frequency and duration of crying in children compared with the sublingual route or to nasal sufentanil. Many children who have received this drug will not accept it again when they come for a second procedure.

Rectal

The rectal route of administering drugs is more acceptable to patients and their families in Europe than in the USA. Blood levels after rectal administration are erratic because of variable absorption. The venous blood supply of the rectum drains into the superior hemorrhoidal vein, which opens into the portal circulation, and into the inferior hemorrhoidal vein, which does not open into the portal circulation. Consequently, a variable first-pass hepatic effect occurs after rectal absorption. Optimal results are achieved with rectal doses of 0.3 to 0.5 mg/kg of midazolam, but the onset of action is slower than with the intranasal route. Rectal diazepam, doses of 0.7 mg/kg, provides less effective sedation than midazolam in pediatric dental patients. With the decrease in concerns about residual gastric volumes and potential aspiration during induction, the oral route remains a more acceptable method.

Intramuscular

The initial preparation of diazepam in propylene glycol was absorbed erratically from intramuscular sites, and caused pain on injection, leading to a recommendation not to administer this drug by the intramuscular (IM) route. In contrast, midazolam is water soluble and has been administered by the intramuscular route with satisfactory sedation achieved with doses of 0.1 to 0.2 mg/kg IM. This mode of delivery in children has been questioned because of the associated pain on injection. A Biojector jet injector has been used to avoid the use of needles, but dose-related pain and crying on injection remained a problem. A different jet injector (Hingson's) was used in another study that claimed that a dose of 0.2 mg/kg of midazolam provided rapid, pain-free and stress-free sedation. However, others have reported respiratory depression with IM doses of 0.1 to 0.2 mg/kg.

Intravenous

Benzodiazepines have also been administered by the intravenous route (0.05 to 0.1 mg/kg) in pediatric patients. The advantage is ease of titration, whereas the disadvantage is the need to insert an intravenous line in a fearful and potentially uncooperative child. The older preparations of diazepam were formulated in propylene glycol, which was irritating to the veins, causing pain on injection. A new lipid-based formulation of diazepam (Diazemules) has been introduced with the advantage of being less irritating to the veins. However, the longer half-life of diazepam makes it less attractive than midazolam for outpatient procedures.

AVAILABLE PREPARATIONS (SEE CHAPTER 26)

INDICATIONS

The major indication for the use of benzodiazepines in the outpatient setting is sedation and anxiolysis for diagnostic and therapeutic procedures. In the United States, oral midazolam has become the most popular anxiolytic, both preprocedure and preanesthesia. Separation from parents is easier and occurs optimally at 20 to 45 minutes after oral ingestion of 0.5 mg/kg, although in one study separation was possible as early as 10 minutes after ingestion. In comparisons with the older sedative drugs used as premedication (ketamine; trimeprazine; droperidol; combinations of meperidine, atropine, and pentobarbital; meperidine, promethazine, chlorpromazine), midazolam was noted to be associated with more satisfactory behavior, more rapid recovery, and decreased respiratory depression.

These drugs are clinically useful in obtaining anxiolysis during procedures that are not inherently painful. Because benzodiazepines do not have analgesic effects, some other form of analgesia must be used during painful procedures (e.g., local anesthetics, nonsteroidal analgesics, or opioids).

CONTRAINDICATIONS AND PRECAUTIONS

Adverse Effects

Major side effects include cardiorespiratory depression, paradoxical excitement, and emergence delirium. These adverse effects are dose-related and vary with the route of administration. Although hypotension and bradycardia can occur with IV midazolam, respiratory depression occurs more often, particularly after rapid IV administration.

Although respiratory depression does not occur with the usual doses of intranasal midazolam (0.2 to 0.4 mg/kg), higher doses (0.6 mg/kg) may lead to prolonged elimination, delayed recovery, and respiratory depression. Some practitioners have been concerned about the possibility of direct neurotoxicity of nasally administered drugs, which may travel along the olfactory nerves to the central nervous system. High blood levels of midazolam (160 ng/mL at 10 minutes) were reported in an infant who received 0.2 mg/kg intranasally and developed apnea. This confirms the need for close monitoring of any child who receives a sedative drug via the intranasal route. No case reports exist of serious respiratory depression with oral midazolam (0.5 mg/kg) except when other sedative drugs are administered concomitantly.

Paradoxical excitement has been reported in 10 to 15% of patients after oral, intravenous, and rectal administration of midazolam and may appear in the recovery phase. The incidence of disinhibition reactions were higher in patients receiving 0.45 mg/kg rectally in one study. This complication is disturbing for family members and health caretakers because the effect is diametrically opposite of the desired effect when the drug was administered. Reports of sedation, amnesia, hallucinations, bizarre behavior, and agitation in adults who have received long-term therapy with triazolam have led to concerns about its use for sedation in the outpatient setting.

Drug Interactions

The combination of midazolam and systemic opioids causes synergistic respiratory depression, and a lower dose of midazolam should be given if systemic opioids are also administered. In some situations, particularly with ASA class III or IV patients, it may be safer to arrange for a general anesthetic in the operating room where the airway can be secured and inhalation agents can be used, rather than to continue to administer additional doses of sedatives in less than ideal conditions.

There are case reports of increased duration of effect when benzodiazepines have been administered to patients who are also receiving erythromycin, cimetidine, or antifungal agents.

Relative Contraindications

Midazolam affects the tone of upper airway muscles and delays cricopharyngeal relaxation. This may exacerbate swallowing difficulties and cause hypoxemia from upper airway obstruction, particularly in children with sleep disorders. Sedation of patients with airway obstruction or abnormal central nervous system control of respiration can be hazardous.

SUGGESTED READING

Bahal-O'Mara N, Nahata MC, Murray RD, et al. Sedation with meperidine and midazolam in pediatric patients undergoing endoscopy. European J Clin Pharmacol 1994;47:319–323.

Battan FK, Harley JR, Brownstein D, et al. A randomized controlled trial of intranasal midazolam as sedation for laceration repair. Pediatr Emerg Care 1990;6:222.

Committee on Drugs. Guidelines for monitoring and management of pediatric patients during and after sedation for diagnostic and therapeutic procedures. Pediatrics 1992;89:1110.

Davis CO, Wax PM. Flumazenil associated seizure in an 11-month-old child. J Emerg Med 1996;14:331–333.

Davis PJ, Tome JA, McGowan FX Jr, et al. Preanesthetic medication with intranasal midazolam for brief pediatric surgical procedures. Effect on recovery and hospital discharge times. Anesthesiology 1995;82:2–5.

Doyle WL, Perrin L. Emergence delirium in a child given oral midazolam for conscious sedation. Ann Emerg Med 1994;24:1173–1175.

Elder JS, Longenecker R. Premedication with oral midazolam for voiding cystourethrography in children: safety and efficacy. AJR 1994;1229–1232.

Greenberg RS, Maxwell LG, Zahurak M, et al. Preanesthetic medication of children with midazolam using the Biojector jet injector. Anesthesiology 1995;83:264–269.

Hamid RKA, Lake CL, Rice LJ, et al, eds. Pediatric Premedication. St. Louis: CV Mosby, 1998;15:227–289.

Hennes HM, Wagner V, Bonadio WA, et al. The effect of oral midazolam on anxiety of preschool children during laceration repair. Ann Emerg Med 1990;19:1006–1009.

Jones RD, Visram AR, Kornberg JP, et al. Premedication with oral midazolam in children—an assessment of psychomotor function, anxiolysis, sedation and pharmacokinetics. Anaesth Intensive Care 1994;22:539–544.

Karl HW, Milgrom P, Domoto P, et al. Pharmacokinetics of oral triazolam in children. J Clin Psychopharmacol 1997;17:169–172.

Malinovsky JM, Populaire C, Cozian A, et al. Premedication with midazolam in children. Effect of intranasal, rectal and oral routes on plasma midazolam concentrations. Anaesthesia 1995;50:351–354.

McMillan CO, Spahr-Schopfer IA, Sikich N, et al. Premedication of children with oral midazolam. Can J Anesth 1992;39;545–550.

Negus BH, Street NE. Midazolam-opioid combination and postoperative upper airway obstruction in children (letter). Anaesth Intensive Care 1994;22:232–233.

Nicolson SC, Schreiner MS, Watcha MF. Preoperative preparation of the child for anesthesia. Am J Anesthesiol 1996;23:157–162.

Patel D, Meakin G. Oral midazolam compared with diazepam-droperidol and trimeprazine as premedicants in children. Paediatr Anaesth 1997;7:287–293.

Peterson MD. Making oral midazolam palatable for children. Anesthesiology 1990;73:1053.

Reves JG, Fragen RJ, Vinik HR, et al. Midazolam: pharmacology and uses. Anesthesiology 1985:63:310–324.

Theroux MC, West DW, Corddry DH, et al. Efficacy of intranasal midazolam in facilitating the suturing of lacerations in preschool children in the emergency room. Pediatrics 1993;91: 624–627.

Yealy DM, Ellis JH, Hobbs GD, et al. Intranasal midazolam as a sedative for children during laceration repair. Ann J Emerg Med 1992;10:584–587.

Zsigmond EK, Kovacs V, Fekete G. A new route, jet-injection for anesthetic induction in children: I. Midazolam dose-range finding studies. Int J Clin Pharmacol Ther 1995;33:580–584.

Classic

Feld LH, Negus JB, White PF. Oral midazolam preanesthetic medication in pediatric outpatients. Anesthesiology 1990;73:831–834.

Roelofse JA, van der Bijl P. Comparison of rectal midazolam and diazepam for premedication in pediatric dental patients. J Oral Maxillofac Surg 1993;51:525–529.

Sandler E, Weyman C, Connor K, et al. Midazolam versus fentanyl as premedication for painful procedures in children with cancer. Pediatrics 1992;89:634.

Weldon BC, Watcha MF, White PF. Oral midazolam in children: effect of time and adjunctive therapy. Anesth Analg 1992;75:51–55.

Reviews

Giovannitti JAJ. Regimens for pediatric sedation. Compendium 1993;14:1002–1006.

Perry HE, Shannon MW. Diagnosis and management of opioid- and benzodiazepine-induced comatose overdose in children. (Review) (36 refs) Curr Opin Pediatr 1996;8:243–247.

Philip BK. Drug reversal: benzodiazepine receptors and antagonists. J Clin Anesth 1993;5(6 Suppl 1):46S–51S.

Rego MMS, Watcha MF, White PF. Changing role of monitored anesthesia care in the ambulatory setting. Anesth Analg 1997;89:1020–1036.

Whitman JG. Flumazenil and midazolam in anaesthesia. Acta Anaesthesiolg Scand (Suppl) 1995;108:15–22.

Chapter 5
Barbiturates

Shobha Malviya

Barbituric acid was first synthesized in 1864. Subsequently, many hypnotic barbiturates with slow onset and prolonged duration of action were introduced between 1903 and 1932. In the early 1930s, the short-acting barbiturates hexobarbital and thiopental were introduced, but because of limited understanding of their pharmacokinetics, their inappropriate use led to disastrous results, including multiple deaths. However, improved understanding of its pharmacokinetics have made thiopental the standard drug for induction of anesthesia, with which all newer induction agents are compared.

The ideal sedative drug for diagnostic and therapeutic procedures should have a quick onset and short duration of action, with minimal effects on respiratory drive, protective airway reflexes, and hemodynamic status of the patient. No drug in the pharmacopoeia of procedural sedation meets all these criteria. With an increasing need for efficient use of health care resources, there has been a resurgence of interest in the use of barbiturates for these procedures because these drugs reliably produce adequate sedation with short induction times and quick recovery. These drugs, however, can produce loss of protective airway reflexes and respiratory depression and they have the potential to cause hemodynamic instability.

GENERAL INDICATIONS

The predominant clinical uses of barbiturates in the outpatient setting are for induction of anesthesia, sedation for diagnostic and therapeutic procedures, and anticonvulsants.

MECHANISM OF ACTION

Gamma-aminobutyric acid (GABA) is the principal inhibitory neurotransmitter in the mammalian central nervous system (CNS). At clinical drug concentrations, barbiturates decrease the rate of dissociation of GABA from the $GABA_A$ receptor complex, thereby increasing chloride conductance through the chloride ion channels. This results in hyperpolarization and inhibition of postsynaptic neurons. The result is a depression of the reticular activating system, which is important in the maintenance of wakefulness. At higher concentrations, barbiturates directly activate chloride channels even in the absence of GABA. Enhancement of GABA may be responsible for the sedative-hypnotic effects, whereas the direct effect on the chloride channels is likely responsible for the anesthetic effects of barbiturates.

PHARMACOKINETICS

Pharmacokinetics vary with the molecular structure and with the route of administration of each of these drugs. The thiobarbiturates (thiopental and thiamylal) have a sulfur atom at the number five carbon position of the barbituric acid ring. These drugs are more lipid soluble than their oxybarbiturate analogues (pentobarbital, secobarbital), and therefore have a more rapid onset but shorter duration of action.

Absorption

When administered orally, most barbiturates are rapidly and almost completely absorbed. The sodium salts are more rapidly absorbed than the free acids. The onset of action after oral administration ranges from 10 to 60 minutes. If the intramuscular route is required, sodium salts must be injected deep into large muscles to minimize pain and possible tissue necrosis.

Distribution

Barbiturates are distributed in the body on the basis of their lipid solubility, protein binding, and the extent to which they are ionized. In addition to these factors, tissue blood flow also plays an important role in the delivery of barbiturates to various tissues. The effect of some of the short-acting barbiturates is terminated by redistribution of the drug rather than elimination. An intravenous dose of thiopental is rapidly distributed by blood flow and molecular diffusion throughout the tissues of the body, particularly to highly perfused tissues like the brain, where high initial concentrations of thiopental result in the induction of anesthesia. Subsequently, concentrations of thiopental in the blood and highly perfused tissues rapidly decrease as the drug is redistributed to less perfused tissue such as muscle and adipose tissue.

Elimination

Barbiturates are metabolized by oxidation primarily in the endoplasmic reticulum of the hepatocytes. In addition, thiobarbiturates are broken down to a small extent in extrahepatic sites including the kidneys and the central nervous system. The metabolites are water soluble and excreted via the kidneys.

ROUTES OF ADMINISTRATION/AVAILABLE PREPARATIONS (TABLE 5.1)

INDICATIONS

Induction of Anesthesia

Thiopental and methohexital, by virtue of their lipid solubility, act in one arm-brain circulation time when injected intravenously with a peak effect in 1 minute. Methohexital use is associated with a more rapid recovery than thiopental; however, it also causes an increased incidence of involuntary skeletal muscle movements in a dose-dependent manner.

Procedural Sedation (See Chapters 21 and 26)

The onset and duration of action of barbiturates varies depending on the route of administration. For example, thiopental or methohexital that are categorized as "ultra short-acting," have a longer duration of action after rectal or intramuscular administration. These properties make them popular as sedatives for procedures of intermediate duration (15 to 60 minutes) such as CT and MRI scans. Pentobarbi-

Table 5.1. Available Preparations and Routes of Administration

Pharmacologic Agent (Generic Name)	Routes of Administration	Dosage (mg/kg)	Available Preparations
Methohexital (Brevital)	IV, PR	IV: 1–1.5 mg/kg[a] (Induction of GA) IM: 10 mg/kg PR: 20–30 mg/kg	500 mg vial Water soluble powder
Thiopental (Pentothal)	IV, PR	IV: 3–6 mg/kg[a] (Induction of GA) PR: 25–50 mg/kg	0.5, 1 gm vials
Pentobarbital (Nembutal)	PO, IM, IV, PR	IV: 2–6 mg/kg[b] IM: 4–6 mg/kg PO: 2–6 mg/kg PR: 2–6 mg/kg	Elixir 20 mL/5 mL Caps 30, 50, 100 mg Supp 30, 60, 120, 200 mg Inj 50 mg/mL

GA, general anesthesia; IM, intramuscular; IV, intravenous; PO, oral; PR, rectal.
[a]As there are no studies on the use of IV thiopental or IV methohexital for procedural sedation in children, the IV route for these drugs is not generally recommended for procedural sedation.
[b]Should be titrated in 1–2 mg/kg increments to achieve desired effect.

tal, a longer-acting barbiturate, is perhaps the most popular sedative agent for radiologic investigations.

Rectal thiopental, rectal methohexital, and IV pentobarbital have been extensively used for sedating children for radiologic procedures. Of these drugs, pentobarbital is perhaps the most popular because it reliably achieves adequate sedation within 30 to 60 seconds after the initial IV dose. The use of pentobarbital for sedation, however, is associated with a 3 to 7.5% incidence of significant oxygen desaturation.

Rectal methohexital (10% solution, 20 to 30 mg/kg, maximum 500 mg) has been extensively used to facilitate anesthetic induction in children. With these doses, Liu, et al demonstrated sleep induction times of 7 to 8 minutes in 80 to 90% of patients. Loss of consciousness with rectal methohexital has been shown to correlate well with plasma concentrations of the drug (mean plasma concentration 4.4 [g/mL at sleep onset time]). A comparison study of methohexital and chloral hydrate for imaging procedures demonstrated adequate sedation in both groups but a significantly shorter induction time and quicker recovery with methohexital. Another study compared the use of rectal thiopental (25 mg/kg) with intramuscular meperidine, promethazine, and chlorpromazine for sedation before local anesthetic infiltration for suturing of lacerations in the emergency department. Sedation was adequate in both groups, but the thiopental group had shorter induction and recovery times. There were no adverse events in either group.

Anticonvulsant

Both thiopental and phenobarbital have been shown to abruptly stop seizures refractory to other anticonvulsant drugs. Thiopental has a low ratio of anticonvulsant to hypnotic action; therefore, its use is restricted to emergency treatment of seizures refractory to other measures.

CONTRAINDICATIONS AND PRECAUTIONS

Adverse Reactions

Injection Complications Injection of barbiturates may be associated with transient hives on the upper torso and face and may rarely cause anaphylactoid manifestations, including hives, bronchospasm, and cardiovascular collapse. Both thiopental and methohexital cause pain on intravenous injection (2 and 5% incidence respectively). When extravasated, thiopental causes a local tissue reaction ranging from pain, edema, and erythema to tissue necrosis.

Inadvertent intra-arterial injection of the thiobarbiturates results in intense arterial spasm and excruciating pain along the distribution of the artery. Intense vasoconstriction is manifest by decreased or absent pulses and blanching or cyanosis of the extremity, and may even progress to gangrene and permanent nerve damage. These changes occur secondary to a chemical endarteritis as thiopental crystals form in the arterioles and capillaries. The treatment of this condition requires attempts to dilute the drug, relieve arterial spasm, and maintain adequate blood flow. These goals may be accomplished by injecting lidocaine, papaverine, or phenoxybenzamine into the affected artery or into a more proximal artery. Direct injection of heparin into the artery and sympathectomy of the extremity by a stellate ganglion block may also be considered.

CNS Effects Barbiturates are administered primarily for their CNS depressant effects. In subanesthetic concentrations, barbiturates may exert antianalgesic effects and cause an exaggerated response to pain. Barbiturates cause restlessness, excitement, and even delirium in the presence of pain. This property makes them unsuitable choices as sole sedative agents for painful procedures. If used for painful procedures, barbiturates must be used in combination with analgesics such as opioids; however, the risk of synergistic respiratory depression must be considered.

Cardiovascular Effects Hemodynamic changes associated with the use of barbiturates depend on the patient's underlying history of heart disease, volume status, resting sympathetic nervous system tone, and the speed of injection of the drug. A standard anesthetic induction dose of thiopental (5 mg/kg) produces a transient mild decrease in blood pressure that is offset by a compensatory mild tachycardia. These changes occur because of venodilation with peripheral pooling and decreased venous return, as well as a modest direct myocardial depressant effect. Barbiturates should therefore be used with great caution in patients with conditions in which an increase in heart rate or decrease in preload would be detrimental, including hypovolemia, ischemic heart disease, and cardiac tamponade.

Respiratory Effects Barbiturates produce a dose-dependent depression of the medullary and pontine respiratory centers. This may lead to apnea, particularly when administered concomitantly with other sedative drugs. While the respiratory pattern may return to normal in a few minutes with the shorter-acting barbiturates, depression of the ventilatory responses to hypercarbia and hypoxia persists for a longer time. Even a small dose of pentobarbital (2 mg/kg) depresses the ventilatory response to hypoxemia.

Other Side Effects Thiopental causes a dose-related histamine release, which accounts for the vasodilatation and pruritus discussed in the previous section.

Acute Toxicity

Acute barbiturate intoxication does not occur frequently. The lethal dose is variable, but severe intoxication occurs with the ingestion of ten times the usual hypnotic dose. Severe intoxication results in coma, respiratory depression and circulatory collapse. Acute renal failure may occur as a result of shock and hypoxia.

Drug Interactions

Barbiturates induce hepatic microsomal enzymes, which accelerate the metabolism of other drugs such as oral anticoagulants, tricyclic antidepressants, and phenytoin that are metabolized by the P-450 system. In addition, when administered in conjunction with other CNS depressants such as ethanol and antihistamines, barbiturates cause greater CNS depression than when given alone.

Relative Contraindications

Rapid intravenous injection of barbiturates in patients with hypovolemia may cause severe hypotension and cardiovascular collapse. (See previous section on cardiovascular effects.)

Absolute Contraindications

Barbiturates are absolutely contraindicated in patients with acute intermittent porphyria or with variegate porphyria because they induce δ-aminolevulinic acid synthetase, a catalyst in the biosynthesis of porphyrins. The use of barbiturates in patients with these conditions may precipitate a widespread demyelination of peripheral and cranial nerves, resulting in life-threatening weakness and paralysis.

SUGGESTED READING

Fragen RJ, Avram MJ. Barbiturates. In: Miller RD, ed. Anesthesia. 4th ed. New York: Churchill Livingstone, 1994;1:229–246.

Hardman JG, Limbird LE, ed. Goodman and Gilman's The Pharmacological Basis of Therapeutics. 9th ed. New York: McGraw-Hill, 1996;321–323, 373–380.

Hirshman CA, McCullough RE, Cohen PJ, et al. Hypoxic ventilatory drive in dogs during thiopental, ketamine, or phenobarbital anesthesia. Anesthesiology 1975;43:628.

Liu LMP, Gaudreault P, Friedman PA, et al. Methohexital plasma concentrations in children following rectal administration. Anesthesiology 1985;62:567–570.

Liu LMP, Goudsouzian NG, Liu PL. Rectal methohexital premedication in children: a dose-comparison study. Anesthesiology 1980;53:343–345.

Manuli MA, Davies L. Rectal methohexital for sedation of children during imaging procedures. AJR 1993;160:577–580.

McCullough RE, Cohen PJ, Weil JV. Effect of pentobarbitone on hypoxic ventilatory drive in man: preliminary study. Br J Anaesth 1975; 47:963.

O'Brien JF, Falk JL, Carey BE, et al. Rectal thiopental compared with intramuscular meperidine, promethazine, and chlorpromazine for pediatric sedation. Ann Emerg Med 1991;20(6): 644–647.

Stoelting RK. Barbiturates. In: Stoelting RK, ed. Pharmacology and Physiology in Anesthetic Practice. 2nd ed. Philadelphia: JB Lippincott Company, 1991;102–117.

Strain JD, Campbell JB, Harvey LA, et al. IV Nembutal: safe sedation for children undergoing CT. AJR 1988;151:975–979.

Young GB, Blume WT, Bolton CF, et al. Anesthetic barbiturates in refractory status epilepticus. J Sci Neurol 1980;7:291.

Chapter 6
Sedatives/Hypnotics

Ronald Litman

CHLORAL HYDRATE

General Indications

Chloral hydrate is a sedative/hypnotic agent with no analgesic properties that induces sleep. For several decades, medical and dental practitioners have used chloral hydrate safely for patients who require sedation during anxiety-provoking procedures (especially for neuroimaging in infants and young toddlers) and for patients (especially in the geriatric population) who require assistance in falling asleep. Because chloral hydrate produces a relatively light level of sleep, it is assumed (though no data are available) that protective airway reflexes are maintained. Therefore, fasting guidelines are often liberalized.

Mechanism of Action

Unknown, although the majority of action is probably caused by trichloroethanol.

Pharmacokinetics

Absorption Chloral hydrate is rapidly absorbed from the GI tract after oral administration. Onset of sleep occurs in 15 to 60 minutes, and sleep may last 1 to 4 hours.

Elimination Chloral hydrate is oxidized to trichloroethanol (TCE), an active metabolite, by aldehyde dehydrogenase in the liver and is then reduced to trichloroacetic acid (TCA), an inactive metabolite, via alcohol dehydrogenase. TCE is responsible for the majority of the sedative/hypnotic effects. TCE can be further metabolized via conjugation with the glucuronic acid in the liver as TCE-G and, subsequently, eliminated in the urine because this compound is water-soluble. TCA also is water-soluble and eliminated in the urine.

Routes of Administration (Tables 6.1 and 6.2)

Available Preparations

Chloral hydrate is available orally in the form of capsules (250 and 500 mg) or solution (250 mg and 500 mg/5 mL). It is available rectally in the form of suppositories (325, 500, and 650 mg).

Indications

Chloral hydrate is most useful for inducing sleep in children who are undergoing nonpainful procedures that do not require strict immobility. These procedures

Table 6.1. Strong Memorial Hospital Fasting Guidelines for Chloral Hydrate for Elective Procedures

	Solids and Milk Products	Breast Milk	Clear Liquids
Dose < 50 mg/kg and child > 40 kg		No restrictions	
All other doses and weights	4 h	2 h	May be given immediately before chloral hydrate administration

Table 6.2. Strong Memorial Hospital Guidelines for Administration, Dosing, and Monitoring of Children Receiving Chloral Hydrate

Monitoring	Dose	Weight
1:1 RN	≥ 75 mg/kg	< 40 kg
1:1 RN extender and q 15 min formal RN assessments for at least 1 h	50–75 mg/kg	> 40 kg
Continuous pulse oximetry	> 50 mg/kg	All
Standard observation by RN extender for first hour after chloral hydrate administration	< 50 mg/kg	> 40 kg

General dosing guidelines: Dose = 25–100 mg/kg. Maximum total dose 100 mg/kg or 2 gm (whichever is less). May administer a second dose in 20–30 minutes if necessary (up to maximum dose). Maximum dose of 75 mg/kg for infants < 10 kg.

All children with significant developmental delay and/or potential for upper airway problems require continuous oximetry, continuous observation by a nurse or extender, and a vital signs check q 15 minutes regardless of dose administered.

RN, registered nurse.

include electroencephalography, echocardiography, and electrocardiography. Chloral hydrate is also useful for sedation during radiologic imaging such as MRI or CT scans. Chloral hydrate is not a useful sedative for use during painful procedures because it lacks analgesic properties and is not potent enough to reliably maintain sleep during physical stimuli. In fact, it may produce excitement or delirium in the presence of pain.

Contraindications and Precautions

Adverse Reactions The adverse reactions of chloral hydrate are as follows:

Respiratory depression (dose related)
Hypotension (especially in neonates—mechanism unknown)
Disorientation/dysphoria/ataxia/dizziness
Prolonged sedation
Headache
Rash
Gastric and esophageal irritation
Nausea/vomiting/diarrhea
Leukoplakia
Eosinophilia

Chloral hydrate is considered to be one of the safest sedative agents available but has the potential for causing unexpectedly deep levels of sedation as well as upper airway obstruction in susceptible patients. These susceptible patients include young infants, children with preexisting upper airway obstruction (e.g., enlarged tonsils, sleep apnea, laryngomalacia), and children who have received other sedatives concomitantly.

Other contraindications and precautions that should be considered include the following:

- Children with developmental delay may have an exaggerated or dysphoric reaction to chloral hydrate (mechanism unknown); lower doses should be considered.
- Chloral hydrate causes decreases in oxyhemoglobin saturation in infants with bronchiolitis. This effect is presumably caused by depression of central nervous system respiratory drive, resulting in a lower respiratory rate and decreased use of accessory muscles of respiration.
- Chloral hydrate should be used with caution in neonates (especially premature)—elimination times are longer than for older children, and prolonged use is associated with hyperbilirubinemia.
- Chloral hydrate is less efficacious in children older than 3 years of age (mechanism unknown).

- Because chloral hydrate is a metabolite of trichloroethylene, an industrial solvent, there are theoretical concerns about the carcinogenicity of chloral hydrate with chronic exposure. The American Academy of Pediatrics has issued a position paper on the safety of chloral hydrate in the acute setting.
- Chloral hydrate crosses the placenta.

Acute Toxicity
- Excessive sedation may result in toxicity.
  - -Large doses of chloral hydrate shorten the cardiac refractory period and depress myocardial contractility. Chloral hydrate is believed to sensitize the myocardium to catecholamines, which results in arrhythmias. This explains why the administration of epinephrine to patients with acute chloral hydrate toxicity may be detrimental. In addition, there is a high incidence of arrhythmias in children who are given chloral hydrate and are receiving concomitant infusions of pressors.
- Gastric irritation may occur.
- Hepatitis may result.

Drug Interactions Chloral hydrate may potentiate the effects of warfarin, CNS depressants, and alcohol. Concomitant use with IV furosemide may result in flushing, diaphoresis, and hypotension. The mechanism of this is unknown but it is postulated that furosemide displaces TCA from albumin, causing an increase in free thyroxin (by an unknown mechanism), which causes a hypermetabolic state.

Relative Contraindications
- Concomitant use of pressors
- Significant renal or hepatic impairment
- Gastritis, esophagitis, ulcers
- Pregnancy
- Extreme prematurity
- Bronchiolitis/asthma

Absolute Contraindications
- Known hypersensitivity
- Severe cardiac disease

PROPOFOL

General Indications

Propofol is an intravenous sedative/hypnotic, with no analgesic properties, that has become popular in recent years because of its rapid onset and offset, easy titratability, and lack of emetogenic effects. Propofol is commonly used to induce general anesthesia; however, in lower doses, propofol provides transient unconsciousness during painful medical procedures in children, and is used as a continuous infusion for sedation in the intensive care unit (ICU).

Mechanism of Action

The mechanism of action of propofol is unknown.

Pharmacokinetics

Absorption Propofol follows a three-compartment linear model represented by the plasma, rapidly equilibrating tissues, and slowly equilibrating tissues. After an IV dose, the plasma concentration rapidly equilibrates with the brain concentration, resulting in the rapid onset of hypnosis/unconsciousness. Plasma levels fall quickly as a result of redistribution and metabolic clearance, thus causing a rapid offset of effect. Higher doses for prolonged periods will result in tissue saturation and a slower offset when discontinued. Pediatric patients require greater doses of propofol than adults to achieve the same desired effect, probably because of a greater volume of distribution.

Elimination Propofol is conjugated in the liver to inactive metabolites that are eliminated in the kidney.

Routes of Administration

Propofol is administered intravenously only (Table 6.3).

Table 6.3.   Propofol Dosing Guidelines

Indication	Dosing Regimen
Induction of general anesthesia	Bolus: 3–5 mg/kg given over 30–60 sec.
Maintenance of general anesthesia	Continuous infusion: 150–200 $\mu g^{-1}kg^{-1}min$. Titrate to maintain heart rate and blood pressure within 20% of baseline.
Procedural sedation	Intermittent bolus: 0.5–1 mg/kg. Repeat as necessary. Continuous infusion: 50–150 $\mu g^{-1}kg^{-1}min$. Titrate to maintain heart rate and blood pressure within 20% of baseline.
Sedation after endotracheal intubation	Continuous infusion: 50–100 $\mu g^{-1}kg^{-1}min$. Titrate to maintain heart rate and blood pressure within 20% of baseline.

Available Preparations

Propofol preparations are available as 10 mg/mL (1%).

Indications

- *Operating room:* induction and maintenance of general anesthesia.
- *ICU:* continuous infusion for maintenance of sedation/unconsciousness during mechanical ventilation and for brief procedures.
- *Outpatient setting:* maintenance of sedation/unconsciousness in children undergoing painful procedures, such as bone marrow aspiration, lumbar punctures, and dislocation reductions.
- *Radiology:* maintenance of sedation/unconsciousness during radiologic imaging studies.
- *Postoperative and chemotherapy-induced emesis:* acts as a weak antiemetic and has been used successfully in small doses (10 to 20 mg) when traditional antiemetics have failed.
- *Pruritus:* treatment of pruritus from various causes.
- *Emergency department:* Propofol would be ideal for the sedation of children during painful procedures in the emergency setting (rapid onset, short duration). However, its use has been limited because of the concern for blunting protective airway reflexes. Studies are needed to demonstrate the safety and efficacy of propofol for children in the emergency department.

Contraindications and Precautions

Adverse Effects The adverse effects of propofol include the following:

- Plasma levels of propofol that result in unconsciousness may also cause apnea, hypoventilation, and loss of protective airway reflexes.
- Bradycardia and hypotension may result even at doses that preserve spontaneous ventilation. This effect is rare and may be caused by interactions with concomitant sedatives.
- Myoclonic movements resembling seizures may result after bolus dosing. These are self-limiting.
- Dysphoric reactions may occur at low doses that preserve consciousness. These are not paradoxical reactions but are dose-related and probably caused by central inhibition. Increasing the dose (decreasing consciousness) will ameliorate this phenomenon.
- Administration of propofol causes severe pain at the injection site. This can be minimized by injecting into a large (antecubital) vein or by mixing the propofol with lidocaine, 0.5 mg/kg (equal to 0.05 mL/kg of a 1% lidocaine preparation). The lidocaine may be given as a pretreatment or mixed with the propofol in the same syringe.
- Patients have developed sepsis from bacterial contamination of propofol. There-

fore, strict aseptic technique must be followed during handling and administration. The intralipid solution is an excellent medium for bacterial growth.

Acute Toxicity Toxicity may result in cardiorespiratory collapse.

Drug Interactions The potential for respiratory and cardiac depression is greatly increased when propofol is given in combination with other CNS depressants, which include, but are not limited to, barbiturates, opioids, and benzodiazepines.

Contraindications The contraindications of propofol are as follows:

- Known hypersensitivity to propofol or any of its constituents (soybean oil, egg lecithin [yolk], glycerol, and disodium edetate).
- Preexisting airway obstruction or anatomical abnormalities that would result in airway occlusion with the onset of unconsciousness.
- Increased intracranial pressure or pulmonary hypertension. Hypoventilation resulting in hypercarbia can lead to worsening of these conditions.

SUGGESTED READING

Chloral Hydrate

American Academy of Pediatrics. Use of chloral hydrate for sedation in children. Pediatrics 1993;92:471–473.

Biban P, Baraldi E, Pettenazzo A, et al. Adverse effect of chloral hydrate in two young children with obstructive sleep apnea. Pediatrics 1993;92:461–463.

Graham SR, Day RO, Lee R, Fulde GWO. Overdose with chloral hydrate: a pharmacological and therapeutic review. Med J Austral 1988;149:686–688.

Hershenson M, Brouillette RT, Olsen E, et al. The effect of chloral hydrate on genioglossus and diaphragmatic activity. Pediatr Res 1984;18:516–519.

Hirsch IA, Zauder HL. Chloral hydrate: a potential cause of arrhythmias. Anesth Analg 1986;65:691–692.

Hunt CE, Hazinski TA, Gora P. Experimental effects of chloral hydrate on ventilatory response to hypoxia and hypercarbia. Pediatr Res 1982;16:79–81.

Jastak JT, Pallasch TJ. Death after chloral hydrate sedation: report of a case. J Am Dent Assoc 1988;116:345–348.

Lambert GH, Muraskas J, Anderson CL, et al. Direct hyperbilirubinemia associated with chloral hydrate administration in the newborn. Pediatrics 1990;86:277–281.

Lees MH, Olsen GD, McGilliard KL, et al. Chloral hydrate and the carbon dioxide chemoreceptor response: a study of puppies and infants. Pediatrics 1982;70:447–450.

Litman RS, Kottra JA, Verga KA, et al. Chloral hydrate sedation: the additive sedative and respiratory depressant effects of nitrous oxide. Anesth Analg 1998;86:724–728.

Mallol J, Sly PD. Effect of chloral hydrate on arterial oxygen saturation in wheezy infants. Pediatr Pulmonol 1988;5:96–99.

Mayers DJ, Hindmarsh KW, Gorecki DKJ, et al. Sedative/hypnotic effects of chloral hydrate in the neonate: trichloroethanol or parent drug? Dev Pharmacol Ther 1992;19:141–146.

Mayers DJ, Hindmarsh KW, Sankaran K, et al. Chloral hydrate disposition following single-dose administration to critically ill neonates and children. Dev Pharmacol Ther 1991;16:71–77.

McCarver-May DG, Kang J, Aouthmany M, et al. Comparison of chloral hydrate and midazolam for sedation of neonates for neuroimaging studies. J Pediatr 1996;128:573–576.

Napoli KL, Ingall CG, Martin GR. Safety and efficacy of chloral hydrate sedation in children undergoing echocardiography. J Pediatr 1996;129:287–291.

Reimche LD, Sankaran K, Hindmarsh KW, et al. Chloral hydrate sedation in neonates and infants—clinical and pharmacologic considerations. Dev Pharmacol Ther 1989;12:57–64.

Yu XQ, Suguihara C, Navarro H, et al. Effects of chloral hydrate on the cardiorespiratory response to hypoxia in newborn piglets. Biol Neonate 1996;69:146–152.

Propofol

Borgeat A, Wilder-Smith OHG, Suter PM. The nonhypnotic therapeutic applications of propofol. Anesthesiology 1994;80:642–656.

Cameron E, Johnston G, Crofts S, et al. The minimum effective dose of lignocaine to prevent injection pain due to propofol in children. Anaesthesia 1992;47:604–606.

Frankville DD, Spear RM, Dyck JB. The dose of propofol required to prevent children from moving during magnetic resonance imaging. Anesthesiology 1993;79:953–958.

Hannallah RS, Baker SB, Casey W, et al. Propofol: effective dose and induction characteristics in unpremedicated children. Anesthesiology 1991;74:217–219.

Havel CJ, Strait RT, Hennes H. A preliminary report of an ongoing randomized double-blind trial of propofol and midazolam for procedural sedation in the pediatric emergency department [abstract]. Acad Emerg Med 1997;4:364.

Kataria BK, Ved SA, Nicodemus HF, et al. The pharmacokinetics of propofol in children using three different data analysis approaches. Anesthesiology 1994;80:104–122.

Lebovic S, Reich DL, Steinberg G, et al. Comparison of propofol versus ketamine for anesthesia in pediatric patients undergoing cardiac catheterization. Anesth Analg 1992;74:490–494.

Mackenzie N, Grant IS. Propofol for intravenous sedation. Anaesthesia 1987;42:3–6.

Martin LD, Pasternak R, Pudimat MA. Total intravenous anesthesia with propofol in pediatric patients outside the operating room. Anesth Analg 1992;74:609–612.

Maxwell LG, Yaster M. The myth of conscious sedation. Arch Pediatr Adolesc Med 1996;150:665–667.

McDowall RH, Scher CS, Barst SM. Total intravenous anesthesia for children undergoing brief diagnostic or therapeutic procedures. J Clin Anesth 1995;7:273–280.

Powers KS, van der Jagt E, Sullivan JS, et al. Safe and effective deep sedation with propofol of children undergoing painful procedures in the outpatient setting (abstract). Pediatrics 1997;100 (Suppl):458.

Rosa G, Conti G, Orsi P, et al. Effects of low-dose propofol administration on central respiratory drive, gas exchanges and respiratory pattern. Acta Anaesthesiol Scand 1992;36:128–131.

Smith I, White PF, Nathanson M, et al. Propofol. An update on its use. Anesthesiology 1994;81:1005–1043.

Swanson ER, Seaberg DC, Mathias S. The use of propofol for sedation in the emergency department. Acad Emerg Med 1996;3:234–238.

Valente JF, Anderson GL, Branson RD, et al. Disadvantages of prolonged propofol sedation in the critical care unit. Crit Care Med 1994;22:710–712.

Chapter 7
Dissociative Agents

Steven Green

Ketamine is the only dissociative agent currently in clinical use, with the street hallucinogen phencyclidine representing the other agent working through a dissociative mechanism. The unique "dissociative state" resulting from ketamine can be defined as: A general trance-like cataleptic state characterized by profound analgesia and amnesia, with retention of protective airway reflexes and independent respirations. Ketamine has been widely used world-wide since its introduction in 1970 and has demonstrated a remarkable safety profile in a variety of settings.

Ketamine is an ideal agent to facilitate short, painful procedures, especially in children. This drug rapidly produces profound analgesia, sedation, amnesia, and immobilization when given parenterally, allowing the performance of such procedures under optimum conditions. Protective airway reflexes are retained, and patients essentially always maintain spontaneous respirations without intubation. Recovery to a degree suitable for outpatient disposition typically occurs in 45 to 120 minutes. Use of ketamine for various applications by both anesthesiologists and nonanesthesiologists has been extensively documented in numerous series containing thousands of patients with outstanding safety and efficacy.

GENERAL INDICATIONS

Ketamine is most commonly used in developed countries to facilitate brief, painful procedures in children in the outpatient setting. This drug has many features that are attractive in the outpatient setting: rapid onset (less than 5 minutes when given IM or IV), consistently effective analgesia and amnesia, airway stability, and an acceptable recovery duration (typical range 45 to 120 minutes). Successful and safe use of ketamine has been reported in settings such as dentistry, emergency departments, pediatric offices, radiation oncology, burn wards, cardiac catheterization, endoscopy, angiography, and pediatric wards.

Endotracheal intubation is unnecessary with ketamine. Muscular tone of the tongue and phanynx are preserved, and spontaneous respirations are essentially always maintained. Protective airway reflexes, such as coughing, sneezing, and swallowing, are not usually repressed and may be slightly exaggerated.

Because of its unique characteristics, ketamine is routinely and regularly used throughout the developing world for both minor and major surgery, especially in areas where an anesthetist is unavailable. Numerous series have described a wide margin of safety, despite monitoring standards that are considered unacceptable in developed countries.

Ketamine's characteristics and efficacy make it ideal for battlefield or disaster situations where the facilities and time are unavailable for general anesthetics. The International Red Cross considers ketamine-assisted surgery without intubation a standard technique for their treatment of surgical war injuries.

MECHANISM OF ACTION

Ketamine produces profound sedation and analgesia while maintaining spontaneous breathing and protective airway reflexes. Unlike all other sedatives, which suppress the reticular activating system, ketamine generates a functional and electrophysiologic dissociation between the cortex and limbic system. The dissociation effectively prevents higher centers from perceiving visual, auditory, or painful stimuli. This resulting trance-like cataleptic state is unique to ketamine and is colorfully described by the expression "The lights are on, but no one's home." Analgesia and amnesia are no less apparent than with inhalational anesthetics; however, unlike these agents, ketamine does not impair laryngeal reflexes or independent airway maintenance. Muscle tone is uninhibited, and purposeful movements unrelated to painful stimuli may occur. The eyes remain open with a "disconnected" stare and nystagmus is typical.

Ketamine differs significantly from essentially all other sedative and analgesic agents in that it lacks the characteristic dose-response continuum to progressive titration. At doses below a certain threshold, ketamine produces solely analgesia and sedation. Once a critical dosage threshold (approximately 1 to 1.5 mg/kg IV or 3 to 4 mg/kg IM) is administered, however, the characteristic dissociative state abruptly appears. This dissociation, once achieved, has no observable levels of depth, and thus the only value of ketamine "titration" is to maintain the presence of the state over time. Administration of further ketamine to a dissociated patient does not enhance sedation in any way and thus is unnecessary. Intentional subdissociative dosing of ketamine has little advantage over opioids and benzodiazepines, because analgesia and amnesia are incomplete.

PHARMACOKINETICS

Absorption

Ketamine is rapidly absorbed parenterally. Peak concentrations occur within 1 minute of intravenous injection, and rapid absorption by the highly perfused central nervous system allows almost immediate initiation of clinical effects. When administered intramuscularly, peak levels and clinical effects occur in approximately 5 minutes.

Elimination

Ketamine slowly redistributes into the peripheral tissues, with a return of coherence averaging 15 minutes if no further injections are given. The elimination half-life of ketamine is 2 to 3 hours in adults and 1 to 2 hours in children. Ketamine is painless and nonirritating after parenteral injection. Ketamine undergoes hepatic metabolism with subsequent renal excretion of degradation products.

ROUTES OF ADMINISTRATION

The preferred routes for ketamine administration are IM and IV. For short procedures, IM administration is simple, effective, and economical. Venous access is unnecessary, and atropine can be concurrently administered in the same syringe. Patients typically cannot recall the injection upon recovery. The dissociative state is produced approximately 5 minutes after IM injection of 3 to 6 mg/kg of ketamine. Dissociation typically lasts 15 to 30 minutes, with coherence and purposeful neuromuscular activity returning in 45 to 120 minutes.

Intravenous administration is attractive because administration is simple, a lower cumulative dose can be used, and recovery is more rapid than with other routes. This technique may be preferable for extremely brief procedures (< 5 minutes), patients who already have IV lines in place, or longer procedures expected to require repeat dosing. The primary caution with this route is that ketamine must be administered slowly (each dose over 1 to 2 minutes) or respiratory depression can occur. The dissociative state usually appears within 1 minute after administration of a loading dose of 1 to 1.5 mg/kg IV. Coherence will begin to return in approximately 15 minutes, and further injections of 0.5 to 1 mg/kg can be given as needed to maintain the dissociative state as long as necessary.

Ketamine undergoes substantial first-pass hepatic metabolism. As a result, oral and rectal administration results in less predictable effectiveness and requires substantially higher doses. Onset is slower than when used parenterally (approximately 20 to 25 minutes), with recovery extending 2 to 4 hours. Oral doses of 6 to 8 mg/kg have been reported to produce the dissociative state in half of children studied, whereas 10 mg/kg has been more consistently effective. Nasal administration has been noted to have inconsistent efficacy and is not always well tolerated.

Available Preparations

Available formulations of ketamine are 10, 50, or 100 mg/mL. The 10-mg/mL solution is preferred for IV administration, and the 100-mg/mL solution is preferred for IM administration in older children to minimize volume-related injection site discomfort.

INDICATIONS

Ketamine is ideal for short, painful procedures that might otherwise require general anesthesia. This drug is also helpful for certain procedures often performed without general anesthesia, especially those requiring immobilization for cosmetic result (e.g., complex facial laceration in a child) or those judged likely to produce excessive emotional disturbance (e.g., sexual assault examination in a child). Other situations in which ketamine can be considered include burn debridement, foreign body removal, abscess incision and drainage, lumbar puncture, fracture reduction, plastic surgery, Steinmann pin placement, and cleaning of extensive contaminated abrasions (i.e., "road-rash").

Sedation for CT or MRI scanning is best performed with benzodiazepines, barbiturates, or chloral hydrate. The dissociative state offers no advantage over pure sedative-hypnotics in this setting, and the occasional random movements typical of ketamine may result in poor quality radiographic studies.

The combative nature of some individuals who are mentally disabled makes the performance of routine procedures (e.g., dental extractions) and evaluations (e.g., pelvic exam) often extremely difficult without pharmacologic adjuncts. Ketamine has been used in these situations with good success.

CONTRAINDICATIONS AND PRECAUTIONS

Adverse Reactions

Respiratory Depression Although ketamine demonstrates mild dose-related respiratory depression, related to shifting of the CO_2 response curve, this has not been shown to be of major clinical significance. Serious respiratory depression is rare, but has been reported when ketamine is pushed by rapid IV bolus, when central nervous system injuries, masses, or abnormalities are present, when administered to ill neonates, or when inadvertent overdoses (22 mg/kg IM or more) occur. It is recommended that IV doses be given over 1 to 2 minutes. Five cases of transient apnea with IM ketamine in healthy children have been reported. When present, these events have occurred 4 to 5 minutes after injection (coinciding with peak central nervous system [CNS] levels) and resolved with brief assisted ventilation.

Neonates and small infants have greater difficulty maintaining a patent airway with ketamine as they similarly do with other sedating agents. This difficulty appears related to differences in airway anatomy and laryngeal excitability peculiar to that age group. For this reason, ketamine is generally considered contraindicated in those less than 3 months of age, and additional caution should be exercised between 3 and 12 months of age.

Airway Malalignment   Occasional airway malpositioning can occur with ketamine because patients will exhibit random purposeless motion and may flex or twist their necks. It is critical that continual attention be paid to airway patency because repositioning of the head or jaw may be necessary if snoring respirations develop.

Hypersalivation   Hypersalivation can occur with ketamine as the drug stimulates salivary and tracheobronchial secretions. Most experts recommend administering a concurrent anticholinergic, such as atropine (0.01 to 0.02 mg/kg, minimum dose 0.1 mg and maximum 0.5 mg) or glycopyrrolate (0.005 mg/kg, maximum dose 0.25 mg), to inhibit these secretions and minimize the necessity of suctioning. Additionally, excessive salivation has been postulated a precipitant of laryngospasm. Despite these concerns, ketamine has been successfully and extensively used without these adjuncts. Atropine and glycopyrrolate are equally efficacious and safe. Either anticholinergic can be combined with ketamine in a single IM injection. Because peak levels of atropine do not occur until 30 minutes after IM injection, its antisialogogue effects will occur during later sedation and recovery.

Laryngospasm   Transient stridor or laryngospasm occasionally have been reported and are probably related to stimulation of hypersensitized laryngeal reflexes. Data pooling of 11,589 ketamine administrations in healthy children revealed laryngospasm requiring intubation in two cases (0.017%). Morbidity was not reported in either circumstance, and one of these episodes was felt to be secondary to apparently unsuctioned hypersalivation. A recent series of 1022 children given IM ketamine for emergency department procedures noted four episodes of laryngospasm (0.4%); all were transient and without sequelae. Ketamine-associated laryngospasm has been reported in children undergoing procedures involving stimulation of the posterior pharynx, and these procedures would appear to be a relative contraindication to this agent.

Laryngospasm associated with inhalational anesthetics has been examined by Olsson in a series of 136,929 patients; the overall incidence was 0.9%. Children less than 10 years of age were more susceptible (1.7%), and infants 1 to 3 months old had a risk over three times higher than average (2.8%). Respiratory infection in children entailed a five-fold increase in risk (9.6%). In their 1197 observed cases of laryngospasm, serious sequelae, such as hypoxia, aspiration, and cardiac arrest, were relatively unusual (3.2%, 1.1%, and 0.5% respectively). The clinician should always be prepared, so that if laryngospasm occurs, the child can be treated with oxygen and assisted ventilation, if necessary, until the episode clears.

Cardiovascular Stimulation   Ketamine is sympathomimetic by inhibiting reuptake of catecholamines and thus can produce mild to moderate increases in blood pressure, heart rate, cardiac output, and myocardial oxygen consumption. Accordingly, ketamine should be used with extreme caution or not at all in individuals with poorly controlled hypertension, elevated pulmonary vascular resistance, congestive heart failure, or coronary artery disease. Ketamine manifests a balance of both direct antidysrhythmic effect and augmented dysrhythmogenicity caused by indirect sympathetic stimulation. Extensive clinical experience has shown that dissociated children consistently maintain stable cardiac rhythms.

Musculoskeletal Effects Skeletal muscle hypertonicity, rigidity, and sometimes myoclonus can be seen with ketamine. Random movement of the head or extremities unrelated to painful stimuli is also frequent; however, this motion is rarely of sufficient intensity to interfere with performance of procedures.

Seizures Although EEG studies 2 decades ago demonstrated that ketamine possesses anticonvulsant properties and more recently that it is an NMDA receptor antagonist, there are several case reports of brief seizures temporally related to ketamine administration in patients with underlying seizure disorders. Accordingly, ketamine should be used with caution in epileptics.

Intracranial Pressure Elevation Ketamine elevates intracranial pressure and increases cerebral metabolism and cerebral blood flow, and thus significant head trauma, hydrocephalus, and central nervous system neoplasms are relative contraindications to its use.

Ataxia Ataxia can be pronounced during recovery from ketamine, and attempts at ambulation must be avoided for several hours after administration until the dysequilibrium subsides. Patients sent home should have close family observation to prevent falls.

Recovery Agitation and Dreaming Ketamine frequently stimulates hallucinations and dreaming during recovery. Manifestations of these experiences are highly variable with vivid reports from adults of psychedelic colors, suspension in mid-air or outer space, floating down a kaleidoscope, rides in space-ships, out of body experiences, or faceless persons walking around the bed. Some patients report the dreams as extremely frightening; others describe them as pleasant, joyful, fascinating, or bizarre. Ketamine is used recreationally by some individuals who enjoy such hallucinatory reactions.

Unpleasant reactions are less common in adolescents than adults and are rare in children under 10 years of age. A recent large emergency department series noted mild agitation (whimpering or light crying) in 17.6% of children and more pronounced agitation in 1.6%. Only 2 of 1022 children had reactions that treating physicians judged severe enough to require treatment, and both children responded promptly to small dosages of midazolam.

Reported risk factors for these hallucinatory reactions include female gender, rapid IV administration, excessive noise or stimulation during recovery, prior personality disorders, or patients who normally dream frequently. Strong psychological factors appear to influence the severity of emergence reactions, and anecdotal evidence suggests that having older children plan topics for their dreaming in advance decreases the likelihood of unpleasant reactions. Attempts should be made to reduce stimuli during the recovery phase (e.g., dim lighting, quiet location, avoid physical contact). Concerns regarding unpleasant recovery reactions in children should not preclude the use of ketamine, because these events are unusual and readily treated with benzodiazepines.

Multiple reports describe success using coadministered benzodiazepines or opioids to both prevent and treat ketamine recovery reactions. These agents slow ketamine metabolism, however, and may prolong recovery time. The use of coadministered benzodiazepines or opioids may also lead to respiratory depression.

Vomiting The incidence of vomiting in children is 6.7%. When present, emesis usually occurs late in the recovery phase when the patient is alert. In almost 30 years of continual use, no documented reports exist of clinically significant ketamine-associated aspiration syndrome in children lacking established contraindications to this drug. Pooled data reveal no apparent association of fasting state with emesis, laryngospasm, or any other complication. Thus, a ketamine fasting requirement for patients lacking other contraindications has no clear substantiation in the literature, and the unique protection of airway reflexes with ketamine may make it preferable to alternative sedatives in such situations.

Other Ketamine may increase intraocular pressure, and based on anecdotal evidence is considered contraindicated in patients with hyperthyroidism, thyroid medications, or porphyria.

Acute Toxicity

The principal adverse event noted in the few reported cases of inadvertent ketamine overdose is prolonged sedation. Respiratory depression can also occur with high doses (e.g., 22 mg/kg IM). No specific treatment is needed other than supportive care.

Drug Interactions

The only potentially dangerous ketamine drug interaction is with thyroid medications, for which the basis is anecdotal. Although ketamine potentiates catecholamines, standard doses of sympathomimetic agents have not been identified as a contraindication. Coadministered benzodiazepines appear to slow the hepatic degradation of ketamine and may prolong recovery.

Contraindications

Standard contraindications are listed in the protocol (see Appendix). Most are based on limited or anecdotal data and, accordingly, most are relative and not absolute. Physicians will need to balance the benefits and potential risks of ketamine sedation in an individualized manner. The listed items most likely to be considered absolute based on the literature are age less than 3 months, pulmonary infection (e.g., pneumonia), severe cardiovascular disease, significant brain injury, abnormal cerebrospinal fluid flow patterns, or underlying psychotic disorder.

SUGGESTED READING

Dachs RJ, Innes GM. Intravenous ketamine sedation of pediatric patients in the emergency department. Ann Emerg Med 1997; 29:146–150.

Green SM, Rothrock SG, Lynch EL, et al. Intramuscular ketamine for pediatric sedation in the emergency department: safety profile with 1,022 cases. Ann Emerg Med 1998;31:688–697.

Parker RI, Mahan RA, Giugliano D, et al. Efficacy and safety of intravenous midazolam and ketamine as sedation for therapeutic and diagnostic procedures in children. Pediatrics 1997;99:427–431.

Petrack EM, Marx CM, Wright MS. Intramuscular ketamine is superior to meperidine, promethazine, and chlorpromazine for pediatric emergency department sedation. Arch Pediatr Adolesc Med 1996;150:676–681.

Pruitt JW, Goldwasser MS, Sabol SR, et al. Intramuscular ketamine, midazolam, and glycopyrrolate for pediatric sedation in the emergency department. J Oral Maxillofac Surg 1995;53:13–17.

Qureshi F, Mellis PT, McFadden MA. Efficacy of oral ketamine for providing sedation and analgesia to children requiring laceration repair. Pediatr Emerg Care 1995;11:93–97.

Classic

Corssen G, Miyasaka M, Domino EF. Changing concepts in pain control during surgery—dissociative anesthesia with CI-581. Anesth Analg 1969;47:746–759.

Green SM, Nakamura R, Johnson NE. Ketamine sedation for pediatric procedures: part 1. A prospective series. Ann Emerg Med 1990; 19:1024–1032.

Jarem BJ, Walker JA, Parks DH, et al. Current practice in anesthesia for pediatric burns. Anesthesiology Review 1978; 5:16–23.

Leppaniemi AK. Where there is no anaesthetist. Br J Surg 1991 Feb;78(2):245–246.

Olsson GL, Hallen B. Laryngospasm during anaesthesia—a computer-aided incidence study in 136,929 patients. Acta Anaesthesiol Scand 1984; 28:567–575.

Phillips LA, Seruvatu SG, Rika PN. Anaesthesia for the surgeon-anaesthetist in difficult situations. Anaesthesia 1970;25:36–45.

Walker AK. Intramuscular ketamine in a developing country. Anaesthesia 1972;27:408–414.

Review Articles

Green SM, Johnson NE. Ketamine sedation for pediatric procedures: part 2. Review and implications. Ann Emerg Med 1990;19:1033–1046.

Reich DL, Silvay G. Ketamine: an update on the first twenty-five years of clinical experience. Can J Anaesth 1989 Mar;36(2):186–97.

Sacchetti A, Schafermeyer R, Gerardi M, et al. Pediatric analgesia and sedation. Ann Emerg Med 1994;23:237–250.

White PF, Way WL, Trevor AJ. Ketamine—its pharmacology and therapeutic uses. Anesthesiology 1982;56:119–136.

APPENDIX

Ketamine Protocol—Loma Linda University Emergency Department
Cited as an example of compliance by the JCAHO
(Care of Patients: Examples of Compliance, ISBN 0–86688–611–7)

Purpose

To define the guidelines for administration, monitoring, and recovery for pediatric patients receiving ketamine for procedural sedation in the emergency department.

Characteristics of the Ketamine "Dissociative State"

1. *Dissociation*—After administration of ketamine, the patient passes into a fugue state or trance. The eyes may remain open but the patient does not respond. "The lights are on, but no one's home."
2. *Catalepsy*—Normal or slightly enhanced muscle tone is maintained. Occasionally, the patient may move or be moved into a position that is self-maintaining. Occasional muscular clonus may be noted.
3. *Analgesia*—Analgesia is typically substantial or complete.
4. *Amnesia*—Total amnesia is typical.
5. *Maintenance of Airway Reflexes*—Upper airway reflexes remain intact and may be slightly exaggerated. Intubation is unnecessary, but occasional repositioning of the head may be necessary for optimal airway patency. Suctioning of hypersalivation occasionally may be necessary.
6. *Cardiovascular Stability*—Blood pressure and heart rate are not decreased and typically are mildly increased.
7. *Nystagmus*—Nystagmus is typical.

Patient Selection

Ketamine is best suited for children aged 12 months to 15 years.
There is an increased risk of airway complications in children less than 3 months of age, and additional caution should be exercised when administering ketamine in children aged 3 to 12 months.

There is an increased risk of unpleasant recovery agitation in patients more than 15 years of age.

Indications

Short, painful procedure, especially those requiring immobilization. Examples:

- Complex facial lacerations
- Reduction of fractures
- Foreign body removal
- Abscess incision and drainage
- Examination judged likely to produce excessive emotional disturbance. Example: pediatric sexual assault examination

Contraindications

Age less than 3 months (use with caution if 3 to 12 months of age)
History of airway instability, tracheal surgery, or tracheal stenosis
Procedures involving stimulation of the posterior pharynx
Active pulmonary infection or disease (including upper respiratory infection)
Full meal within 3 hours of procedure
Cardiovascular disease including angina, heart failure, or hypertension
Head injury associated with loss of consciousness, altered mental status, or emesis
Central nervous system masses, abnormalities, or hydrocephalus
Poorly controlled seizure disorder
Glaucoma or acute globe injury
Psychosis, porphyria, thyroid disorder, or thyroid medication

Environment

Area with suction, oxygen, and equipment for advanced airway management
Physician immediately available who is adept at advanced airway management
WHEN KETAMINE IS ADMINISTERED IM, IV ACCESS IS NOT REQUIRED.
Supplemental oxygen is not required

Presedation

Patients should undergo a presedation assessment in accordance with hospital policy
Educate parents or caretakers regarding the unique characteristics of the dissociative state
Baseline level of consciousness and oxygen saturation will be recorded on the medical record before administration of ketamine
Older children should be informed that they will dream during recovery and should be encouraged to "plan" pleasant dream topics in advance

Ketamine Administration—General

To minimize ketamine-associated hypersalivation, coadministration of atropine
0.01 mg/kg (minimum 0.1 mg, maximum 0.5 mg) or glycopyrrolate (0.005
mg/kg, maximum 0.25 mg) is recommended. Atropine or glycopyrrolate can
either be given IV just before ketamine or mixed with ketamine in the same
syringe for IM injection.

Ketamine is not administered until the physician is ready to begin the procedure
(onset of dissociation is typically within 5 minutes).

Use adjunctive physical restraint if needed to control random motion (occasional).

Use adjunctive local anesthetic if needed for incomplete analgesia (unusual).

Ketamine Administration—IM Route

Use ketamine 4 mg/kg IM, with atropine mixed in the same syringe

Repeat ketamine dose (2 to 4 mg/kg IM without additional atropine) if sedation
is inadequate after 5 to 10 minutes (unusual) or if additional doses required.

Ketamine Administration—IV Route

A ketamine loading dose of 1 to 1.5 mg/kg is administered slowly IV over 1 to 2
minutes.

IV administration more rapidly than over 1 to 2 minutes produces high CNS levels and has been associated with respiratory depression.

Additional incremental doses of ketamine may be given (0.5 mg/kg) if initial sedation is inadequate or if repeated doses are necessary to accomplish a longer
procedure. Repeat doses of atropine are generally unnecessary.

Route of Administration	IM	IV
Advantages	No IV access necessary	Ease of repeat dosing; slightly faster recovery
Peak concentrations and clinical onset	5 min	1 min
Typical duration of effective sedation	15–30 min	10–15 min
Typical time from dose to discharge	60–140 min	50–110 min

Interactive Monitoring

Mandatory close observation of airway and respirations is carried out by an experienced health care professional until recovery is well established.

THE PATIENT IS NEVER LEFT ALONE.

Drapes are positioned such that airway and chest motion can be visualized at all times.

Occasional repositioning of the head may be indicated for optimal airway patency.

Occasional suctioning of the anterior pharynx may be necessary.

Mechanical Monitoring

Continuous pulse oximetry until recovery is well established

Continuous cardiac monitoring until recovery is well established

Potential Side Effects

Airway malalignment requiring repositioning of head (0.7%)

Transient laryngospasm (0.4%)

Transient apnea or respiratory depression (0.3%)

Hypersalivation (1.7%)

Emesis while sedated (0.8%)

Emesis well into recovery (5.9%)

Unpleasant recovery, agitation, or dreams (mild in 17.6%, moderate or severe in 1.6%)

Muscular hypertonicity and random, purposeless movements

Clonus, hiccuping, and/or rash

Recovery Area

Minimal physical contact or other psychic disturbance

Quiet area with dim lighting if possible

Advise parents or caretakers not to stimulate patient prematurely

Discharge Criteria

Return to pretreatment level of verbalization and awareness

Return to pretreatment level of human recognition

Return to pretreatment level of purposeful neuromuscular activity

Discharge Instructions

Nothing by mouth for 2 hours

Careful family observation and no independent ambulation for 2 hours

Chapter 8
Local Analgesia

Constance Houck

Local anesthetics have been available for more than a century to provide reversible sensory blockade of nerve fibers within the skin and mucous membranes. Cocaine was first introduced in 1884 after it was isolated from the leaves of the Erythroxylon coca tree growing in the Andes mountains. Although it has a long track record of success for local anesthesia and vasoconstriction of the mucous membranes and skin, cocaine's central nervous system and cardiovascular effects, high price, and potential for abuse have made the newer synthetic local anesthetics much more attractive for use in both adults and children. The first synthetic local anesthetic, procaine, became available in 1905 and was widely used until 1948 when lidocaine became available. Since that time, and despite the development of a number of new local anesthetics, lidocaine remains the most popular local anesthetic for infiltrative and topical anesthesia. The combination of lidocaine with prilocaine in the base form to make a liquid at room temperature (EMLA), and the use of electricity to drive the charged particles across intact skin (iontophoresis) have made it possible to deliver this local anesthetic topically as well as by infiltration.

The judicious use of local anesthetics can provide profound analgesia for most pediatric procedures and reduce the need for pharmacologic and physical restraint. The use of buffered lidocaine and topical anesthetics can make the administration of local anesthetics much less painful and eliminate the widely held belief among pediatric professionals that the administration of local anesthetics, especially for venipuncture and venous cannulations, can be more painful than the procedure itself.

MECHANISM OF ACTION

Local anesthetics prevent the generation and conduction of nerve impulses in the cell membrane. This is accomplished by decreasing or preventing the increase in permeability of the excitable membranes to Na^+ during depolarization. As the anesthetic action progressively develops in the nerve, the threshold for electrical excitability gradually increases, the rate of rise of the action potential declines, and impulse conduction slows. Although there are several notable exceptions, small unmyelinated nerve fibers are more susceptible to the action of local anesthetics than larger myelinated fibers. Also, sensory fibers are usually more easily blocked than large motor fibers. Clinical effectiveness is enhanced by the fact that within sensory nerves, pain and temperature impulses are abolished first followed by blockade of touch and deep pressure sensations at higher local anesthetic concentrations. The loss of temperature sensation can often be used as a simple and noninvasive test of the initial effectiveness of the local anesthetic.

The time during which the local anesthetic is in contact with the nerve determines the duration of action. Therefore, commercial preparations of local anesthetics often contain a vasoconstrictor to reduce the rate of absorption. Vasoconstrictors serve a dual action by not only localizing the anesthetic at the desired site, but also allowing the rate of clearance in the body to keep pace with the rate at which it is absorbed into the circulation. This serves to reduce systemic toxicity and also allows the use of larger volumes of local anesthetics for infiltration.

PHARMACOKINETICS

Local anesthetics are classified into two distinct categories based on their metabolism. **Amide** local anesthetics (i.e., lidocaine, prilocaine, bupivacaine) are cleared by biotransformation in the liver to either less active or inactive metabolites and are then excreted via the kidneys. **Ester** local anesthetics (i.e., tetracaine, cocaine) are broken down by cholinesterases, which are found principally in the plasma, to inactive metabolites. Although not pharmacologically active, one metabolite, paraaminobenzoic acid (PABA) may be associated with the subsequent, although rare, allergic reactions seen with the ester local anesthetics. Because they are rapidly metabolized in the plasma and do not rely on either hepatic or renal function to become inactive, ester local anesthetics have a shorter duration of action than amides. Metabolism in either case relies on the drug moving away from the site of action and into the plasma. Such factors as local vasoconstriction or trapping of the ions within the stratum corneum, as occurs with the gel form of tetracaine, may increase the duration of action considerably. Further details of the comparative pharmacology of the local anesthetics used for infiltrative and topical anesthesia can be found in Table 8.1.

INFILTRATIVE LOCAL ANESTHESIA

The local anesthetics most frequently used for infiltrative local anesthesia are lidocaine and bupivacaine. To avoid toxicity, no more than 2.0 to 2.5 mg/kg of

Table 8.1. Comparative Pharmacology of Local Anesthetics Used for Infiltration and Topical Anesthesia

Agent	Potency	Onset	Clinical Duration (min)	Maximum Dose in Children (mg/kg)	Protein Binding (%)	Clearance (mL/min/kg)	Elimination Half-life (min)
Amides							
Lidocaine	1	rapid	60–120	5 (7–10 w/EPI)	70	9.2	96
Bupivacaine	4	slow	240–480	2.5–3	95	7.0	144
Prilocaine	1	slow	60–180	5	55		
Esters							
Tetracaine	16	slow	60–180	1	76		
Cocaine		rapid	30–45	3	91	32	48

Data from Stoelting. Pharmacology and Physiology in Anesthetic Practice. Philadelphia: J.B. Lippincott Company, 1987.

bupivacaine or 5 to 7 mg/kg of lidocaine should be administered. This is equivalent to approximately 0.5 mL/kg of 0.5% bupivacaine or 1% lidocaine. More dilute solutions can be used in younger children to provide adequate spread of the anesthetic without exceeding the recommended limits. Epinephrine-containing solutions are desirable in highly vascular areas to slow vascular uptake of local anesthetics and to prolong the duration of effect. However, they should be avoided when procedures are performed on the distal extremities, nose, or penis to avoid ischemic injury to these areas.

Local anesthetics are not soluble unless they are combined with a hydrochloride salt. The hydrochloride salts provide a certain amount of stability especially for ester anesthetics and local anesthetics with added vasoconstrictors and can significantly prolong their shelf life. These salts are mildly acidic, causing pain on subcutaneous injection. This pain can be significantly reduced by adding sodium bicarbonate to the local anesthetic just before injection. A recent study by Palmon and colleagues demonstrated that the addition of 1 mL of 8.4% bicarbonate to 4 mL of lidocaine significantly reduced pain on injection compared with unbuffered lidocaine, even when a small gauge (30 g.) needle was used.

INTRAVENOUS REGIONAL ANESTHESIA

Intravenous regional anesthesia (Bier block) can provide analgesia for brief but painful extremity manipulations or more extensive hand or forearm lacerations. The technique is simple and does not require extensive knowledge of neural blockade techniques. Two intravenous catheters are placed, one to administer fluids and medications in a separate extremity and the other to administer the local anesthetic block. A tourniquet is placed to isolate the local anesthetic within the extremity to be blocked. Before the tourniquet is inflated, the extremity is exsanguinated with an Esmarch bandage. The local anesthetic is then administered through the previously placed intravenous line. Duration of the block is independent of the type of local anesthetic used, but is determined by the length of time the tourniquet is inflated. After release of the tourniquet, the local anesthetic is diluted by the increase in blood flow, and normal sensation and skeletal muscle tone return rapidly. Prilocaine is especially suited for this type of block because of its low incidence of thrombophlebitis and rapid metabolism. Slow release of the tourniquet is essential to decrease the likelihood of a rapid rise in plasma local anesthetic concentrations.

IONTOPHORESIS OF LOCAL ANESTHETICS

Iontophoresis is a drug delivery system that employs an electrical field to drive charged ions, such as local anesthetics, through the epithelial surface. This system has a much shorter onset time than most topical anesthetics for intact skin and can produce cutaneous analgesia in as little as 10 minutes.

The most commonly used anesthetic by this route is 2% lidocaine with 1:100,000 epinephrine. Although a mild tingling sensation occurs during drug delivery, this is generally well tolerated. Deeper levels of dermal anesthesia can be achieved with iontophoresis compared with EMLA, and depth of analgesia can exceed 7 mm. This can provide significant analgesia of both skin and veins, making venous cannulation less painful.

The duration of application to achieve sufficient analgesia depends on the amount of current used. With higher currents (i.e., 4 μAmps), there is more tingling of the skin, but analgesia can be achieved in 10 minutes. Longer application times (approximately 25 to 30 minutes) are needed when lower currents are used, but the tingling sensation can be made almost undetectable. Many centers have allowed older children to adjust the current themselves based on their tolerance of the electrical current.

CONTRAINDICATIONS AND PRECAUTIONS

In addition to blocking peripheral nerves, local anesthetics interfere with conduction in all major organs in which transmission of nerve impulses occurs. Therefore, effects are noted within the central nervous system (CNS), autonomic ganglia, and myocardium. The earliest effect and most common CNS side effect of local anesthetics is drowsiness, although dysphoria and euphoria have occasionally been noted with lidocaine blood concentrations below 5 μg/mL. As plasma concentrations reach higher levels, stimulation of the central nervous system occurs, initially causing restlessness, muscle twitching, and tremor. Adults and older children often report feelings of tremulousness or agitation, which can easily be overlooked or misinterpreted in younger children who are already frightened and cannot express these sensations. Therefore, in infants and young children, generalized seizure activity may be the first clear cut indication of CNS toxicity. Rarely, when serum concentrations reach high levels rapidly, loss of consciousness and respiratory arrest can occur without signs of CNS stimulation.

Local anesthetics decrease electrical excitability, conduction rate, and contraction force within the myocardium. Hypotension also can result from relaxation of arteriolar smooth muscle and direct myocardial depression. The conduction and inotropic effects are only seen with high systemic concentrations of local anesthetics and after CNS effects are produced. One notable exception is bupivacaine, which may be associated with selective cardiac toxicity. Inadvertent intravascular injection of therapeutic doses of bupivacaine have been associated with precipitous hypotension, cardiac dysrhythmias, and atrioventricular heart block. This selective cardiac toxicity is most likely caused by the slow rate of dissociation of this highly lipidsoluble local anesthetic from the sodium channels.

Few individuals may manifest a hypersensitivity reaction to local anesthetics. Less than 1% of all adverse reactions to local anesthetics are caused by an allergic mechanism. Hypersensitivity occurs most commonly with ester local anesthetics, but reactions may occur to the preservatives within amide local anesthetics. A careful history should be obtained from patients who report allergic reactions to local anesthetics because untoward symptoms can be associated with inadvertent intravascular injection or epinephrine added to the local anesthetic to prolong block duration. Patients reporting syncope, palpitations, hypertension, or dysrhythmias in association with local anesthetic administration are manifesting one of these other types of reactions.

Adverse effects of local anesthetics are short-lived and require only supportive treatment. Initial treatment focuses on the maintenance of adequate oxygenation, ventilation, and cardiac support. Rapid control of seizures is also important, because even brief convulsions can cause hypercarbia, acidosis, and increased brain uptake of local anesthetic agents. Benzodiazepines are effective in suppressing local anesthetic-induced seizures because these drugs can facilitate the inhibitory neurotransmitter gamma-aminobutyric acid (GABA). Cardiac depression caused by high plasma levels of bupivacaine can be reversed with bretylium (20 mg/kg), which will also elevate the threshold for ventricular tachycardia.

SUGGESTED READING

Arvidsson SB, Ekroth RH, Hansby MC, et al. Painless venipuncture. A clinical trial of iontophoresis of lidocaine for venipuncture in blood donors. Acta Anethesiol Scand 1984; 28:209–210.

Ashburn MA. The iontophoresis of lidocaine with epinephrine: an evaluation of the depth and duration of skin anesthesia following short drug delivery times. Anesthesiology 1994;81:A391.

Ashburn M, Gauthier M, Love G, et al. Iontophoretic administration of 2% lidocaine HCL and 1:100,000 epinephrine in man. Clin J Pain 1997;13:1322–1326.

Ashburn MA, Stephen RL, Ackerman E, et al. Iontophoretic delivery of morphine for postoperative analgesia. J Pain Symptom Manage 1992;7:27–33.

Banga AJ, Chien YW. Iontophoretic delivery of drugs: fundamentals, developments and biomedical applications. J Controlled Release 1988;7:1–24.

Bartfield JM, Ford DT, Homer PJ. Buffered versus plain lidocaine for digital nerve blocks. Ann Emerg Med 1993;22:216–219.

Bartfield JM, Gennis P, Barbera J, et al. Buffered versus plain lidocaine as a local anesthetic for simple laceration repair. Ann Emerg Med 1990;19:1387–1389.

Berde CB. Toxicity of local anesthetics in infants and children. J Pediatr 1993;122:S14–S20.

Bjerring D, Arendt-Nielson L. Depth and duration of skin analgesia to needle insertion after topical application of EMLA cream. Brit J Anesthesiol 1990;64(2):173–177.

Christoph RA, Buchanan L, Begalla K, et al. Pain reduction in local anesthetic administration through pH buffering. Ann Emerg Med 1988;17:117–120.

Garrison JC. Histamine, Bradykinin, 5-Hydroxytryptamine, and Their Antagonists. In: Goodman and Gilman, eds. The Pharmacological Basis of Therapeutics. 8th ed. New York: Pergamon Press, 1990:575–581.

Gibson LE, Cooke R. A test for the concentration of electrolytes in sweat in cystic fibrosis of the pancreas utilizing pilocarpine by iontophoresis. Pediatrics 1959;23:545–549.

Grossman M, Jamieson MJ, Kellog DL et al. The effect of iontophoresis on the cutaneous vasculature: evidence for current-induced hyperemia. Microvasc Res 1995;50(3):444–452.

Irsfield S, Klement W, Lipfert P. Transdermal local anesthesia: comparison of EMLA cream with iontophoretic local anesthesia. Brit J Anesthesiol 1993;71:375–378.

Jay SM, Ozolins M, Elliot C, et al. Assessment of children's distress during painful procedures. Health Psych 1983;2(2):133–147.

Klein EJ, Shugerman RP, Leigh-Taylor K, et al. Buffered lidocaine: analgesia for intravenous line placement in children. Pediatrics 1995;95:709–712.

Koren G. Use of eutectic mixture of local anesthetics in young children for procedure related pain. J Pediatr 1993;122:S30–S35.

Leduc S. Electronic Ions and Their Use in Medicine. Liverpool: Rebman Ltd, 1908.

Li LC, Scudds RA. Iontophoresis: an overview of mechanisms and clinical application. Arthritis Care Res 1995;8(1):51–61.

Mader TJ, Playe SJ, Grab JL. Reducing the pain of local anesthetic infiltration: warming and buffering have a synergistic effect. Ann Emerg Med 1994;23:550–554.

Maloney JM, Bezzant JL, Stephen RL, et al. Iontophoretic administration of lidocaine anesthesia in office practice: an appraisal. J Dermatol Surg Oncol 1992;18:937–940.

Petelenz T, Axenti I, Petelenz TJ, et al. Mini set for iontophoresis for topical analgesia before injection. Int J Clin Pharmacol Ther Toxicol 1984;22(3):152–155.

Ross DM, Ross SA. Childhood pain: the schoolaged child's viewpoint. Pain 1984; 20:179.

Scott J, Huskisson EC. Vertical or horizontal visual analogue scales. Ann Rheum Dis 1979;38:560.

Singh J, Maibach HI. Topical iontophoretic drug delivery in vivo: historical development, devices and future perspectives. Dermatology 1993;187(4):234–238.

Theib U, Kuhn I, Lucker PW. Iontophoresis—is there a future for clinical application? Meth Find Exp Clin Pharmacol 1991;13(5):353–359.

Zeltzer L, Regalado M, Nichter LS, et al. Iontophoresis versus subcutaneous injection: a comparison of two methods of local anesthesia delivery in children. Pain 1991;44:73–78.

Chapter 9
Topical Analgesia

Michael Shannon

Much of the pain and anxiety associated with painful procedures in children is the sight of a needle and the discomfort of the first injection. Even though the pain of dermal infiltration with local anesthetics can be reduced by buffering lidocaine with sodium bicarbonate or by nonpharmacologic interventions, the combination of anticipation, sight, and sensation can make the most calm and cooperative child anxious, frightened, and uncontrollable. Therefore, it was of monumental importance when Pryor in 1980 showed that local anesthesia for laceration repair could be achieved through the topical application of a combination anesthetic solution containing tetracaine, adrenaline, and cocaine (TAC). This finding initiated an explosion of clinical research on topical anesthetics for cleansing and repair of broken skin, as well as performance of painful percutaneous procedures (e.g., venipuncture, lumbar puncture, bone marrow aspiration). A rapidly growing list of effective topical anesthetics now permits completion of painful procedures with a minimum of restraint and little to no sedation. These agents have a broad profile of safety coupled with a high degree of efficacy. Now, with an extensive list of options available in topical anesthesia, initial application of such an agent should be considered the cornerstone of management when conducting painful procedures in children.

PHARMACOKINETICS

The relevant pharmacology of topical anesthetics has been described in Chapter 8, Local Analgesia. These agents have in common the ability to provide temporary insensitivity of local pain receptors to noxious stimuli. Topical anesthetics in current use contain, singly or in combination, one of the following agents: a local anesthetic amide or ester class; a local vasoconstrictor, which acts to potentiate the activity of the anesthetic; and cocaine. Many of the newer topical agents have begun to remove the cocaine component, substituting equally effective but safer anesthetics. Also, in an effort to facilitate drug penetration through intact skin, unique drug delivery vehicles have been created.

AVAILABLE PREPARATIONS

The growing versatility of topical anesthetics permits their use on virtually any body surface, ranging from broken to intact skin and from epidermal to mucosal surfaces (Table 9.1).

Eutectic Mixture of Local Anesthetics

For use on intact skin, eutectic mixture of local anesthetics (EMLA) has become the most popular agent. EMLA can be considered for any painful percutaneous procedure, including intravenous cannulation and arterial puncture. EMLA has the disadvantages of a relatively long onset of action (45 to 60 minutes) and a moderate cost (approximately $4.90 per 5 g tube). EMLA may also produce a mild elevation in methemoglobin.

Vapocoolant

An alternative to EMLA is a vapocoolant spray (ethyl chloride or Fluori-Methane). These agents produce local hypothermia, which results in transient ($<$ 1 minute) anesthesia. The vapocoolant sprays are as safe and effective in children, if not more effective than EMLA, at a fraction the cost (Fluori-Methane costs approximately $14 per 3 oz bottle). Ethyl chloride, unlike Fluori-Methane, has the disadvantage of being highly combustible.

Tetracaine, Adrenaline, and Cocaine

Topical anesthetics for use on broken skin have received the most attention because wounds are so common in children. The most popular of these have become preparations containing the combination of tetracaine, adrenaline, and cocaine (TAC). TAC provides significant local anesthesia at only 5 to 10 minutes after application on broken skin; it is ineffective on intact skin. TAC has undergone various reformulations to contain a lower concentration of cocaine and to create a viscous preparation that won't run when applied on a wound. Under current protocols, TAC is applied directly to a wound for 10 to 20 minutes. TAC should not be placed within 0.5 cm of a mucosal surface (nares, mouth) or the conjunctivae, or at any site that receives an end-arteriolar blood supply (ear, tip of nose, penis, fingers) because of the risk of excessive vasoconstriction and loss of adequate perfusion. When not used properly, adverse effects from TAC have been significant, primarily consisting of agitation; however, seizures have also been reported. A fatality occurred in a child who had the solution placed too close to the mouth. TAC also has the disadvantages of containing a controlled substance that is relatively expensive and requires refrigeration to optimize its shelf life.

Table 9.1. Common Topical Anesthetics

	Agent	Constituents	Potential ADR	Typical Dose	Comments
For intact skin	EMLA	Lidocaine (2.5%), prilocaine (2.5%)	Methemoglobinemia	2–2.5 g	45–60-minute onset
	Vapocoolant sprays				
	Ethyl chloride	same	Combustion hazard	qs	Rapid onset, ultra-short duration
	Fluori-Methane	same	none	qs	Rapid onset, ultra-short duration
For broken skin	TAC	Tetracaine, adrenaline, cocaine (11.8%)	Cocaine toxicity	1–3 mL	Controlled substance, expensive, requires refrigeration
	LET	Lidocaine, epinephrine, tetracaine	None reported	1–3 mL	Inexpensive room temperature storage
	2% lidocaine	same	Lidocaine toxicity (seizures)	2–7 mg/kg	Weight-based dose restrictions
	PP	Prilocaine, phenylephrine	None reported	1–3 mL	Alternative to LET
	PLP	Prilocaine, lidocaine, Phenylephrine	None reported	1–3 mL	Alternative to LET
For nasal or oral mucosa	Cetacaine	2% butamben/ 2% tetracaine	Allergic reaction	qs	Ester-class anesthetic
	4% cocaine	Same	Cocaine toxicity	1–2 mg/kg	Controlled substance, expensive, dose restrictions
	Viscous lidocaine	Same	Lidocaine toxicity	2–7 mg/kg	Dose restrictions
	Dental creams	Benzocaine	Allergic reaction, Methemoglobinemia		
Ophthalmic preparations	0.5% proparacaine	Same	Allergic reaction	1–2 drops	Ester-class anesthetic

ADR, adverse drug reaction; *qs*, quantity sufficient to produce desired effect.

Lidocaine, Epinephrine, and Tetracaine

The combination of lidocaine, epinephrine, and tetracaine (LET) has been one of the most important advents to topical anesthesia for open wounds since TAC was first used. With the replacement of cocaine by lidocaine, LET remains effective and offers the advantages of low cost (comparable doses of $3 versus $35 for TAC), room storage, use without controlled substances documentation, and relative safety on mucous membranes. With the availability of LET, the place of TAC in wound management is no longer clear.

Lidocaine

Lidocaine alone has been used for topical anesthesia, e.g., the cleansing of abrasions. It offers significant anesthesia but, having a narrow therapeutic index, lidocaine carries the risk of lidocaine toxicity if doses are excessive. Because the absorption of lidocaine from open wounds can be unpredictable, excessive application of lidocaine to large abrasions is potentially hazardous. However, if the quantity is dosed in the 3- to 7-mg/kg range, toxicity would not be expected.

Newer combinations of topical anesthetics for broken skin continued to be identified, and additional agents will likely appear. These agents will need to exceed the profile of cost, safety, and efficacy that has been achieved by LET.

Cocaine, Cetacaine, and Viscous Lidocaine

Topical anesthesia of ocular and mucosal surfaces was first achieved in the 19th century with the discovery of cocaine. Cocaine remains one of the most effective drugs for local anesthesia of these specialized surfaces. Also, cocaine not only confers local anesthesia but also a vasoconstrictive action, which potentiates its own anesthetic properties. Unfortunately, the efficacy of this drug must be balanced by a substantial toxicity if doses are exceeded. Alternatives to cocaine for anesthesia of the oral mucosa include Cetacaine and viscous lidocaine. Cetacaine, like most topical anesthetics used in dentistry, contains benzocaine in concentrations as high as 14%. Being an anesthetic of the ester class, benzocaine is associated with the risk of allergic reaction. Amide anesthetics, such as lidocaine and tetracaine, do not have such an allergic potential. Also, excessive use of benzocaine can produce methemoglobinemia in susceptible hosts. In the case of lidocaine, its excessive application on mucosal surfaces has been associated with significant toxicity.

SUGGESTED READING

Bonadio WA, Wagner V. Efficacy of TAC topical anesthetic for repair of pediatric lacerations. AJDC 1988;142:203–205.

Bonadio WA, Wagner V. Half-strength TAC topical anesthetic for selected dermal lacerations. Clin Ped 1988;27:495–498.

Dailey RH. Fatality secondary to misuse of TAC solution. Ann Emerg Med 1988;17:159–160.

Daya MR, Burton BT, Schleiss MR, et al. Recurrent seizures following mucosal application of TAC. Ann Emerg Med 1988;17:646–648.

Ernst AA, Marvez E, Nick TG, et al. Lidocaine adrenaline tetracaine gel versus tetracaine adrenaline cocaine gel for topical anesthesia in linear scalp and facial lacerations in children aged 5 to 17 years. Pediatr 1995;95:255–258.

Halperin DL, Koren G, Attias D, et al. Topical skin anesthesia for venous, subcutaneous drug reservoir and lumbar punctures in children. Pediatr 1989;84:281–284.

Hess GP, Walson PD. Seizures secondary to oral viscous lidocaine. Ann Emerg Med 1988;17:725–727.

Pryor G, Kilpatrick W, Opp D. Local anesthesia in minor lacerations: topical TAC vs. lidocaine infiltration. Ann Emerg Med 1980;9:568–571.

Reis EC, Holubkov R. Vapocoolant spray is equally effective as EMLA cream in reducing immunization pain in school-aged children. Pediatrics (electronic pages) 1997;100: URL:http://www.pediatrics.org/cgi/content/full/100/6/e5.

Schilling CG, Bank DE, Borchert BA, et al. Tetracaine, epinephrine (adrenaline), and cocaine (TAC) versus lidocaine, epinephrine, and tetracaine (LET) for anesthesia of lacerations in children. Ann Emerg Med 1995;25:2–3–208.

Schubert CJ, Wason S. Cocaine toxicity in an infant following intranasal instillation of a four percent cocaine solution. Pediatr Emerg Care 1992;8:82–84.

Smith GA, Strausbaugh SD, Harbeck-Weber C, et al. New non-cocaine-containing topical anesthetics compared with tetracaine-adrenaline-cocaine during repair of lacerations. Pediatr 1997;100:825–830.

Chapter 10
Systemic Analgesia

Tamiko Long, Navil Sethna

Opioids, especially the short-acting agents fentanyl and sufentanil, occupy a central role in the pharmacopoeia of procedural sedation and analgesia. Controlling pain, whether from the primary injury or secondary to a short but painful therapeutic procedure required to treat that injury, is imperative. Opioids can be used alone or in combination with a sedative/anxiolytic for analgesia and sedation during procedures. Depending on the nature of the injury and the procedure required, analgesia may be administered topically, locally, or systemically. This chapter focuses on the systemic opioid (morphine, meperidine, fentanyl, sufentanil) and nonopioid (ketorolac) analgesics commonly used for procedural sedation and analgesia.

DEFINITION OF TERMS

The word opioid is preferred to narcotics (which means numb) or opiates (derivatives of the poppy plant) because it is a broader term that includes endogenous peptides as well as exogenous drugs with morphinelike attributes. Opioids include the following:

1. Naturally occurring opium alkaloids (e.g., morphine, codeine)
2. Semisynthetics opioids (e.g., hydromorphone, hydrocodone, oxycodone)
3. Synthetic narcotics analgesics such as phenylpiperidine derivatives (e.g., meperidine, fentanyl, sufentanil)

MECHANISM OF ACTION

Derivatives of morphine are produced by substitution at the phenolic (responsible for potency property) or the alcoholic hydroxy (responsible for central nervous system side effects action) groups. In general, modification at the phenolic position produces a decrease in both analgesic activity and side effects. Analgesic activity and side effects are also determined by receptor subtypes. Mu_1 receptors are concentrated in the brain and spinal cord and opioids produce analgesia by acting at these receptors. Mu_2 type receptors are located in brainstem, gastrointestinal tract, and spinal cord. Opioid-induced respiratory depression and increased gastrointestinal tract transit time occurs with stimulation of this subtype receptor.

Cardiovascular System

When a patient is in supine position, therapeutic doses of opioids (except meperidine) have little effect on the blood pressure, heart rate, or rhythm. When a patient is in sitting or standing position, gravitational shift may produce hypotension because of peripheral venodilatation and arteriolar dilatation. Morphine is believed to cause vasodilatation from histamine release. Opioids produce dose-dependent bradycardia caused by central stimulation of the vagal nucleus in the medulla, which can be antagonized by atropine. Meperidine produces tachycardia because of its structural resemblance to atropine. Meperidine also may produce negative inotropic effects at doses of 2 mg/kg or in lower doses in the presence of compromised cardiac function. Meperidine should therefore be avoided in presence of cardiac disease.

Gastrointestinal System

Opioids can produce the following effects on the gastrointestinal (GI) tract:

- Increase resting tone of smooth muscles of the small and large intestine and ileocecal valve and the anal, Oddi, and pyloric sphincters
- Reduce motility of the small and large intestines
- Increase gastric emptying time
- Inhibit gastric, biliary, and pancreatic secretions
- Increase transit time through the bowel, increase water absorption, and cause desiccation of bowel content leading to constipation

Genitourinary Effects

Opioids increase the tone and amplitude of contractions in the bladder and its sphincter, which may present clinically as urinary retention, particularly in men.

PHARMACOKINETICS

Morphine

Morphine is primarily metabolized via glucuronidation (conjugation with glucuronide acid) in the liver. The major metabolites are morphine-3-glucuronide and morphine-6-glucuronide. The latter has significant analgesic activity and may contribute to the analgesic effect of the parent drug. Hepatic dysfunction occasionally impairs metabolism of morphine, and morphine can be used safely until end-stage failure. Excreted in the urine are 85 to 90% glucuronide metabolites and 5 to 10% free morphine, and less than 10% is excreted in biliary excretion. Renal failure does not diminish excretion of the morphine metabolites, but the active metabolite morphine-6-glucuronide can accumulate in the presence of impaired renal function and produce prolonged analgesia and may predispose to respiratory depression. Therefore, morphine should be used cautiously in patients with impaired renal failure.

Meperidine

Predominant metabolism is in the liver; 90% of a dose is biodegraded by N-demethylation to normeperidine and hydrolysis to normeperidine acid. The elimination half-life of meperidine is 3 to 4 hours. A large dose or repeated doses of meperidine may cause nervous system excitation consisting of tremor, muscle twitches, and seizures. The excitatory effects become apparent when the daily dose exceeds 25 mg/kg (or 50 mg/h) and are unaffected by the tolerance. Normeperidine is about one-half as active as an analgesic but twice as active as a convulsive agent as meperidine. Normeperidine has a long elimination half-life of 15 to 40 hours. Renal or hepatic failure aggravates normeperidine CNS toxicity by prolonging the elimination half-life from 3 to 4 hours in healthy individuals to 24 hours in hepatic failure and 35 hours in renal failure.

The duration of analgesia with meperidine is shorter than morphine, and the dose may be repeated every 2 to 3 hours. Intramuscular injection of meperidine 1 mg/kg in children 7 to 13 years is rapidly absorbed and peak levels are reached within 10 minutes.

Fentanyl

Like meperidine, fentanyl is a derivative of the phenylpiperidine family and is approximately 100 times more potent than morphine. Rapid onset and short analgesic duration (30 to 45 minutes) occur because of high lipid solubility and rapid distribution to highly perfused tissues such as the brain. The effects of fentanyl in the CNS are terminated by the rapid decline of plasma concentrations caused by redistribution to body fat and muscle depots. However, with repeated doses or continuous infusion, fentanyl may saturate these depots, raise plasma concentrations, and eventually prolong the pharmacologic effect. Fentanyl is completely metabolized in the liver to the inactive metabolites norfentanyl and despropionylnorfentanyl, which are excreted in the bile and urine. The hepatic metabolism of fentanyl is minimally affected by liver disease, has no active metabolites, and thus is safely used in patients with hepatic and renal disease.

Fentanyl is a potent analgesic and CNS depressant. Rapid administration can produce respiratory depression and, with large doses, muscle rigidity. Like most opioids, fentanyl produces bradycardia but does not produce peripheral vasodilatation or release histamine.

Sufentanil

Sufentanil is 5 to 10 times more potent than fentanyl. The pharmacologic effect of sufentanil is similar to fentanyl but it is more sedating than fentanyl. The pharmacokinetic profile of sufentanil resembles that of fentanyl but it has a slightly more rapid onset of effect, a smaller volume of distribution, and a shorter elimination half-life and duration of action because it is highly lipid soluble and diffuses rapidly to the CNS. Sufentanil has a short analgesic duration when administered in small doses because of its rapid redistribution out of the CNS to inactive body tissues. It is primarily metabolized in the liver to inactive metabolites that are excreted in urine and bile in equal proportions. Sufentanil should be used with caution in patients with renal dysfunction because significant amounts of both conjugated and active metabolites may accumulate.

Sufentanil is only used in the intranasal route for procedural sedation. Delivered intranasally, sufentanil enters the systemic circulation directly and eventually achieves plasma concentrations similar to those with intravenous administration. A range of doses of intranasal sufentanil (0.75 to 4.5 µg/kg) have been investigated in children ages 6 months to 10 years. These doses produce relaxation, drowsiness, or rarely somnolence. Doses of 2 µg/kg or greater are associated with a high incidence of oxygen desaturation. The higher dose of 4.5 µg/kg is associated with increased incidence of vomiting and seizures. The safety and efficacy of sufentanil can be improved by decreasing its dose and combining it with an anxiolytic such as midazolam.

Intranasal administration of sufentanil is relatively easy, pain-free, acceptable to most children, and reduces pain and anxiety associated with mild to moderately painful procedures. After administration, children are less anxious, willing to separate from their parents, and less objectionable to procedures that normally invoke pain and/or fear such as local anesthetic infiltration, insertion of intravenous catheters, or application of face mask for induction of anesthesia. The combination of intranasal sufentanil (0.75 µg/kg) and midazolam (0.20 mg/kg) has been shown to effectively relieve the pain and anxiety associated with laceration repair in children. The recommended dose of intranasal sufentanil alone in children ages 6 months to 10 years for blunting the distress response to painful procedures is 1.5 to 2 µg/kg.

Ketorolac Tromethamine

Ketorolac is a pyrrole acetic acid derivative nonsteroidal anti-inflammatory drug. Like other nonsteroidal anti-inflammatory drugs (NSAIDs), ketorolac inhibits cyclooxygenase (prostaglandin synthetase) enzymes. These enzymes catalyze the conversion of arachidonic acid to precursors of prostaglandins. The popularity of ketorolac stems from its suitability for parenteral administration, effectiveness for mild to moderate pain control, potentiation of opioid analgesia, and lack of depression of cardiovascular and respiratory systems. Onset of analgesic effect occurs at approximately 10 minutes after intramuscular and intravenous injections, with the mean peak effect within 40 to 60 minutes, lasting approximately 6 hours. Ketorolac is metabolized primarily in the liver by conjugation with glucuronic acid, and a small amount undergoes parahydroxylation to hydroxyketorolac, which has minimal analgesic and anti-inflammatory activity. After administration of intravenous ketorolac (0.5 mg/kg) to children over the age 4 years, the volume of distribution at steady state (0.26 ± 0.1 L/kg) and plasma clearance (0.7 ± 0.14 mL/kg/minute) were estimated approximately two times higher than those in adults, but the mean elimination half-life (6 ± 2 hours) was similar. Therefore, an intravenous or intramuscular ketorolac dosing regimen (every 6 hours) is the same in children and adults and the duration of therapy is not to exceed 5 days.

A preliminary unpublished report of pharmacokinetics of ketorolac in infants more than 3 months suggests that the average half-life of elimination is comparable to older children. In children over 5 years of age, analgesic efficacy of a single intravenous dose of ketorolac at 0.9 mg/kg is comparable to intravenous morphine of 0.1 mg/kg. Intramuscular ketorolac in a dose of 0.75 mg/kg provides analgesia comparable to intramuscular meperidine 1 mg/kg. When used in combination with opioids, ketorolac significantly enhances analgesia and reduces opioid consumption.

The routine use of ketorolac in children under the age of 3 years should be discouraged until detailed data on pharmacokinetics are available. Recommended doses for children over the age 3 years is 0.25 to 0.5 mg/kg. Recently, a lower dose of ketorolac 0.25 mg/kg with a total daily dose less than 60 mg in adults is reported to have a low risk of serious gastrointestinal bleeding and may be equally effective as the initially recommended dose of 0.5 mg/kg, particularly when used as a coanalgesic with an opioid. Parenteral administration of ketorolac appears to have little effect on the GI tract in the clinically recommended doses and when analgesic therapy is used for less than 5 days after surgery.

ROUTES OF ADMINISTRATION

Systemic analgesics are administered by various routes, which include intravenous, intramuscular, subcutaneous, intraosseous, transdermal, and intranasal. Subcutaneous and intramuscular routes are unsuitable for pain control in children because these routes are painful, render the child uncooperative, onset is slow, absorption is unpredictable, and there is five- to seven-fold variation in blood levels. With the exception of sufentanil (which is only used in the intranasal route in procedural sedation), the intravenous route has many advantages including the following:

1. Rapid onset of drug action, which produces prompt relief of severe pain and anxiety
2. More predictable optimal concentrations and fast peak effects, which allows titration of drug dosage to match individual patient's need
3. Blood concentration and drug effect progressively decline, which limit the time of toxic effects if they occur
4. Duration of action is relatively short as the plasma concentrations of the drug decline rapidly because of uptake by body tissues and elimination from the body by biotransformation and excretion

Available Preparations and Dosing (Table 10.1)

ADVERSE EFFECTS

Opioids produce dose-dependent analgesia and other adverse effects irrespective of the route of administration. Most opioids produce a similar degree of analgesia and side effects at analgesic dose equivalents. There are some differences in side effects among opioids related to differences in chemical structures (Fig. 10.1).

Central Nervous System Effects

Dose-related sedation, somnolence, reduced level of consciousness, inability to concentrate, and slurred speech can occur.

Respiratory Depression

Appropriately administered opioids rarely cause clinically significant respiratory depression. Pain acts as an antagonist to respiratory depression. All opioid agonists have similar depressant effect on the brain stem respiratory center at equianalgesic doses. After administration of therapeutic doses the following may occur:

Table 10.1. Available Preparations and Dosing for Procedural Sedation/Analgesia

	Available IV Preparations	Dosing
Fentanyl	IV: 50μg/mL	1–5 μg/kg IV
Sufentanil	IV: 100 μg/mL	0.7–1.0 μg/kg IN
Morphine	IV: 5 mg/mL	0.05–0.15 mg/kg IV
Meperidine	IV: 50 mg/mL	0.5–1.0 mg/kg IV
Ketorolac	IV: 15, 30 mg/mL	0.25–0.5 mg/kg IV/IM
		Maximum dose
		30 mg/dose (IV)
		60 mg/dose (IM)

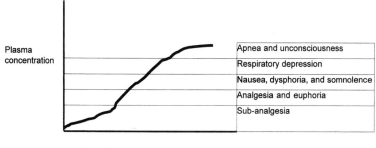

Figure 10.1. Opioid response and adverse effects.

- Initial decrease in respiratory rate occurs and compensatory increase in tidal exchange occurs; but the compensation is incomplete and eventually the minute volume decreases and arterial carbon dioxide tension rises.
- Maximum respiratory depression occurs within 7 to 10 minutes after intravenous administration, within 20 to 30 minutes after intramuscular administration, and within 90 minutes after subcutaneous administration. However, respiratory function tests can reveal abnormalities for as long as 4 to 5 hours.
- Depression of the pontine and medullary respiratory centers' response to increased blood carbon dioxide tension results in prolonged pauses between breaths, delayed exhalation, periodic breathing, and eventually apnea.
- An important clue to the presence of opioid-induced respiratory depression is the presence of miosis.

Medical conditions associated with an increased risk of respiratory depression after opioid administration include the following:

1. Decreased opioid clearance
   a. Moderate to severe renal and hepatic dysfunction
   b. Infants under the age of 3 months
2. Abnormal ventilatory control
   a. Premature infants less than 60 weeks postconceptual age
   b. Intracranial disorders—central apnea, Arnold-Chiari malformation, intracranial hypertension, etc.
   c. Concomitant use of sedative/hypnotics
3. Airway compromise
   a. Narrowing of the airways by anatomic distortion such as enlarged tonsils, enlarged tongue, cystic hygromas and vascular anomalies, subglottic stenosis, vascular ring, mediastinal masses, etc.

4. Decreased pulmonary reserve
   a. Neuromuscular disorders
5. Cardiorespiratory disease and hemodynamic instability

Opioids can be used safely in these children provided that the initial standard recommended doses are reduced and gradually increased stepwise to individual patient's response while monitoring the patient closely.

Excitatory Effects

Miosis (pupillary constriction) is caused by stimulation of the oculomotor nerve nucleus and can be antagonized by atropine. Unlike other opioids, meperidine causes mydriasis because of its atropinelike action.

Myoclonus and Seizure

Central nervous system hyperexcitability and myoclonus are infrequent side effects of opioid therapy for acute pain. Seizures have been reported with high doses (above the dosing range used for procedural sedation) of fentanyl, sufentanil, and meperidine. Myoclonic jerks and seizure have been reported with chronic administration or with high doses of meperidine because of accumulation of normeperidine metabolite, interaction with other drugs, or because of a patient's renal insufficiency.

Nausea and Vomiting

Nausea occurs frequently after intravenous administration of opioids and is produced by stimulation of chemoreceptor trigger zone dopamine receptors in the medulla, a change in vestibular function, and an inhibitory effect on gastrointestinal motility. Nausea and vomiting occur more frequently with an escalating dose, an intravenous route, and in ambulating patients. Commonly used intravenous antiemetics for treatment of opioid-induced nausea and vomiting include the following:

a. Ondansetron 0.1 mg/kg, maximum dose 4 mg/kg
b. Diphenhydramine 1 mg/kg, maximum dose 50 mg
c. Metoclopramide 0.1 to 0.2 mg/kg, maximum dose 10 mg
d. Droperidol 0.03 to 0.075 mg/kg, maximum dose 1.25 mg
e. Perphenazine 15 to 25 mg/kg, maximum dose 1 mg

Most of these drugs cause sedation and may limit the use of effective opioid doses safely.

Skin Reactions

Morphine, meperidine, and codeine produce histamine release and manifest as venodilation or local urticaria along the injected vessel. This should not be mistaken for an allergic reaction. Generalized release of histamine manifests as flushed skin which may be relevant when administered to patients with asthma. Morphine is a relative contraindication in patients with asthma. Fentanyl and sufentanil do not release histamine.

Pruritus

Systemic opioid therapy can be associated with pruritus, particularly with morphine because of histamine release, but can occur with any opioids caused by central effect.

DRUG INTERACTIONS

Meperidine

The coadministration of the following medications may also enhance meperidine toxicity:

1. Phenothiazines (promethazine [Phenergan], chlorpromazine, prochlorperazine [Compazine], perphenazine [Trilafon]) have been shown to lower the seizure threshold, and may contribute to the seizures.
2. Meperidine has anticholinergic activity, which can be exacerbated by coadministration of drugs with similar action, such as atropine, doxepin hydrochloride, and cimetidine, and may culminate in seizures.
3. Coadministration of monoamine oxidase (MAO) inhibitors has resulted in severe hemodynamic instability.
4. Hepatic N-demethylation enzyme-inducing agents such as loperamide (a piperidine derivative and congener of meperidine) and carbamazepine may increase the formation of normeperidine.
5. Hyponatremia may also aggravate normeperidine neurotoxicity.

CONTRAINDICATIONS

Ketorolac

1. Ketorolac may prolong bleeding time and should not be used in patients with hemostatic defects. Although ketorolac increases bleeding time, it appears to have little clinical significance in patients with normal hemostatic function.
2. Ketorolac should not be used in patients with a history of peptic ulcer disease or upper gastrointestinal bleeding.
3. Ketorolac should not be used in patients with impaired renal function. All

NSAIDs, including ketorolac, can cause renal insufficiency by inhibiting synthesis of renal prostaglandins. Ketorolac has no or little potential for renal toxicity in patients with normal volume status and normal renal function.

4. Ketorolac should not be used during states in which activation of renin-angiotensin system occurs and are dependent on prostaglandins to maintain renal blood flow such as congestive heart failure, hypovolemia, renal function impairment, or hepatic cirrhosis. Inhibition of renal prostaglandin synthesis in these conditions by ketorolac may result in renal arteriolar constriction and renal insufficiency.

SUGGESTED READING

Bates BA, Schutzman SA, Fleisher GR. A comparison of intranasal sufentanil and midazolam to intramuscular meperidine, promethazine, and chlorpromazine for conscious sedation in children. Ann Emerg Med 1994;24:646–651.

Bilmire DA, Neale HW, Gregory RO. Use of IV fentanyl in the outpatient treatment of pediatric facial trauma. J Trauma 1985;25:1079–1080.

Christensen ML, Wang WC, Harris S, et al. Transdermal fentanyl administration in children and adolescents with sickle cell pain crisis. J Pediatr Hematol Oncol 1996;18(4):372–376.

Chudnofsky CR, Wright SW, Dronen SC, et al. The safety of fentanyl use in the emergency department. Ann Emerg Med 1989;18:635–639.

Davis PJ, Cook DR. Clinical pharmacokinetics of the newer intravenous anaesthetic agents. Clin Pharmacokinet 1986:11;18–35.

Dickenson AH. Mechanisms of the analgesic actions of opiates and opioids. Br Med Bull 1991;47(3):690–702.

Ferrante FM. Opioids. In: Ferrane FM, VadeBoncouer TR, eds. Postoperative Pain Management. New York: Churchill Livingstone, 1993.

Jeal W, Benfield P. Transdermal fentanyl. A review of its pharmacological properties and therapeutic efficacy in pain control. Drugs 1997;53(1):109–38.

Karl HW, Keifer AT, Rosenberger JL, et al. Comparison of the safety and efficacy of intranasal midazolam or sufentanil for preinduction of anesthesia in pediatric patients. Anesthesiology 1992;76(2):209–15.

Kart T, Christrup LL, Rasmussen M. Recommended use of morphine in neonates, infants and children based on a literature review: Part 1—pharmacokinetics. Paediatr Anaesth 1997;7(1): 5–11.

Kart T, Christrup LL, Rasmussen M. Recommended use of morphine in neonates, infants and children based on a literature review: Part 2—clinical use. Paediatr Anaesth 1997;7(2):93–101.

Olkkola KT, Leijala MA, Maunuksela EL. Paediatric ventilatory effects of morphine and buprenorphine revisited. Paediatr Anaesth 1995;5(5):303–335.

Pokela ML, Olkkola KT, Koivisto M, et al. Pharmacokinetics and pharmacodynamics of intravenous meperidine in neonates and infants. Clin Pharmacol Ther 1992;52(4):342–349.

Santeiro ML, Christie J, Stromquist C, et al. Pharmacokinetics of continuous infusion fentanyl in newborns. J Perinatol 1997;17(2):135–139.

Smith TC. Pharmacology of respiratory depression. Int Anesth Clin 1971;199:464–468.

Stimmel B. Pain, Analgesia, and Addiction: The Pharmacologic Treatment of Pain. New York: Raven Press, 1983.

Chapter 11
Nitrous Oxide

Keira Mason, Babu Koka

> *Said Syntax, "I have often heard*
> *Philosophers of high regard*
> *Speak of this nitrous inhalation*
> *And its gay exhilaration."*

Nitrous oxide (N_2O) was first discovered in 1772 by Priestley and shortly thereafter its properties for pain relief and mood exhilaration were recognized. Clinical use of nitrous oxide as an anesthetic agent dates back to 1844. Nitrous oxide has been used in the outpatient setting as a sedative, amnestic, and analgesic since the 1950s. In 1960, emergency medical services began to offer patients the opportunity to self-administer nitrous oxide during transport to the hospital.

GENERAL INDICATIONS

Nitrous oxide is the most commonly used anesthetic agent in patients undergoing surgical procedures under general anesthesia. In addition, nitrous oxide is used in various outpatient settings, which include the dental office, endoscopy suite, and the emergency department. Concentrations of 40 to 50% nitrous oxide in the emergency department have been shown to provide effective analgesia for laceration repairs in children over 8 years old. The analgesia attained from nitrous oxide in children who are less than 8 years of age, however, does not show statistically significant results as compared to placebo. Nitrous oxide has also been shown to be an effective analgesia for reduction of fractures in children in the emergency department, with a short recovery period and greater patient acceptance. Nitrous oxide in the outpatient setting in the United States is used exclusively through a demand valve mask, which precludes its use in children less than 5 years of age. Other countries, especially in Europe, administer nitrous oxide as a free-flowing gas, which allows its use in children as young as 2 years old.

MECHANISM OF ACTION

The mechanism of action of nitrous oxide is unclear. Nitrous oxide has analgesic properties, and some studies indicate that nitrous oxide works at the opioid receptor and may stimulate the release of opioid agonists. Nitrous oxide acts directly at the mu and delta sites and possibly at the kappa, sigma, and epsilon sites.

Effects on Circulation

Nitrous oxide activates the sympathetic nervous system and may cause a small increase in cerebral blood flow and intracranial pressure. In both infants and adults, nitrous oxide acts as a mild depressant on systemic hemodynamics. Specifically, when 50% nitrous oxide was administered to infants, the average heart rate decreased by 9%, the mean arterial blood pressure decreased by 12%, and cardiac index decreased by 13%. Pulmonary artery pressure and pulmonary vascular resistance was unaltered, regardless of preexisting pulmonary hypertension. Although the depression in systemic hemodynamics is real, it is unlikely that nitrous oxide would have a clinically significant effect, unless administered to a child with severely compromised cardiovascular reserve.

Effects on Respiration

Nitrous oxide may depress the ventilatory response to arterial hypoxemia. Nitrous oxide does not, however, alter the ventilatory response to carbon dioxide. Thus, there should be no respiratory depression when breathing spontaneously with nitrous oxide. Some studies indicate that at concentrations as low as 20%, nitrous oxide may stimulate ventilation, with an increase in tidal volume and a decrease in inspiratory time.

PHARMACOKINETICS

Nitrous oxide has the lowest molecular weight of any inhaled anesthetic. The pharmacokinetics of inhalational agents are determined by four factors:

1. Uptake from the alveoli to the pulmonary circulation
2. Distribution throughout the body into tissues of the brain, muscle, and fat
3. Metabolism
4. Elimination via the lungs

The partition coefficient describes the concentration of inhaled anesthetic that is distributed between the two phases at equilibrium. With its low blood:gas solubility coefficient, nitrous oxide is poorly soluble in blood. Because of its negligible solubility, nitrous oxide concentration increases at a rapid rate at the alveoli, regardless of changes in alveolar ventilation. Nitrous oxide does not bind to any carrier proteins in the blood. Because of its low solubility in blood and tissues, nitrous oxide is quickly exhaled at the conclusion of its administration. Most of nitrous oxide is exhaled in its original state. Only 0.004% of an absorbed dose of nitrous oxide is actually metabolized to nitrogen at the level of the gastrointestinal tract. Anaerobic bacteria participate in this reductive metabolism.

METHOD OF ADMINISTRATION

Nitrous oxide is odorless and nonflammable. Although nonflammable, it can support combustion. Nitrous oxide is administered with modern anesthesia equipment mixed with oxygen at concentrations of 50 to 70 %. This mixture often produces a state of analgesia and pain relief.

For self-administration of oxygen/nitrous oxide, the mask should be held over the nose or the mouth. Adequate mental facilities and muscle coordination are needed to perform this task. When adequate sedation and analgesia is achieved, the patient should invariably loosen his or her grip on the mask. The mask is equipped with an "on-demand" valve, which generally requires a negative pressure of 1 to 5 cm H_2O to activate. With the release of the mask, the demand valve of the delivery system no longer delivers nitrous oxide, which is similar to a fail-safe mechanism. The demand valve not only prevents the patient from becoming oversedated, but also reduces the nitrous oxide pollution in the ambient setting.

CONTRAINDICATIONS AND PRECAUTIONS

Diffusion Hypoxia

Diffusion hypoxia has been described after the cessation of nitrous oxide. Because nitrogen is approximately 33 times less soluble in blood than the nitrous oxide that replaces it, nitrous oxide is excreted faster than nitrogen is taken up. As a consequence, nitrous oxide continues to diffuse into the alveoli and dilute the alveolar oxygen even after nitrous oxide is discontinued. This phenomenon is known as diffusion hypoxia. The first 3 to 5 minutes after nitrous oxide is discontinued is the time of greatest risk for diffusion hypoxia. It is for this reason that 100% oxygen is routinely administered after nitrous oxide is discontinued. Some studies indicate that diffusion hypoxia is of no clinical consequence when nitrous is administered in concentrations of less than 50%. In healthy children in the dental setting who were exposed to 40% nitrous oxide, there was no clinically significant desaturation after nitrous was discontinued.

Nausea and Vomiting

It is unclear whether there is an association between nitrous oxide administration and adverse consequences of nausea and vomiting. A retrospective study of 3,000 pediatric patients in the outpatient setting who were exposed to 50 to 60% nitrous oxide revealed a 0.3% incidence of vomiting. Another study had similar results: in more than 3500 patients, there was a 0.3% incidence of vomiting in patients receiving 30 to 40% nitrous oxide. A double-blind study of 780 patients postoperatively revealed no association between nitrous oxide and postoperative nausea and vomiting.

Sleep Apnea-Like Syndrome

An association may exist between nitrous oxide inhalation and a sleep apnea-like syndrome. Specifically, when healthy adults with normal breathing patterns during sleep were exposed to 30 to 50% nitrous oxide, some alterations in respiratory patterns occured. These respiratory disturbances only occurred when the EEG demonstrated a sleep pattern. The respiratory events were consistent with obstructive and central sleep apnea. This report suggests that the usual vigilance should be paid to the respiratory pattern/behavior of children exposed to nitrous oxide during spontaneous ventilation.

Diffusion into Air-Containing Body Cavities

The high partial pressure of nitrous oxide in blood, coupled with its low blood:gas solubility coefficient, causes it to diffuse rapidly into air-filled cavities. Nitrous oxide should be considered as contraindicated in patients with head injuries, pneumothoraces, emphysematous blebs, and bowel obstruction.

SUGGESTED READING

American Academy of Pediatrics, Committee on Drugs, Section on Anesthesiology. Guidelines for the elective use of conscious sedation, deep sedation, and general anesthesia in pediatric patients. Pediatrics 1985;76:317–321.

Beydon L, Goldenberg F, Heyer L, et al. Sleep apnea-like syndrome induced by nitrous oxide inhalation in normal men. Respiration Physiology 1997;108:215–224.

Burton JH, Auble TE, Fuchs SM. Effectiveness of 50% nitrous oxide/50% oxygen during laceration repair in children. Acad Emerg Med 1998;5:112–117.

Cheng E, Nimphius N, Kampine J. Anesthetic drugs and emergency departments. Anesth Analg 1992;74:272–275.

Crocker D, Koka BV, Filler RM, et al. Tissue uptake and excretion of nitrous oxide in pediatric anesthesia. Anesth Analg (Cleve) 1974;53:779–785.

Dahan A, Ward D. Effect of 20% nitrous oxide on the ventilatory response to hypercapnia and sustained isocapnic hypoxia in man. Br J Anaesth 1994;72:17–20.

Dunn-Russel T, Adair SM, Sams DR, et al. Oxygen saturation and diffusion hypoxia in children following nitrous oxide sedation. Pediatr Dent 1993;16:88–92.

Etzwiler LS, Fleisher G, McGravey A. Safety and effectiveness of nitrous oxide for sedation and analgesia in the pediatric emergency department. Pediatr Emerg Care 1990;6:225.

Evans JK, Buckley SL, Alexander AH, et al. Analgesia for the reduction of fractures in children: a comparison of nitrous oxide with intramuscular sedation. J Pediatr Orthop 1995;15:73–77.

Gamis AS, Knapp JF, Glenski JA. Nitrous oxide analgesia in a pediatric emergency department. Ann Emerg Med 1989;18:177–181.

Gillman MA. Analgesic (subanesthetic) nitrous oxide interacts with the endogenous opioid system: a review of evidence. Life Sci 1986;39:1209–1211.

Gillman MA. Nitrous oxide an opioid addictive agent. Am J Med 1986;81:97–102.

Gregory PR, Sullivan JA. Nitrous oxide compared with intravenous regional anesthesia in pediatric forearm fracture manipulation. J Pediatr Orthop 1996 16:187–191.

Griffin G, Campbell V, Jones RL. Nitrous oxide-oxygen sedation for minor surgery: experience in a pediatric setting. JAMA 1983;245:2411–2413.

Guidelines for monitoring and management of pediatric patients during and after sedation for diagnostic and therapeutic procedures. Pediatrics 1992;89:1110–1115.

Guidelines for the elective use of pharmacologic conscious sedation and deep sedation in pediatric dental patients. Pediatr Dent 1993;15:297–301.

Hennrikus WL, Simpson RB, Klingelberger CE, et al. Self-administered nitrous oxide analgesia for pediatric fracture reductions. J Pediatr Orthop 1994 14:538–542.

Hennrikus WL, Shin AY, Klingelberger CE. Self-administered nitrous oxide analgesia combined with hematoma block for outpatient reductions of fractures in children. J Bone Joint Surg 1995 77:335–339.

Hickey PR, Hansen DD, Stafford M, et al. Pulmonary and systemic hemodynamic effects of nitrous in infants with normal and elevated pulmonary vascular resistance. Anesthesiology 1986;65:374–378.

Hong K, Trudell JR, O'Neil JR, et al. Metabolism of nitrous oxide by human and rat intestinal contents. Anesthesiology 1980;52:16–19.

Houpt MI, Kupietzky A, Tofsky NS, et al. Effects of nitrous oxide on diazepam sedation of young children. Pediatr Dent 1996;18(3):236–241.

Litman RS, Berkowitz RJ, Ward DS. Levels of consciousness and ventilatory parameters in young children during sedation with oral midazolam and nitrous oxide. Arch Pediatr Adolesc Med 1996;150:671–675.

Malamed S. Sedation—A Guide to Patient Management. St. Louis: CV Mosby Co, 1985: 149–266.

McCann W, Wilson S, Larsen P, et al. The effects of nitrous oxide on behavior and physiological parameters during conscious sedation with a moderate dose of chloral hydrate and hydroxyzine. Pediatr Dent 1996;18(1):35–41.

McKinnon K. Pre-hospital analgesia with nitrous oxide/oxygen. Can Med Assoc J 1982;125: 836–840.

Muir JJ, Warner M, Offord K, et al. Role of nitrous oxide and other factors in postoperative nausea and vomiting. Anesthesiology 1987;66:513–518.

Notini-Gudmarsson AK, Dolk A, Johansson C. Nitrous oxide: a valuable alternative for pain relief and sedation during routine colonoscopy. Endoscopy 1996;28:283–287.

Sacchetti A, Schafermeyer R, Gerardi M, et al. Pediatric analgesia and sedation. Ann Emerg Med 1994;23:237–250.

Saunders BP, Fukomoto M, Halligan S, et al. Patient-administered nitrous oxide/oxygen inhalation provides effective sedation and analgesia for colonoscopy. Gastrointest Endosc 1994;40:418–421.

Stewart RD. Nitrous oxide sedation/analgesia in emergency medicine. Ann Emerg Med 1985;4:139–148.

Stoelting RK. Pharmacology and physiology in anesthetic practice. 1991.

Wattenmaker I, Kasser JR, McGravey A. Self-administered nitrous oxide for fracture reduction in children in an emergency room setting. J Orthop Trauma 1990;4:35–38.

Wilson S. A survey of the American Academy of Pediatric Dentistry membership: nitrous oxide and sedation. Pediatr Dent 1996;18:287–293.

Wright W. Doctor Syntax in Paris, 46 Fleet Street, London, 1820.

Chapter 12
Benzodiazepine and Opioid Antagonists

Holly Perry

Reversal agents (i.e., opioid and benzodiazepine antagonists) have enhanced the safety of sedation and analgesia in the outpatient setting in both the adult and pediatric populations. Reversal of sedation and analgesia may be attained safely and effectively by administration of competitive antagonists. A competitive antagonist displaces an agonist from receptor sites in the central nervous system (CNS) but does not itself produce a physiologic response. Competition is stoichiometric with administration of larger amounts of antagonist displacing more agonist and resulting in more complete reversal of agonist effect. The opioid receptor antagonists include naloxone and nalmefene, although flumazenil is the only available benzodiazepine receptor antagonist. There is no cross-reactivity among agents: flumazenil does not reverse sedation from opiates nor do naloxone and nalmefene reverse sedation from benzodiazepines.

Naloxone was introduced in 1960, flumazenil in 1987, and nalmefene in 1995. Since their introduction, these agents have been shown to be both safe and efficacious when used to reverse general anesthesia or sedation and analgesia for painful procedures. These agents are also approved for empiric use in patients with a suspected drug overdose, although use of flumazenil and nalmefene in this setting is controversial. In the setting of acute drug overdose, nalmefene may result in a prolonged period of symptoms of acute opioid withdrawal while flumazenil may unmask seizures in mixed drug overdoses. Although serious adverse events have been reported after naloxone and flumazenil administration, these are rare. In the case of flumazenil, careful selection of appropriate patients lowers the risk even further.

OPIOID ANTAGONISTS: NALOXONE AND NALMEFENE

Mechanism of Action

Opioids produce analgesia, sedation, and respiratory depression by binding to three subtypes of opioid receptors in the CNS. Agonist binding at the mu receptor subtype produces miosis, analgesia, euphoria, and respiratory depression. Binding at the kappa receptor results in only analgesia and sedation and binding at the sigma receptor produces psychogenic effects such as dysphoria. Naloxone and nalmefene are competitive antagonists at each of these receptor subtypes, with highest affinity for the mu receptor subtype, and thus reversing the effects of opioids. They have no agonist activity, and administration of large doses does not cause sedation or respiratory depression. Additionally, naloxone has been hypothesized to produce catecholamine release, which could explain rare adverse events such as ventricular tachycardia after its administration.

Although either naloxone or nalmefene will reverse opioid-induced analgesia, naloxone is the preferred agent. In the emergency department setting, short-acting opioids such as fentanyl are commonly used and, therefore, administration of a reversal agent with a prolonged duration of action such as nalmefene does not confer any additional benefit.

Pharmacokinetics (Table 12.1)

Naloxone and nalmefene differ primarily in duration of action, with nalmefene having a significantly longer duration than naloxone. Both are lipid soluble and are rapidly distributed to the brain. Both are primarily metabolized in the liver by glucuronidation, and the inactive metabolites are excreted by the kidney.

Routes of Administration

Both naloxone and nalmefene may be given either intravenously, intramuscularly, or subcutaneously, although the preferred route is intravenously.

Available Preparations

Naloxone is available in a neonatal preparation of 0.02 mg/mL in 2 mL ampules and in adult preparations of 0.4 mg/mL and 1.0 mg/mL in either multiple dose vials or 2 mL ampules. Naloxone should be given in small, incremental doses every 2 to 3 minutes until the desired effect is attained. Incremental administration may obviate rare adverse reactions. The dose for adults is 0.4 to 2 mg (depending on the degree of respiratory depression) and for children it is 0.1 mg/kg for children weighing less than 20 kg and 2.0 mg for children weighing more than 20 kg. In contrast to approved labeling that states that the dose for neonates should be 0.005 to 0.01 mg/kg, the American Academy of Pediatrics recommends that neonates be treated with 0.1 mg/kg (the same dose as older children) to ensure adequate opiate reversal.

Table 12.1. Pharmacokinetics of Reversal Agents

Agent	Antagonist	Route	Dose	Frequency	Maximum Per Dose	Onset	Duration
Naloxone	Opioids	IV (preferred) IM, subq	Adults: 0.1–0.4 mg Children: < 20 kg: 0.05–0.1 mg/kg > 20 kg: 1–2 mg	q 2–3 min	2.0 mg	1–2 min (IV) 15 min. (IM, subq)	30–60 min
Nalmefene	Opioids	IV (preferred) IM, subq	0.25 µg/kg	q 2–5 min	1 µg/kg	5 min (IV) 15–20 min (IM, subq)	210 min
Flumazenil	Benzodiazepines	IV	0.02 mg/kg (0.2 mg maximum initial, single dose)	q 1 min	1.0 mg	1–2 min (IV)	20–60 min

Nalmefene is supplied as Revex and is available in two concentrations: 100 μg /mL and 1.0 mg/mL. It should be given in incremental doses of 0.25 μg/kg every 2 to 5 minutes until the desired effect is attained.

Contraindications and Precautions

Opioid antagonists are generally safe. Mild side effects such as nausea, vomiting, paranoia, dizziness, and chills occur in 1 to 18% of patients. Nausea is the most commonly reported adverse reaction. Serious adverse effects are rare. There have been isolated case reports of sudden cardiac death, ventricular fibrillation, and pulmonary edema in healthy young adults receiving either naloxone or nalmefene after general anesthesia. There have been no reports of sudden cardiac death after reversal of analgesia with naloxone or nalmefene in the outpatient setting. The only absolute contraindication to the use of opioid antagonists is administration to a neonate delivered to a narcotic-dependent woman because it may precipitate life-threatening opiate withdrawal.

BENZODIAZEPINE ANTAGONIST: FLUMAZENIL

Mechanism of Action

Gamma-aminobutyric acid (GABA) is one of the two primary inhibitory neurotransmitters in the CNS. Agents that enhance GABA activity produce CNS depression and those that antagonize it cause CNS excitation. Benzodiazepines produce sedation and anxiolysis through enhancement of GABA activity at the $GABA_A$ receptor. Agents such as ethanol and barbiturates also produce some of their clinical effects by enhancement of GABA binding at this receptor through binding sites distinct from benzodiazepine receptors. Flumazenil is a competitive antagonist at this receptor and reverses benzodiazepine-induced sedation without necessarily reversing anxiolysis. Clinically important antagonists (i.e., agents that diminish GABA binding at the $GABA_A$ receptor) include cyclic antidepressants.

Flumazenil has been shown to be both safe and efficacious in a number of double-blind placebo-controlled trials when used to reverse benzodiazepine sedation after a variety of painful procedures. It has also been studied systematically in the pediatric population where it has been shown to be safe and efficacious. Flumazenil has been used safely in the newborn period.

Pharmacokinetics

The onset of action is 1 to 2 minutes, maximal effect occurs by 6 to 10 minutes, and effects last for approximately 40 to 80 minutes. Flumazenil is metabolized in the liver primarily by glucuronidation and excreted as the inactive metabolite by the kidney.

Routes of Administration

Flumazenil is only recommended for intravenous use. This agent has been shown to work effectively via the sublingual and rectal routes, although the onset is considerably delayed making these routes impractical. Extensive first-pass metabolism limits its oral efficacy.

Available Preparations

Flumazenil is supplied as Romazicon in a single preparation of 0.01 mg/mL in multiple-use vials. Flumazenil should be given in increments so that the clinician can assess the effect of the medication. The initial dose is 0.02 mg/kg (maximum 0.2 mg) infused intravenously over 15 seconds. Additional doses may be given every minute until response occurs or a maximum of 1.0 mg has been reached. The patient should be observed for 2 hours after reversal. If resedation occurs, the patient may be treated with an additional dose of flumazenil.

Contraindications and Precautions

Adverse reactions to flumazenil have a 1 to 6% incidence. The most common adverse reactions are crying, agitation, aggressive behavior, headache, nausea, and dizziness. Rarely, flumazenil has been associated with serious adverse effects such as hypotension and seizures, although this is much more common when flumazenil is given to patients with an unknown drug overdose. Seizures or cardiac dysfunction are unlikely if high-risk patients are excluded.

Resedation   Flumazenil is effective in reversing benzodiazepine sedation. Resedation has been reported to occur in as many as 7% of pediatric patients after flumazenil was used to reverse midazolam. Resedation has only been reported in patients 5 years of age and younger. On average, resedation occurs at 25 minutes, with a range of 19 to 50 minutes. A higher rate of resedation may occur with benzodiazepines with a longer half-life than midazolam.

Paradoxical Reactions   Flumazenil is also effective in reversing paradoxical reactions to benzodiazepines. A paradoxical reaction is characterized by inconsolable crying, combativeness, disorientation, agitation, and restlessness and has been reported in as many as 1.4% of children receiving midazolam intravenously before endoscopy. These reactions have also been reported with intramuscular, intranasal, or rectal administration of benzodiazepines. Administration of flumazenil brings about clinical improvement, generally within 15 minutes.

Administration of flumazenil is contraindicated in several situations. Flumazenil should not be given to patients who are on benzodiazepines as part of therapy for a seizure disorder. Furthermore, it should be given cautiously to patients who are on medications known to lower the seizure threshold, such as tricyclic antidepressants, theophylline, isoniazid, lithium, propoxyphene, and cyclosporine. Use of flumazenil in these patients could precipitate a seizure.

SUGGESTED READING

American Academy of Pediatrics Committee on Drugs. Naloxone dosage and route of administration for infants and children: addendum to emergency drug doses for infants and children. Pediatrics 1990;86:484–485.

Andree RA. Sudden death following naloxone administration. Anaesth Analg (Cleve) 1980;59:782–784.

Barsan WG, Seger D, Danzl DF, et al. Duration of antagonistic effects of Nalmefene and Naloxone in opiate-induced sedation for emergency department procedures. Am J Emerg Med 1989;7:155–161.

Chudnofsky CR, for the Emergency Medicine Conscious Sedation Study Group. Safety and efficacy of flumazenil in reversing conscious sedation in the emergency department. Acad Emerg Med 1997;4:944–950.

Evans JM, Hogg MIJ, Rosen M. Reversal of narcotic depression in the neonate by naloxone. Br Med J 1976;2:1098.

Anon. Reversal of central benzodiazepine effects by flumazenil after intravenous conscious sedation with diazepam and opioids; report of a double-blind multicenter study. The flumazenil in intravenous conscious sedation with diazepam multicenter study group II. Clin Ther 1992;14:910–923.

Gaeta TJ, Capodano RJ, Spevack TA. Potential danger of nalmefene use in the emergency department. Ann Emerg Med 1997;29:193–194.

Glass PSA, Jhaveri RM, Smith R. Comparison of potency and duration of action of nalmefene and naloxone. Anesth Analg (Cleve) 1994;78:536–541.

Handal KA, Schauban JL, Salamone FR. Naloxone. Ann Emerg Med 1983;12:438–445.

Henderson CA, Reynolds JE. Acute pulmonary edema in a young male after intravenous nalmefene. Anesth Analg (Cleve) 1997;84:218–219.

Heniff MS, Moore GP, Trout A, et al. Comparison of routes of flumazenil administration to reverse midazolam-induced respiratory depression in a canine model. Acad Emerg Med 1997;4:1115–1118.

Longnecker DE, Grazis PA, Eggers GWN. Naloxone for antagonism of morphine-induced respiratory depression. Anesth Analg (Cleve) 1973; 52:447–453.

Massanari M, NovitskyJ, Reinstein LJ. Paradoxical reactions in children associated with midazolam use during endoscopy. Clin Pediatr 1997;36:681–684.

Nalmefene-a long acting injectable opioid antagonist. Med Lett 1995;37:97– 98.

Prough DS, Roy R, Bumgarner J, et al. Acute pulmonary edema in healthy teenagers following conservative doses of intravenous naloxone. Anesthesiology 1984;60:485–486.

Richard P, Autret E, Bardol J, et al. The use of flumazenil in a neonate. Clin Toxicol 1991;29:137–140.

Shannon M, Albers G, Burkhart K, et al. Safety and efficacy of flumazenil in the reversal of benzodiazepine-induced conscious sedation. J Pediatr 1997;131:582–586.

Spivey WH. Flumazenil and seizures: analysis of 43 cases. Clin Ther 1992;14:292–305.

Sugarman JM, Paul RI. Flumazenil: a review. Pediatr Emerg Care 1994;10:37–43.

Taft RH. Pulmonary edema following naloxone administration in a patient without heart disease. Anesthiology 1983;59:576–577.

White PF, Shafer A, Boyle WA 3d, et al. Benzodiazepine antagonism does not provoke a stress response. Anesthesiology 1989; 70:636–639.

Part Two

Principles and Management Strategies

Chapter 13
General Principles for Procedural Sedation and Analgesia

Thomas Terndrup

Practitioners who care for children in the outpatient setting (emergency physicians, pediatricians, anesthesiologists, family physicians, dentists, general and plastic surgeons, and orthopedists) must be constantly on the look out for painful conditions in considering measures to actively control pain and anxiety. This is especially the case in preverbal infants, those with depressed mental states, and those who are mentally challenged. Pain or observable distress is the most common reason why patients, including children, present for emergency care. Despite recent enthusiasm for pain research, it remains true that infants and children often remain undertreated for their painful conditions. Our challenge in emergency pediatric care is to recognize that pain or distress exists and to appropriately manage that pain and distress while establishing a diagnostic impression. A wide array of clinical issues will dictate how the individual patient will be managed. Key factors to consider include the patient's severity of pain or anxiety, the patient's clinical cardiorespiratory and neurological stability, and the anticipated depth of sedation and analgesia required for an intended procedure. The duration of the procedure, relative contraindications to certain agents, and the presence or absence of an intravenous catheter will dictate which agents should be used and by how they can best be administered.

In the outpatient setting, there are widespread indications for analgesia and sedation in children. The indications can be viewed as a function of the patient's clinical condition (e.g., fractured radius), apparent severity of pain or distress (e.g., variable pain associated with various types of pharyngitis, from mild sore throat to severe peritonsillar abscess), and mechanism of injury or insult (e.g., a fall while playing vs. struck by car). Other indications include patients with anticipated pain, especially in those cases where the duration of pain associated with the performance of painful procedures is prolonged (e.g., reducing a both-bones forearm fracture vs. nursemaid's elbow), known or expected effects of clinical conditions or therapies, or the need to control distress or poor cooperation to establish a diagnostic impression or perform a life-saving procedure before establishing a firm diagnostic impression.

The general indications for procedural sedation are listed in Table 13.1. The majority of children requiring analgesia alone are those with minor infections or trauma. For children who are undergoing procedures associated with little additional pain, sedation may be required to reduce anxiety and improve patient cooperation. These patients include those with uncomplicated lacerations and younger patients undergoing neuroimaging procedures. When the anticipated procedure may produce more than minor pain, as in the case of some complex laceration repairs or a difficult foreign body extraction, analgesia should also be provided. Common indications for routinely providing sedation plus analgesia are for fracture reductions, abscess incision and drainage, and burn wound debridement.

DEFINITION OF TERMS

General Considerations

Pain is defined by the International Association for the Study of Pain as "an unpleasant sensory and emotional experience associated with actual or potential tissue damage, or described in terms of such damage." Pain-control measures include

Table 13.1. Indications for Procedural Sedation and Analgesia

Sedation (Alone)	Analgesia (Alone)	Sedation/Analgesia
Cooperation	Pain Control	Relaxation, Analgesia
Neuroimaging	Pharyngitis	Fracture reduction
Laceration repair	Otitis media	Dislocation reduction
Sexual abuse examination	Burns	Foreign body, deep
Barium enema	Abscess drainage	Bone marrow aspiration
Slit lamp examination		Joint aspiration
Lumbar puncture		Hernia reduction
Foreign body, superficial		Cardioversion
Central line placement		
Chest tube placement		
Thoracentesis		
Endotracheal intubation		

Note: Sedation often enhances analgesic efficacy, and opioids have sedative effects. More severe conditions dictate that more potent medications be used. Local and regional anesthesia and psychological measures should be used whenever possible to reduce systemic medication requirements.

psychological and medicinal techniques used to produce analgesia (i.e., to relieve or reduce nociception) and sedation (i.e., to induce a state of reduced awareness). In recognition of the frequent need to produce both sedative and analgesic effects in children with painful or acute conditions, the 1998 Current Procedural Terminology book includes codes for sedation alone and that with analgesia (99141 for intravenous, intramuscular, and inhalation; 99142 for oral, rectal, and nasal), with respect to procedures being performed by medical practitioners.

Levels of Sedation

Many children with emergency or urgent conditions will have such a heightened sense of anxiety as to benefit from anxiolysis. Some may view the reduction of anxiety as sedation without analgesia, but perhaps it is most akin to the preinduction phase of anesthesia, where anxiolytics are given to reduce the distress associated with parental separation or a mask induction. Regardless of semantics, there is a gradation in the level of sedation beginning with an anxious/frightened, alert child, moving to an alert and calm state, continuing with hypnotic agents that induce sleep, and ultimately progressing to that of general anesthesia. These varying levels of sedation (and consciousness) represent a continuum of responses to medications that may progress from alert/awake to hypoventilation/apnea in a nonlinear fashion. This "slippery slope" phenomenon in sedation and analgesia is especially true in children and requires constant vigilance on the part of the clinician. Furthermore, children have varying responses to analgesic and sedative agents (especially benzodiazepines) depending on the child's age and the time of day the medication is administered. Clinicians administering analgesia and sedation for procedures should be familiar with and able to recognize the varying manifestations of levels of sedation in children.

Traditional Terminology

Several clinical guidelines have suggested that conscious and deep sedation be used to describe the intended or expected effects of certain pharmaceutical agents. **Conscious sedation** has been defined as a "minimally depressed level of consciousness that retains the patient's ability to maintain a patent airway independently and continuously, and respond appropriately to physical stimulation or verbal command." **Deep sedation** has been defined as a "controlled state of depressed consciousness or unconsciousness from which the patient is not easily aroused, which may be accompanied by a partial or complete loss of protective reflexes. This includes the inability to maintain a patent airway independently and respond purposefully to physical stimulation or verbal command." **General anesthesia** is a medically controlled state of unconsciousness induced by potent sedative/analgesic or anesthetic agents and accompanied by loss of protective reflexes, typically produced to perform invasive body cavity surgery. This terminology has been widely criticized, and more recent recommendations have abandoned the use of the term "conscious sedation." In May 1998, the American College of Emergency Physicians came out with a new designation of "procedural sedation" defined as:

> *A technique of administering sedatives or dissociative agents with or without analgesics to induce a state that allows the patient to tolerate unpleasant procedures while maintaining cardiorespiratory function. Procedural sedation and analgesia are intended to result in a depressed level of consciousness but one that allows the patient to maintain airway control independently and continuously. Specifically, the drugs, doses, and techniques used are not likely to produce a loss of protective airway reflexes. (American College of Emergency Physicians: Clinical policy for procedural sedation and analgesia in the emergency department. Ann Emerg Med 1998;31:663–677.)*

In general, light sedation may be viewed as a condition in which the patient may sleep, but remains able to respond to mild tactile or verbal stimulation, whereas deeper sedation produces a condition where responsiveness to mild stimulation is lost or reduced. Light sedation is performed for relatively painless procedures, like neuroimaging, where enhanced cooperation or reduced movement is desired. For the more painful procedures, like fracture reduction, deeper sedation is sought and seems appropriate to the expected requirement for the patient's condition. The implication is that patients expected to become more sedated or those who are sicker (e.g., neurologically or hemodynamically unstable) will require more vigilant monitoring to assure their safety because they may lose basic protective reflexes or achieve a state of unintended general anesthesia, which carries additional attendant risks. Consultation with an anesthesiologist should be sought for elective procedures in American Society of Anesthesiologists (ASA) class III, IV patients (see Chapter 17).

Setting Specific Modifications

Although some have questioned the applicability of clinical guidelines for outpatient sedation to emergency medicine practice, they should certainly be viewed as appropriate minimum standards for nonelective procedures. These general outpatient guidelines were intended to improve the clinician's adherence to proper safety measures and to remind them in the outpatient setting of the inherent risks associated with administration of analgesic or sedative agents. Appropriate revisions are needed in the general guidelines that allow for adjustment of the guidelines to meet the unique needs of each outpatient setting (emergency department, office practice, dental practice, radiology).

For example, many practitioners would regard as liberal NPO (nothing by mouth) guidelines the requirement of at least 4 hours without milk or solids and no intake of clear liquids less than 2 hours before sedation. Yet a further liberalization was safely used in some recent publications for *elective cases* without apparent hazard, but not without criticism. For emergency patients requiring nonelective procedures, an assessment of food and fluid intake should precede medication. The risks of sedation must be weighed against the benefits and "the lightest effective sedation" used. The benefits of delaying a procedure because of recent food intake is often difficult to judge, because prolonged delays in certain clinical situations (e.g., hip dislocation, certain supracondylar elbow fractures, and even certain lacerations) are strongly associated with a worsened outcome or prognosis.

Is it acceptable or even desirable to delay a both-bone fracture of the forearm reduction until sufficient time has passed to minimize the risks of aspiration from effective sedation with analgesia? Patients in pain have unreliable gastric emptying, and waiting will still not guarantee an empty stomach. Clinicians must look for less risky but effective methods for achieving rapid orthopedic treatment, allowing manipulation to occur without unnecessary pain. Alternative approaches to immediate reduction of such a forearm fracture might include local or regional anesthesia associated with 50% nitrous oxide in oxygen, splinting and reduction after at least 4 hours after oral intake, or proceeding to the operating room or general anesthesia with full upper airway protection. Given the safety profile of nitrous oxide, this alternative seems safer than the combination of a potent opioid and benzodiazepine. Arguably, the adoption of effective agents with the best safety profiles, augmented with excellent local or regional anesthesia, may assist in minimizing the risks to patients who have recently eaten. The routine adoption of potent sedatives for managing uncomplicated laceration repairs is unwarranted and risks sedation disasters by virtue of ever-increasing numbers of children undergoing sedation. Accordingly, children undergoing simple laceration repair with topical anesthesia should only be considered for sedation when they are overtly anxious or grossly uncooperative during the procedure.

MONITORING (SEE CHAPTERS 3 AND 15)

The level of sedation and analgesia required for most children is a function of the patient and the intended procedure. The intensity of monitoring is dictated by the expected depth of sedation, whereas the duration of monitoring is dictated by the activity of the agents used and the patient's clinical condition. The vast majority of children who appear to require sedatives for procedural assistance require either anxiolysis or light sedation, allowing minimally or mildly painful procedures to be carried out such as neuroimaging studies or already locally anesthetized lacerations.

A quote from the 1993 Joint Commission on Accreditation of Healthcare Organizations guidelines illustrates the interpretation required to build satisfactory or even well-written guidelines:

". . . sedation (with or without analgesia) for which there is reasonable expectation that in the manner used, the sedation/analgesia will result in the loss of protective reflexes for a significant percentage of a group of patients."

Unfortunately, neither a "reasonable expectation" nor what constitutes a "significant percentage" of patients is defined in these guidelines. Without further clarification, the clinical validation of sedation guidelines must depend on further scientific investigation in establishing under what clinical conditions, dosages, and agents loss of protective reflexes occurs. As new data are obtained, clinicians must be prepared to alter their clinical practice so that it is consistent with new, and presumably better, ways of providing sedation and analgesia.

PERSONNEL (SEE CHAPTERS 3, 17, AND 18)

Continuous availability of appropriately trained and equipped health care professionals is essential wherever sedation is performed in children. Optimal configurations are unclear, but minimum standards have been defined for resuscitation equipment and life support training backgrounds. Children receiving deeper levels of sedation or provided greater levels of analgesia will require greater attention from individual personnel (as well as more careful monitoring). Personnel trained in airway management and resuscitation should be immediately available. Nonintubating personnel assigned to direct clinical observation should be at least capable of performing evaluation of vital signs, interpreting bedside monitoring parameters, and initiating basic life support. In the emergency department or other settings where physicians in training are working, every child undergoing sedation should be known to the supervising or attending physician, and therapeutic plans should be clarified with this individual before performing sedation.

TITRATION PRINCIPLES

Routes of Administration

Traditional routes of drug administration are oral (PO) or rectal (PR) for mild pain and anxiety problems and intramuscular (IM) or intravenous (IV) routes for moderate to severe pain and titratable sedation. Other routes of administration include transmucosal (either sublingual or nasal), inhalational, transdermal, and intraosseous. Although PO administration is painless and convenient, the absorption reliability and relative contraindications (e.g., head injury) may limit applicability to hemodynamically and neurologically stable children with mild pain or anxiety who are not vomiting. Although less convenient, administration of mild analgesics and potent sedatives may be effective PR. Diazepam, midazolam, methohexital, acetaminophen, and thiopental can be reliably given PR. Although IM medication remains the most common route of administration of potent analgesics, it is painful and may result in unreliable absorption. Transmucosal administration of sedatives and analgesics has become popular and has been used successfully with ketamine, fentanyl, sufentanil, and midazolam.

The preferred method of rapid, titratable drug delivery is intravenously. IV administration facilitates the rapid onset of activity and controlled titration of effects. However, insertion of an IV line in a struggling toddler may be much more distressful than a single IM injection. Many children requiring sedation are appropriately treated without the need to establish vascular access, such as those needing anxiolysis to undergo a laceration repair. For children likely to require deep sedation or those in severe pain, an IV catheter allows titration of clinical effects, repeated dosing, and emergency access in case of complications. Single, IM injections may be used for children who will likely not require further parenteral analgesia or sedation or in whom waiting until vascular access can be obtained will extend the period of suffering excessively. Once an IV catheter is in place, there is no need to administer sedative or analgesic medications by other routes of administration.

Reversal Agents (see Chapter 12)

Other considerations for using sedative and analgesic pharmacotherapy in children include the ability to reverse serious side effects, dosing based on a measured weight, and the question of whether local or regional anesthesia will suffice over systemic analgesics or sedatives. Reversal of central nervous system (CNS) and respiratory depression from opioids and benzodiazepines is a specific and effective therapy that enhances the safety profile of these agents.

Assessing Risks and Benefits

When choosing sedative and analgesic agents, the clinician must keep in mind the dual objectives of safety and efficacy. Although potent sedative and analgesic agents are widely available, their routine use at doses producing significant cardiorespiratory depression for minor procedures, such as uncomplicated laceration repair, appears unwarranted. The beneficial effects of these agents must be weighed against their potential complications and also weighed in relation to the objective and endpoint of sedation and analgesia for each child. Clinical experience and literature clearly indicate that sound environmental and psychological management contribute substantially to the beneficial aspects of emergency care for children.

Pain Measurement

Monitoring of analgesia and sedation should also incorporate a measurement of the efficacy of the sedation. Safe but ineffective sedation, with or without analgesia, is inconsistent with clinical practice goals and does not meet the needs of patients. Methods have been suggested for age-appropriate pain or distress assessment (pain rating scales, behavioral scales, self-report scales). Although these scales represent a significant improvement in pain assessment over traditional empiric observations, the content validity (i.e., whether the scale actually measures pain severity), repeatability, precision, and accuracy of these scales must be studied further in the outpatient setting before specific recommendations for their use can be made.

SUGGESTED READING

Algren JT, Algren CL. Sedation and analgesia for minor pediatric procedures. Pediatr Emerg Care 1996;12:435–441.

American Academy of Pediatrics, Committee on Drugs. Guidelines for monitoring and management of pediatric patients during and after sedation for diagnostic and therapeutic procedures. Pediatrics 1992;89:1110–1115.

American Pain Society. Principles of analgesic use in the treatment of acute pain and chronic cancer pain (2nd ed.). Clin Pharm 1990;9:601.

Anon. Practice guidelines for sedation and analgesia by non-anesthesiologists. Anesthesiology 1996;84:459–471.

Bailey PL, Pace NL, Ashburn MA, et al. Frequent hypoxemia and apnea after sedation with midazolam and fentanyl. Anesthesiology 1990;73:826–830.

Baktai G, Szekely E, Marialigeti T, et al. Use of midazolam and flumazenil in paediatric bronchology. Cur Med Res Opin 1992;12:552–559.

Benedetti C. Acute pain: a review of its effects and therapy with systemic opioids. In: Benedetti C, Chapman CR, Giron G, eds. Advances in Pain Research and Therapy. Vol 14. Opioid Analgesia: Recent Advances in Systemic Administration. New York: Raven Press, 1990.

Cheng EY, Kampine JP. Anesthetic drugs and non-anesthesiologists. Anesth Analg 1997; 72:S37.

Cote CJ, Rolf N, Liu LMP, et al. A single-blind study of combined pulse oximetry and capnography in children. Anesthesiology 1991;74:980–987.

Cote CJ. Sedation protocols—why so many variations? Pediatrics 1994;94:281–283.

Farrell RG, Swanson SL, Walter JR. Safe and effective IV regional anesthesia for use in the emergency department. Ann Emerg Med 1985;14:239.

Friesen RH, Alswang M. End-tidal PCO2 monitoring via nasal cannulae in pediatric patients: accuracy and sources of error. J Clin Monitor 1996;12:155–159.

Hart LS, Berns SD, Houck CS, et al. The value of end-tidal CO2 monitoring when comparing three methods of conscious sedation for children undergoing painful procedures in the emergency department. Pediatr Emerg Care 1997;13:189–193.

Holzman RS, Cullen DJ, Eichhorn JH, et al. Guidelines for sedation by nonanesthesiologists during diagnostic and therapeutic procedures. J Clin Anesth 1994;6:265–276.

Jones RD, Lawson AD, Andrew LJ, et al. Antagonism of the hypnotic effect of midazolam in children: A randomized, double-blind study of placebo and flumazenil administered after midazolam-induced anaesthesia. Br J Anaesth 1991;66:660–666.

Kain ZN, Mayes LC, O'Connor TZ, et al. Preoperative anxiety in children: predictors and outcomes. Arch Pediatr Adolesc Med 1996;150:1238–1245.

Maxwell LG, Yaster M. The myth of conscious sedation. Arch Pediatr Adolesc Med 1996;150:665–667.

Parker RI, Mahan RA, Giugliano D, et al. Efficacy and safety of intravenous midazolam and ketamine as sedation for therapeutic and diagnostic procedures in children. Pediatrics 1997;99:427–431.

Sacchetti A, Schafermeyer R, Gerardi M, et al. Pediatric analgesia and sedation. Ann Emerg Med 1994;23:237–250.

Schecter NL. The undertreatment of pain in children: an overview. Pediatr Clin North Am 1989;36:781.

Selbst SM, Henretig FM. The treatment of pain in the emergency department. Pediatr Clin North Am 1989;36:965.

Shane SA, et al. Efficacy of rectal midazolam for the sedation of preschool children undergoing laceration repair. Ann Emerg Med 1994;24:1065.

U.S. Department of Health and Human Services, Public Health Service, Agency for Health Care Policy and Research, Acute Pain Management in Infants, Children, and Adolescents. Operative and medical procedures. Quick reference guide for clinicians, DHHS Pub. No. (AHCPR) 92–0019. Silver Spring, MD: AHCPR Clearinghouse, 1992.

Vade A, Sukhani R, Dolenga M, et al. Chloral hydrate sedation of children undergoing CT and MR imaging: safety as judged by American Academy of Pediatrics guidelines. Am J Roentgenol 1995;165:905–909.

Walco GA, Cassidy RC, Schechter NL. Pain, hurt, and harm: the ethics of pain control in infants and children. N Eng J Med 1994;331:541–544.

Yamamoto LG, Young LL, Roberts JL. Informed consent and parental choice of anesthesia and sedation for the repair of small lacerations in children. Am J Emerg Med 1997;15: 285–289.

Chapter 14

Nursing Principles in the Management of Sedated Patients

Fran Damian, Mary Fallon Smith

Nurses play a key role in the care of children undergoing procedural sedation. They are responsible for patient safety; providing support and reassurance to the patient and their family; discharge evaluation; and teaching parents about proper care at home before patient discharge. The family's perception of the experience is shaped in large part by the quality of nursing care their child receives. Nurses can offer a supportive presence that decreases fear and anxiety for both the child and family, as well as provide ongoing explanations and reassurance during all stages of the procedure.

Psychosocial considerations are essential components in planning nursing interventions for children. Medical procedures are stressful experiences for both children and their parents. The many unfamiliar stimuli in health care environments intensify normal childhood fears. The suddenness or seriousness of the child's condition also impacts the child and family's response to the experience. Nurses can diminish anxiety by applying principles of child and family development to interventions requiring sedation. Stress-reducing strategies that are specific to a child's developmental stage can easily be incorporated into the presedation plan. For example, offering an infant a pacifier or allowing a toddler to hold a favorite toy during the procedure are simple and effective strategies for minimizing stress. Interventions that promote a sense of control will enhance cooperation and decrease fear.

ESTABLISHING SEDATION GUIDELINES

Several factors should be considered before establishing a pediatric sedation program. The preparatory process encompasses education and training, medical equipment acquisition, drug preparation, and communication. Nurses who assist in procedural sedation must be knowledgeable about the pharmacology of agents used, competent in establishing intravenous (IV) access in children, and able to provide advanced life support in the event of a serious complication.

Institutions must develop guidelines, policies, and procedures for staff who use procedural sedation in outpatient settings. Adherence to policies and monitoring adverse events are key. The Emergency Nurses Association (ENA) and the American Association of Critical Care Nurses (AACN) have published policy statements on the role of nursing in the sedation of patients. The American Academy of Pediatrics (AAP) and the American College of Emergency Physicians (ACEP) have also published similar documents.

The following sections discuss the roles and responsibilities of the nurse in the process of procedural sedation from presedation preparation to monitoring during the procedure to recovery and discharge teaching (Table 14.1).

PREPROCEDURE INTERVENTIONS

Behavioral

This is the period in which the nurse can set the tone for the child's experience by creating a nonthreatening environment. A variety of techniques can be used with children and families to lower their anxiety level before the procedure. For toddlers, the procedure room is a strange environment filled with unfamiliar equipment, which can be frightening for this age group. Anxiety-provoking equipment, such as needles and syringes, should be kept out of view at all times. Permitting children to handle some of the equipment in the room and demonstrating how some of the monitoring equipment works on someone else, such as the parents, is reassuring. Allowing the child to make choices whenever possible, such as which finger the oxygen saturation probe should go on, gives the child a sense of mastery and control.

Anxiety-provoking words such as "shot," "needle," or "hurt" should be avoided if possible. If IV access is required, it should be explained using terms that minimize the anticipation of pain as much as possible. Any other sensations that the child may experience during the procedure should be explained using familiar and emotionally neutral or positive terms.

Everyone involved in the procedure should be introduced to the patient because personnel assisting with the procedure appear as strangers to the young child. Terms such as "helpers" or "friends" to describe roles are more easily understood than formal job titles. Parents should be allowed to stay in the room during the procedure unless they request otherwise or their level of anxiety is escalating the child's anxiety.

The nurse can explore with the parents several ways that they can help their child during the procedure such as holding hands with their child or singing a favorite song. Having a plan ahead of time ensures that everyone involved is clear on the parents' role in maintaining a calm environment.

Table 14.1.   Nursing Role in Pediatric Sedation

	Behavioral Interventions	Monitoring Interventions	Pharmacologic Interventions
Preprocedure	• Set the tone • Create a non-threatening environment • Explain the procedure of resuscitation	• Set up monitoring equipment/alarms • Set up appropriate size bag-valve-mask • Set up suction • Verify availability of resuscitation equipment	• Calculate drug dosages • Verify orders/doses with second RN • Draw up drugs and flushes • Calculate doses of reversal agents • Establish IV access
During procedure	• Use distraction techniques • Involve parents • Explain progress of procedure • Monitor patient/family response to procedure	• Continuously monitor O_2 saturation • Monitor vital signs q 5 min • Document on medical record	• Ensure patency of IV • Administer drugs
Postprocedure	• Maintain quiet/calm environment • Involve parents in helping child during recovery • Talk soothingly to child • Provide parents with individualized discharge teaching and instructions	• Assess discharge criteria parameters q 15 min • Determine discharge score q 15 min • Alert physician to adverse responses • Document on medical record	• Monitor for adverse effects of sedation drugs • Discontinue IV access

Monitoring and Room Preparation (see Chapter 3)

Special medical equipment designed for use in pediatrics is required for a safe environment. Bedside equipment must include monitoring equipment, various size bag-valve-mask ventilation devices, and a suction set up with tonsil suction. Nurses must be familiar with the proper use of this equipment and how to select the correct size for individual patients. Use of bag-valve-mask equipment can be practiced with a child size CPR mannequin. A 500 mL Ambu bag is the recommended size for full term infants up to age 1. A 1 L Ambu bag may be used on children over 1 year. Mask selection is based on which size best fits the patient's face. The narrow portion of the mask should not cover the eyes but fit well over the nose; the wide portion should fit as snugly as possible to the child's face. Oxygen supply and tubing must be checked for ample supply and proper connections. Suctioning equipment for all patients must be attached to a large tonsil suction device in the event that vomiting occurs.

Monitoring equipment for procedural sedation includes a cardiorespiratory monitor, a pulse oximeter, a noninvasive blood pressure monitor, and a capnograph, if available. This equipment should be preprogrammed with pediatric parameters and come equipped with pediatric accessories. The nurse should ensure that the alarm parameters are set to the normal range for the patient.

Pediatric resuscitation equipment should be readily available in any department in which children receive procedural sedation. This includes pediatric-size laryngoscope handles and blades, endotracheal tubes, and stylets. Drugs used in pediatric advanced life support should be located in the same area. A quick-reference with information on calculating pediatric resuscitation drugs and determining correct sizes of airway management equipment should also be available.

Pharmacologic

Once the equipment needed for the procedure is set up and checked for proper functioning, the nurse obtains the ordered medications. The orders must be verified for accuracy by a second nurse, following institutional policy. All syringes containing medications must be clearly labeled. Reversal agents should be readily available in the room with their dosages calculated ahead of time. It is not necessary to draw them up until they are actually needed.

If the medications are to be administered intravenously, equipment required for IV access should be set up ahead of time out of the child's view. A local anesthetic such as EMLA may be applied to the site if time allows. An assistant must be readily available to help hold the patient for insertion of the IV catheter. The IV insertion should be done as quickly and calmly as possible. Behavioral techniques for preparing a child for procedures can be used here as well.

Presedation preparation also applies to situations in which children are going to be sedated in areas outside the department for a procedure. An area where this is commonly done is radiology. A preestablished checklist for these situations is helpful for nurses to use before leaving the department with the patient (Fig. 14.1).

INTERVENTIONS DURING THE PROCEDURE

Behavioral

Once the procedure is underway, a child can be distracted in a variety of ways that can keep the focus on the distraction rather than the procedure. If the hands

1. **Medications**
   - ☐ Drawn-up
   - ☐ Labeled
   - ☐ Adequate number of saline flushes or running IV

2. **Monitoring equipment**
   - ☐ Checked and in working order

3. **Personnel**
   - ☐ Nurse
   - ☐ Designated physician (fellow or attending)[a]

4. **Supplemental equipment**
   - ☐ Oxygen (check amount in tank)
   - ☐ Proper sized ventilatory bag
   - ☐ Proper sized mask
   - ☐ Appropriate stretcher to transport sedated patient postprocedure
   - ☐ Other airway equipment (as needed)—ETT, laryngoscope
   - ☐ Extra syringes

5. **Communication with radiology**
   - ☐ Are they ready for the patient?
   - ☐ Have they checked the procedure room to make sure oxygen and suction are available and in working order?

6. **Sedation plan**
   - ☐ Has the ED physician reviewed the sedation plan with you?
   - ☐ Is the plan appropriate for this procedure and this patient? (Discuss with attending if plan seems inappropriate.)
   - ☐ Are the dosing regimens correct? (Double check in ACEP Guidelines for Pediatric Procedural Sedation Handbook.)

[a]In the rare event that an attending or fellow cannot accompany the patient, the attending will discuss this with the charge nurse and assign an appropriate resident.

Figure 14.1. Sedation of emergency department patients in radiology.

are free, the child can color in a coloring book or draw a picture on a pad of paper. The nurse can ask the child to recite the alphabet, count to 100, or sing a favorite song. School-aged children love to talk about their favorite activities such as sports they participate in or musical instruments they play. These are simple yet effective ways the nurse can engage the child during the procedure. Parents can assist in distracting the child by reading to them or keeping them focused on discussing their favorite topics. The parents can also be cued by the nurse to try another preplanned distraction technique if the one being used is no longer effective.

Patient Monitoring

The nurse oversees all aspects of the procedure, continuously monitors the patient and family's response to the procedure, and readily communicates any adverse responses to the physician. Baseline vital signs including blood pressure and oxygen saturation are obtained before sedating the patient. Once the procedure has begun, the nurse continuously monitors oxygen saturation and assesses vital signs and mental status every 5 minutes. The frequency of monitoring blood pressure is determined collaboratively with the physician because inflation of the cuff during the procedure may be stimulating enough to disrupt a young child who is lightly sedated. Perfusion status may be assessed alternatively by monitoring heart rate, skin color, and mental status throughout the procedure.

POSTPROCEDURE INTERVENTIONS (SEE CHAPTER 18)

Behavioral

Nurses assist patients recovering from procedures by creating the familiar, safe, and comfortable environment needed for a smooth and gentle emergence and recovery. Family members should be at the bedside with the child's toys or personal belongings. Nurses can encourage family members to talk to the child and tell the child stories to help him or her awaken and to decrease fears.

Monitoring

Postprocedure Assessment The nurse assesses the following criteria to determine if a patient is ready to be safely discharged:

- The airway and vital signs are stable.
- The child is able to follow age-appropriate commands.
- The child is arousable, returns to baseline in ability to talk, and is able to sit unaided.
- The child is adequately hydrated.

As long as a child meets the criteria described above, he or she does not need to be able to walk steadily to be safely discharged. Sometimes a child may require extended observation and monitoring if discharge criteria are not satisfactorily met. In some cases, overnight hospitalization may be indicated.

Discharge Scoring A discharge scoring system is an organized approach to tracking recovery. The system uses the same principles as an Apgar score or Glasgow coma score, in which specific criteria are measured at frequent intervals using a numeric value to indicate the level of patient response. Although there are many ways to design a discharge scoring system, any system must include five essential components: respirations, blood pressure, motor activity, oxygen saturation on room air, and level of consciousness (Fig. 14.2).

The recovery period begins immediately when the procedure is complete. Each criterion is measured and assigned a numeric value. The nurse continues to monitor each parameter every 15 minutes until the child achieves a satisfactory score. Once the child is ready for discharge, the nurse reviews the discharge instructions with the parents and assesses the level of comfort and care the child will need at home.

Discharge Teaching

Individualized discharge instructions specifying care of the child who received procedural sedation are extremely important. Key components of discharge teaching include diet, activity, sleeping, when to call the doctor, and when to return to the ED. Instructions must be individually tailored to reflect time of day, normal routines for the child, and developmental level. The following provides an example of information useful to parents whose child has been sedated.

Activity Level

Based on time of day, restrict activities that require physical coordination for up to 12 hours. Older children should avoid bike riding, skateboarding, or similar

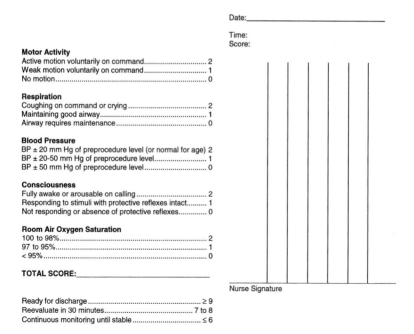

Date:_____

Time:
Score:

Motor Activity
Active motion voluntarily on command............................... 2
Weak motion voluntarily on command............................... 1
No motion.. 0

Respiration
Coughing on command or crying 2
Maintaining good airway... 1
Airway requires maintenance... 0

Blood Pressure
BP ± 20 mm Hg of preprocedure level (or normal for age) 2
BP ± 20-50 mm Hg of preprocedure level.......................... 1
BP ± 50 mm Hg of preprocedure level............................... 0

Consciousness
Fully awake or arousable on calling 2
Responding to stimuli with protective reflexes intact.......... 1
Not responding or absence of protective reflexes.............. 0

Room Air Oxygen Saturation
100 to 98%.. 2
97 to 95%.. 1
< 95% 0

TOTAL SCORE:_____

Nurse Signature

Ready for discharge .... ≥ 9
Reevaluate in 30 minutes... 7 to 8
Continuous monitoring until stable .... ≤ 6

Figure 14.2. Sample discharge scoring system.

activities that require coordination and concentration. Parents must pay especially close attention to toddlers and should be strongly encouraged to provide a high level of vigilance when the child returns home.

Diet

Wait until the child is fully awake before giving solid foods. Begin by offering the child clear liquids and advance the diet if the child does not experience nausea or vomiting.

Sleep

Instruct parents to wake the child once 2 hours after the child has fallen asleep. If the child responds as usual, he or she may sleep the remainder of the night or for the duration of the nap.

When to Call the Doctor

Instruct parents to call the child's doctor or take the child to the emergency department if the child experiences any breathing difficulty or changes in skin color or if the child is difficult to wake up.

SUGGESTED READING

Bernardo LM, Conway AE. Pain assessment and management. In: Soud TE, Rogers JS. Manual of Pediatric Emergency Nursing. St. Louis: Mosby-Year Book, 1998.

Damian FJ, Smith MF, Krauss BS. Conscious sedation roundtable: a collaborative practice model for problem solving in the emergency department. J Emerg Nurs 1997;23(2)153–155.

Chapter 15

Risk Management and Medicolegal Aspects of Procedural Sedation

Steven Selbst

The majority of children who receive sedation and analgesia in the outpatient setting have a good outcome and benefit from the efforts to reduce pain and anxiety during a procedure. Occasionally, there is a preventable or unavoidable complication. Those providing care to sedated children must take steps in advance of a procedure and vigilantly monitor the child during the procedure to minimize potential adverse outcomes. This chapter will discuss the specific steps that should be taken to allow appropriate defense of litigation.

Administration of sedative and analgesic agents to children always carries some risk to the patient, and thus potential liability for the provider. Several settled cases have involved problems with sedation of children. For example, a 2-year-old boy was brought to a Texas emergency department (ED) for treatment of a tongue laceration that he suffered while playing. The boy was given midazolam and morphine for sedation to repair the laceration and naloxone after completion of the procedure. The patient was discharged from the ED 8 hours after the procedure, apparently still asleep. He never woke up at home, and was pronounced dead. The parents sued the hospital and the treating physician, claiming that the medication was given inappropriately and the child was not properly monitored. The hospital settled for $975,000. The action against the physician is pending.

Use of topical analgesics are generally safe in the pediatric ED; however, the Oregon Poison Center reported a 5-year-old boy suffered recurrent seizures 10 minutes after a pledget soaked with tetracaine, epinephrine, cocaine (TAC) was applied to the wound and then sucked into the posterior pharynx. It is well known that TAC can cause seizures and death.

A 4-year-old given intramuscular (IM) ketamine for sedation to remove a foreign body from the ear suffered respiratory arrest. The child recovered with no apparent ill effects. The case illustrated the need for adequate monitoring and preparation for emergency intervention when using ketamine in the ED. Respiratory arrest has also been reported in a 14-month-old given intravenous (IV) midazolam and fentanyl for sedation before a bone marrow aspiration. The patient recovered after administration of naloxone and there were no long-term sequelae. This case reminds us that many sedation injuries occur from lack of appreciation of drug interactions.

Whenever a child has a bad outcome after receiving procedural sedation, it is possible that a malpractice suit will follow. This does not necessarily reflect poor care by the health professional, but that care will certainly be scrutinized. The health professional should take precautions to prevent adverse outcomes and subsequent litigation.

REQUIREMENTS AND GUIDELINES

Many organizations have published guidelines to assist health care professionals in sedating children in a safe manner (see Chapter 16). The American Academy of Pediatrics (AAP) published guidelines for sedation in 1985. These guidelines were revised in 1992 when the AAP noted that there had been an increase in the use of sedatives and general anesthetic agents for invasive procedures involving pediatric patients outside the operating room setting. The AAP guidelines defined three levels of sedation: conscious sedation, deep sedation, and general anesthesia. These definitions provide the basis for varying levels of precautions and monitoring when caring for sedated children.

A clinician should not mislabel a child who is in a state of deeper sedation (e.g., as "conscious sedation") to reduce the level of staffing needed to monitor a patient within the AAP guidelines. The needs of the provider or the institution must not be placed ahead of the safety or comfort of the patient. Instead, the clinician must recognize that many children who are sedated for a painful procedure reach a level of deeper sedation, if the attempt is to be successful. Appropriate precautions should be taken.

The AAP advises that the clinician who uses procedural sedation should have the facilities, personnel, and equipment immediately available to manage emergency situations. Possible complications such as vomiting, seizures, anaphylactic reactions, and cardiopulmonary impairment or arrest should be anticipated. A plan for back-up emergency services should be clearly identified. For nonhospital facilities, an emergency assist system with ready access to ambulance service should be established.

Other organizations besides the AAP have offered guidelines on pediatric sedation and analgesia. The American College of Emergency Physicians (ACEP) published a policy that states that each ED should develop its own guidelines for monitoring, providing adequate support personnel, discharge instructions, and a continuous quality improvement program. The ACEP Committee on Pediatrics published a paper with recommendations similar to the AAP in terms of monitoring, personnel, and equipment for sedation in an emergency setting.

The Joint Commission on Accreditation of Healthcare Organizations (JCAHO) has recognized that there is significant variation in the level of care provided to children depending on where the sedation is administered in the same institution (emergency department, clinic, radiology suite, etc.). The JCAHO recently mandated that each institution develop its own specific protocols for patients receiving sedation that carries the risk of loss of protective airway reflexes. JCAHO also specifies that the standard of care be the same for all sedated patients throughout the hospital. The institution must standardize its documentation process in terms of history, physical examination, and events of the procedure and recovery phase. Furthermore, monitoring guidelines and skills of the personnel who are providing care for the sedated child must be uniform as well. JCAHO provides a sample of a policy and procedure for conscious sedation, but allows institutions to modify this or develop its own.

How will these organizational guidelines affect malpractice litigation with regard to adverse outcomes and the use of procedural sedation in children? The answer remains largely unknown. The guidelines may highlight errors in practice or they may define exemplary care. They may help to defend a physician who follows them, or they may be used against a doctor who doesn't.

A guideline does not automatically become the standard of care. The "standard of care" is defined as "that which a reasonable physician, in that same specialty, would have done under the same circumstances." A guideline must be widely accepted by a specialty before it is used as the standard of care in a malpractice case. A study published in 1990 found that only 42% of respondents said their ED complied with the 1985 AAP recommendation to have one designated person to monitor sedated children continuously. It was hypothesized that limited staff was then available to monitor sedated children for up to 1 or 2 hours as needed for most procedures. Moreover, only 18% of EDs had written discharge protocols for sedated children. Obviously the guidelines had not then become the standard of care. Since JCAHO has recently required hospitals to set uniform standards for sedation, it seems more likely that a majority of hospitals will now comply with sedation policies. This may ultimately redefine the standard of care.

Following recommended guidelines does not guarantee a good outcome. However, guidelines may improve the chances of successful defense of a litigation case. As with most guidelines, a practitioner can deviate as long as there is reasonable justification.

DOCUMENTATION

Careful documentation of the use of sedatives and analgesics is extremely important (see chapters 17 and 18). The child's chart may be the first item reviewed by an attorney and a consulting expert physician in determining whether a complication was the result of negligence. A complete and thorough record may prevent a lawsuit. Certainly, it will help the health care provider to defend such action. Often, there is an extended length of time between the patient encounter and a subsequent malpractice suit. A complete, well-prepared record will then prove helpful when the practitioner's recall of the event has faded. The chart should reflect a neat, professional appearance and should be maintained as if it were a public document.

If an inpatient or outpatient chart already exists, repeating the information previously documented is not necessary. However, a brief note to indicate that the chart was reviewed is recommended. A note indicating the child's presedation status is generally helpful. A notation should be made that the patient's condition hasn't changed since arrival or since the last examination in the record.

When using sedatives and analgesics, a well-designed record is essential. A *separate form or checklist* is particularly useful as a supplement to the main hospital or outpatient note. The checklist may improve efficiency and may serve to remind the caregiver to ask specific questions or perform a specific part of the physical examination. The ACEP Committee on Pediatrics published a sample form that will permit a time-based record. Figure 15.1 represents a sample flow sheet that can be modified to meet the desires of a particular institution and the AAP recommendations listed below.

Documented *history* should include the child's age and abnormalities of the airway (snoring, sleep apnea) or other relevant diseases. Details of the last oral intake are important. A review of systems, previous hospital admissions, and relevant family history should also be documented. The record should indicate any history of allergies or adverse drug reactions and any medications used before sedation. It is important to place this information near the section for writing the sedation orders so they can be reviewed when medications are ordered.

The *physical examination* should focus on the airway and cardiovascular system. The patient's weight must be carefully recorded and reviewed at the time of treatment. Dosing errors are the leading category of mishaps involving medications, and approximately 10% of these are related to the child's weight that was obtained or recorded incorrectly. The weight should be written in an obvious location in the record, and it is best to record this consistently in kilograms. Baseline vital signs should be documented and recorded intermittently (every 5 minutes for children undergoing deeper sedation) until awake. Every 10 to 15 minutes may suffice for those with only light sedation or recovering from a procedure.

A time-based record should include all *drugs and doses* administered and the routes of administration. The inspired oxygen and use of inhalation sedation agents, including the duration of their administration, should be documented if used. Any adverse effects should be recorded. The findings while monitoring, such as pulse oximetry readings, should be recorded. It is also helpful to document the child's level of consciousness during the procedure, e.g., how he or she responds to verbal commands or tactile stimulation. Before discharge, note the patient's level of consciousness.

Discharge instructions must be reviewed with the child's guardian before the patient is allowed to go home. They may be preprinted and include a reminder to parents that the child should not be involved in play for 24 hours that requires coordination such as bike riding or skating. Adult supervision should be recommended for at least 8 hours. Unsupervised bathing or use of electrical devices or other possibly dangerous items should not be permitted for at least 8 hours. The family should be told to call their doctor or return to the ED if the child does not appear well at home. A 24-hour telephone number for the practitioner or the ED should be provided for the family.

Finally, it is never wise to *alter the record* or make a late entry after an adverse event has occurred. Errors in charting should be appropriately corrected with a single line placed through the error, and the correction dated and initialed. The clinician should not attempt to cover up the mistake by blacking out words or phrases because this will likely arouse suspicion. Should litigation ensue, it is usually easier to defend missing facts or a poor record than one that has been altered.

CONSENT

The family of a child who receives sedation is entitled to information about the procedure and the medications to be used. Parents have the right to know about the risks and benefits of the treatment for their child and any alternatives available. Their consent should be given before administration of any agents. Whether consent is obtained in writing or verbally depends on local, state, and institutional requirements. A general consent form signed at the time of arrival to the outpatient facility does not usually imply consent for use of sedation and analgesics. Separate consent for sedation is advised. Pennsylvania law defines informed consent as giving the consenting person a description of the procedure and the risks and alternatives such that a "reasonably prudent person" would be able to make an informed decision about whether to undergo the procedure. This "modern" patient-focused concept of informed consent is followed by most states. The parents could conceivably bring a lawsuit against a physician for failing to obtain informed consent if they are not told of a risk of the treatment and the child suffers harm from the sedation. The parents would have to prove that reasonable people, properly advised, would not have consented to the procedure had they been previously informed. If the physician were subsequently found liable for not obtaining informed consent, he or she would be liable for all subsequent damages, even if they resulted from an unavoidable complication rather than negligence.

Parents should be informed consumers. Information should be given in a clear, straight-forward manner. The care provider should be sure the guardian understands the information given; it may be useful to ask the parent to paraphrase what they have been told. If a serious complication could result from treatment, then the caregiver should inform the family of all but the most remote risks. On the contrary, if the potential for injury is minor, the family only need to be informed of the risks that are common. It is more important to disclose remote risks if alternative treatments with lesser risks exist. No parent should be forced to make a specific decision for a child. However, most parents desire the opinion of the experienced caregiver, and advice from the doctor helps them make a reasonable determination of what is best for the child.

HOSPITAL FOR CHILDREN

Patient Name: _____

Medical Record #: _____

D.O.B. _____ Age: _____

Date: _____

Diagnosis: _____

Procedure Planned: _____   Procedure Location: _____

Attending Physician: _____   Informed Consent Obtained: ☐

Past Medical History:
_____
_____

Past two weeks: ☐ cough cold   ☐ wheezing   ☐ significant snoring
                       ☐ croup   ☐ pneumonia   ☐ sinus infection

Previous Sedation: ☐ No   ☐ Yes   ☐ Any reactions: _____
                                                        _____

Allergies: _____ Latex allergy ☐ Yes   ☐ No

Last meal / solids @: _____   Last clear liquids @: _____

Current medications:
_____
_____

Nursing assessment presedation:
_____
_____
_____

                                       Initials: _____ Signature: _____

Physician assessment presedation:
_____
_____

    H + P in record — no change ☐

    H + P first or change in status   _____
                                       _____

IV access: _____   Time: _____ Needle Size: _____

Patient weight: _____ Kgs

Sedation orders: _____
_____
_____

Physician Signature: _____   Date and Time: _____

Figure 15.1. A. Ambulatory sedation assessment. (*continued*)

Written consent forms have value in educating the guardian with respect to the procedure, and they may provide some protection to the caregiver by documenting the steps taken to inform the family. However, signing a form does not necessarily imply informed consent. The guardian may still claim the risks and benefits were not adequately explained. If a specific consent form is not used, it must be clearly documented in the record as to what the parents were told and that they gave verbal agreement. In a true emergency, informed consent is not needed; it is implied and assumed that a reasonable parent would want immediate necessary care.

Patient Name: _____

HOSPITAL FOR CHILDREN

D.O.B. #: _____ Med. Rec. #: _____

Date: _____ Physician: _____

Flow Sheet

Time Base	Pox	Pulse	Resp	B/P	Color	Medication	Route	Dose	Monitoring RN's Initials	Comments/Interventions Temperature:

Time Study Completed

Sedation Discharge Criteria	Meets Time	Doesn't Meet Time	Plan for Discharge
Respiratory Status Airway Stable			
02 Saturation > 95% or 5% baseline			
Sedation score 6 or baseline			
Vital signs stable			
Pain free or managed			

Discharge Instructions Given To:
_____

Verbalized Understanding   ☐ YES   ☐ NO

Progress Note:
_____
_____
_____
_____
_____
_____

Sedation Scores		Baseline Time	Discharge from protocol Time
Mental Status	Awake 2 Arousable 1 Not arousable 0		
Airway	Talks/cries 2 Breathing easily 1 Airway support 0		
Movement	Purposely 2 Involuntary 1 Not moving 0		
Total			

Discharge Date/Time: _____

Via: ☐ Wheelchair ☐ Ambulatory ☐ Carried

Signature(s): _____**RN**

Initials: _____

Ambulatory Sedation Assessment & Flow Sheet

ORIGINAL - PATIENT RECORD

Figure 15.1—*continued* B. Flow sheet.

COMPLICATIONS

Whenever sedative or analgesic medications are used, there is always a chance for error (see Chapter 19). Medication errors are the second most frequent and second most expensive procedure causing medical liability claims. One study found that medication errors occur at a rate of 3.99 per 1000 medication orders for hospital patients, and many are potentially serious. Opioid analgesics are the drug class that most frequently contributes to the adult patient's death when an error occurs.

Experienced and inexperienced staff, including physicians, nurses, pharmacists, support staff, and others make medication errors. By producing look-alike and sound-alike drugs, sometimes with similar packaging, drug manufacturers are also responsible for some errors. Many of these errors are preventable.

A few of the more serious errors involve a misplaced decimal point, which can result in a tenfold error. Thus, when writing medication orders it is recommended to place a zero before a decimal point to express a number less than one (e.g., 0.5 mL). However, one should not use a terminal zero (e.g., 5.0), because failure to see the decimal point may result in the patient getting ten times the dose desired. Allergic reactions are a complication of using any medication. Preventable errors may also occur when the health care provider fails to obtain an adequate medical history, fails to read the record, or does not obtain old records to document an allergy. Many errors are the result of incorrect computation. Some of these may be preventable by computer technology in which only approved drug doses are accepted by the computer.

When a complication related to sedation has occurred, the hospital Risk Management Office should guide the staff concerning documentation and any further action necessary. Generally, subsequent treatment rendered to the patient should be noted in the medical record. Lengthy details of the problem, however, should not be discussed in the record, but rather documented on an Incident Report. This will allow investigation of the event in a confidential manner. The Incident Report should be written as soon after the adverse event as possible, and the hospital Risk Management Office should receive the only copy. Generally, the Incident Report should contain a description of the incident, names, date, time of the event, clinical impact of the problem, and actions taken. There should not be a written apology or conclusion assigning blame to an individual. Also, do not make self-serving or defensive statements in the medical record. Reference should not be made to the Incident Report in the patient's record because this assures discovery should litigation result.

SUGGESTED READING

ACEP Pediatric Emergency Medicine Committee. The use of pediatric sedation and analgesia-policy statement. Ann Emerg Med 1993;22:626–627.

American Academy of Pediatrics, Committee on Drugs: Guidelines for monitoring and management of pediatric patients during and after sedation for diagnostic and therapeutic procedures. Pediatr 1992;89:1110–1115.

American Academy of Pediatrics, Committee on Drugs, Section on Anesthesiology. Guidelines for the elective use of conscious sedation, deep sedation, and general anesthesia in pediatric patients. Pediatrics 1985;76:317–321.

American Society of Hospital Pharmacists. ASHP guidelines on preventing medical errors in hospitals. Am J Hosp Pharm 1993;50:305–314.

Applebaum PS, Grisso T. Assessing patients' capacities to consent to treatment. N Engl J Med 1988;319:1635–1638.

Barratt K, Schwid B, Schwid M. Don't doctor your records. Wis Med J 1996;95:385–387.

Bates DW, Spell N, Cullen DJ, et al. The costs of adverse drug events in hospitalized patients. JAMA 1997;277:307–312.

Bean RV. Altering records: discrediting your best witness. J Med Assoc Ga 1993;82:63–64.

Botkin JR. Informed consent for lumbar puncture. Am J Dis Child 1989;143:899–903.

Cote CJ. Sedation protocols-why so many variations? (editorial). Pediatrics 1994;94:281–283.

Dailey RH. Fatality secondary to misuse of TAC solution. Ann Emerg Med 1988;17:159–160.

Dava M. Recurrent seizures following mucosal application of TAC. Vet Hum Toxicol 1987;28:6.

Garnick DW, Hendricks AM, Brennan TA. Can practice guidelines reduce the number and costs of malpractice claims? JAMA 1991;266:2856–2860.

Hawk W, Crockett K, Ochsenschlager DW, et al. Conscious sedation for the pediatric patient for suturing: a survey. Pediatr Emerg Care 1990;6:84–88.

Joint Commission on Accreditation of Healthcare Organizations. Comprehensive Accreditation Manual for Hospitals: The Official Handbook. 1997:TX 15–17, 76–80.

Koren G, Barzilay Z, Greenwald M. Tenfold errors in administration of drug doses: a neglected iatrogenic disease in pediatrics. Pediatrics 1986;77:848–849.

Korin JB, Selbst SM. Legal aspects of emergency department pediatrics. In: Fleisher GR, Ludwig S, eds. Textbook of Pediatric Emergency Medicine. Baltimore: Williams & Wilkins, 1993:1544–1564.

Laska L. Medical Malpractice—Verdicts, Settlements and Experts. 1996;12:17.

Leape LL, Bates DW, Cullen et al. Systems analysis of adverse drug events. JAMA 1995;274:35–43.

Lesar TS, Briceland L, Stein DS. Factors related to errors in medication prescribing. JAMA 1997;277:312–317.

Maxwell LG, Yaster M. The myth of conscious sedation. Arch Pediatr Adolesc Med 1996;150:665–667.

Miller LJ. Informed consent. JAMA 1980;244:2347–2351.

Physicians Insurers Association of America. Medication Errors Study. 1993;1–44.

Sacchetti A, Schafermeyer R, Gerardi M, et al. Pediatric analgesia and sedation. Ann Emerg Med 1994;23:237–250.

Selbst SM. Pediatric emergency medicine: legal briefs. Pediatr Emerg Care 1996;12:309.

Smith JA, Santer LJ. Respiratory arrest following intramuscular ketamine injection in a 4 year-old child. Ann Emerg Med 1993;22:613–615.

Thewes J, Fitzgerald D, Salmasy DP. Informed consent in emergency medicine-ethics under fire. Emerg Med Clin North Am 1996;14:245–254.

Wright SW. Conscious sedation in the emergency department: the value of capnography and pulse oximetry. Ann Emerg Med 1992;21:551–555.

Zellar L. Occurrence (incident) reports. In: Henry GL, ed. Emergency Medicine Risk Management—A Comprehensive Review. Dallas, TX: American College of Emergency Physicians, 1991:249–252.

Chapter 16
Establishing Procedural Sedation Guidelines and Policies

Grant Innes, Steven Green

Diagnostic and therapeutic procedures, unavoidable components of patient care, can cause pain and anxiety. Children have more intense physical and emotional responses to pain. Many procedures, even some that cause little discomfort, are simply not possible in unsedated children. Increasingly, health care providers are acknowledging that it is inhumane to perform these procedures without taking steps to limit the associated pain and anxiety. Hopefully, the days of bundling screaming children into rolled sheets or strapping them onto "papoose boards" are over. Today safe and humane pharmacologic and nonpharmacologic alternatives are available to minimize anxiety and maximize cooperation.

The term "conscious sedation" has been widely used to describe the process of providing analgesia, sedation, and amnesia for patients undergoing painful procedures; however, this term is misleading and should be abandoned. A more descriptive term is "procedural sedation and analgesia," which will be referred to as "procedural sedation" in this chapter. Health care reform (budget cutting) and managed care have limited access to hospitals, specialists, and operating rooms, and there is increasing pressure to provide services on an outpatient basis. Procedural sedation and analgesia has become a critical skill in many clinical settings.

Health care providers administer procedural sedation in diverse clinical settings, but the goals of sedation should be identical, regardless of the practitioner or setting:

- To consider patient safety and welfare the first priority
- To provide adequate analgesia, anxiolysis, sedation, and amnesia during the performance of painful and anxiety-producing diagnostic or therapeutic procedures
- To minimize the adverse psychological responses associated with painful or frightening interventions
- To control motor behavior that inhibits the provision of necessary care
- To return the patient, in a time-efficient manner, to a state in which safe discharge is possible

CASE STUDY—A SYNTHESIS OF REAL CASES
KNOWN TO THE AUTHOR

A 2-year-old child presents to a medical clinic with a forehead laceration that requires suturing. Two nurses attempt to restrain the child, but he screams and flails when the physician attempts to inject local anesthetic, and the procedure is aborted. One of the nurses suggests a technique she has seen other doctors use: an injection of Demerol, Phenergan, and Thorazine. The drugs are administered and 30 minutes later the team tries again. The child is less combative, but is not adequately sedated and continues to struggle. This time, with one nurse stabilizing the child's head and another draped over his torso, the physician is able to proceed. He drapes the child's face and begins suturing. Each of the health care providers is focused on their task and 10 minutes later the job is done. The physician pulls back the drape to find a pulseless, apneic child. The nurse looks for a bag-valve-mask, but cannot find one. The other nurse begins mouth-to-mouth ventilation, but moments later the child vomits and aspirates. The physician looks frantically for suction but there isn't any. Someone calls 9-1-1. Paramedics arrive 5 minutes later and intubate the child, but he has suffered an irreversible anoxic brain injury. At the subsequent inquest, several problems are identified:

1. The physician was unfamiliar with the drugs he used and did not have a sedation endpoint in mind.
2. The child was inadequately sedated, so a nurse held him down in a way that impaired ventilation.
3. No one was assigned to watch the child's level of consciousness, ventilation, or vital signs.
4. Observation was hampered by the surgical drapes.
5. No pulse oximeter was used.
6. No reversal drugs were present.
7. No suction, oxygen, or resuscitative equipment was present.
8. The only face mask in the clinic, an adult mask, was in a remote part of the building.
9. The child had a full stomach and vomited and aspirated.
10. The physician was unaware of and not trained to deal with the possible complications.
11. No staff with airway or resuscitation skills were available in the clinic.
12. The clinic had no policy dealing with procedural sedation.

PROCEDURAL SEDATION

Opioids and sedating agents are safe and effective when used by competent people in controlled environments, but tragic misadventures in dental offices, endoscopy suites, and emergency departments have made the use of these agents by nonanesthetists controversial. Although anesthesiologists are uniquely qualified to provide sedation, their availability is often limited by commitments to the operating room. It is, therefore, the reality that nonanesthesiologists will supervise the majority of outpatient procedures.

Some practitioners receive extensive procedural sedation training during their residencies; others receive none. Practitioners work in different settings with different support personnel. They perform different types of procedures requiring different levels of sedation and analgesia. Practitioners have differing degrees of pediatric expertise, differing experiences with analgesics and sedating agents, and differing resuscitation skills. As a result, "safety margins" differ depending on who performs sedation and where it is performed.

Further complicating matters is the fact that different patients have different physiologic reserve and respond differently to drugs. Any sedative or analgesic, in a sufficient dose, can cause cardiorespiratory compromise. Even in the best of hands, patients may unexpectedly progress to deeper than desired level of sedation. Hypoventilation, apnea, hypoxemia, and hypotension may occur at any time during a procedure. Therefore, safety is a critical issue.

Despite the infinite combinations of practitioners, patients, procedures, and settings, appropriate guidelines and policies can enhance patient safety. Recognizing this, several organizations and specialty societies have developed sedation guidelines, each reflecting the perspective of the specific group. Because skills, expertise, procedures, patients, practice environments, definitions, connotations, and perspectives differ from specialty to specialty, no one sedation guideline has been universally accepted.

STANDARDS, GUIDELINES, AND POLICIES

Although these terms are synonymous in the minds of many, they are clearly and critically distinct. The Joint Commission on Accreditation of Healthcare Organizations (JCAHO) defines "standard" as a statement of expectation that defines the structures and processes that must be substantially in place in an organization to enhance the quality of care. Standards are essentially rules—generally accepted minimum requirements for sound practice. Deviation from standards is rarely permissible and might be expected to result in an adverse outcome in a peer review process.

Guidelines are recommendations developed through a formal process that incorporates expert opinion and the best scientific evidence of effectiveness. They are intended to improve health care by helping clinicians adopt a common, "best practice" approach to the condition or process in question. Guidelines are not intended to be standards or requirements, nor are they intended to define the standard of care for malpractice litigation. They may be adopted, modified, exceeded, or rejected, according to specific clinical needs, and are often used as a starting point from which to develop institutional or departmental policies. Guidelines may focus on improving a clinical process or optimizing the use of diagnostic and therapeutic interventions in specific clinical circumstances. They should define the expected changes in health care processes and outcomes. The skills, equipment, and processes recommended should be available and applicable in the target setting. Guidelines should be flexible enough to allow physicians to exercise clinical judgment in applying them.

Guidelines should be developed in collaboration with representatives of those who will be affected by them, including relevant clinician groups, patients, and other health care providers. Practitioners are most likely to accept guidelines developed by people who understand the disease spectrum they see, the skills they possess, the procedures they perform, and the conditions under which they work. Before implementation, guidelines should be reviewed by expert and user groups and tested, if possible. Guidelines must be dynamic and should be revised as medical advances occur and knowledge changes.

Policies are written statements that clearly indicate a facility's or service's position and values on a given subject. Policies generally specify the manner of proceeding in some process. They are developed for use in specified settings and derived with local perspectives, expertise, and needs in mind. Policies can be established for an institution or department and can be tailored to achieve maximal relevance in the setting they are to be applied.

To summarize, health care facilities require written policies to guide clinical activities. Such policies may be derived from appropriate specialty society guidelines and will contain and conform to relevant standards. In the United States, the JCAHO has published specific standards that apply to anesthesia care and sedation wherever they are provided. These standards must be adhered to when establishing sedation policies. Key JCAHO standards for anesthesia care and sedation are summarized in Tables 16.1 and 16.2. The JCAHO has also published a sample sedation policy, which is not a standard, but may serve as a reasonable template for developing an institutional policy.

Table 16.1.   Key JCAHO Standards on Anesthesia Care

- JCAHO standards for anesthesia care apply when patients receive, for any purpose, by any route 1) general, spinal, or major regional anesthesia or 2) sedation which, in the manner used, may be reasonably expected to result in the loss of protective reflexes. Loss of protective reflexes is defined as an inability to handle secretions without aspiration or to maintain an airway.
- Organized anesthesia services are directed by a physician member of the medical staff with appropriate clinical and administrative experience. The director's responsibilities include participating with representatives of other departments/services that provide anesthesia services in the formulation of mechanisms to provide uniform quality of anesthesia services throughout the hospital. The mechanisms are developed by representatives from the surgical, anesthesia, and nursing departments/services and other clinical departments/services that provide surgical and anesthesia services.
- The level of care provided to patients who have been administered anesthesia in areas outside the operating room is comparable to that provided in the operating room.
- Mechanisms are available to assure that each practitioner provides only those services for which he or she has been determined to be competent.

Table 16.2.   Key JCAHO Standards for Sedation Policies

- Each organization develops specific appropriate protocols for the care of patients receiving sedation that carries the risk of loss of protective reflexes. These protocols are consistent with professional standards and address at least the following:
  ⇒Sufficient qualified personnel present to perform the procedure and to monitor the patient
  ⇒Appropriate equipment for care and resuscitation
  ⇒Appropriate monitoring of vital signs—heart and respiratory rates and oxygenation using pulse oximetry equipment ("Monitoring methods depend on the patient's preprocedure status, anesthesia choice, and the complexity of the procedure.")
  ⇒Documentation of care
  ⇒Monitoring of outcomes
- Any patient for whom anesthesia is contemplated receives a preanesthesia assessment.

EXISTING SEDATION GUIDELINES

Practice variability suggests the lack of a standard of care and casts doubt on the quality and scientific validity of medical care. Guidelines bridge the gap between research and practice, limiting practice variability that is not justified by the evidence. Valid guidelines improve the scientific basis of care, optimize clinical processes, reduce practice variation, and enhance patient outcomes.

Because adverse outcomes associated with sedation procedures are rare events, existing sedation guidelines are based primarily on case reports and expert opinion rather than on the results of clinical trials; nevertheless, they have the potential to reduce practice variation, enhance safety, and improve patient outcomes. Sedation guidelines will help clinicians provide the benefits of sedation and analgesia while limiting the associated risks.

Existing sedation guidelines were written from different perspectives for different audiences, but all apply to patients receiving analgesia or sedation for painful or anxiety-provoking procedures. The American Society of Anesthesiologists' (ASA) document targets all nonanesthesiologists who sedate adults or children. The American Academy of Pediatrics' (AAP) document deals with the sedation of children in unspecified settings. The Canadian Association of Emergency Physicians' (CAEP) and the American College of Emergency Physicians' (ACEP) guidelines focus on emergency department sedation, the latter document being specific to children. Other guidelines target the dental office and GI endoscopy suite.

A detailed description of these is beyond the scope of this chapter, but brief discussion is warranted. Although different guidelines have different specific recommendations, all have safety as their underlying theme. All provide definitions of relevant terms, address appropriate patient selection, discuss practitioner skills and knowledge, and define equipment and monitoring requirements. Most specify the need for support personnel, presedation evaluation, pulse oximetry, and discharge criteria. Some discuss selection of agents and practical aspects of sedation.

SEDATION POLICIES

The JCAHO standards for anesthesia care refer specifically to the provision of general anesthesia. However, general anesthesia, "a controlled state of unconsciousness accompanied by a partial or complete loss of protective reflexes, including the inability to independently maintain an airway," is rarely an acceptable endpoint for procedural sedation. Rather, it is an undesirable state to be specifically avoided outside the operating room (OR). In other words, procedural sedation is not general anesthesia, and this fact must be emphasized when institutions establish sedation policies. If all the standards relevant to general anesthesia are simply extended to the provision of sedation, then sedation policies will be inappropriately restrictive and will prevent the humane application of safe sedation techniques to children who need them. Therefore, sedation policies must walk a fine line: They must address the same safety issues that are central to the provision of anesthesia, but must be relevant to the patients, procedures, practitioners, settings, and sedation methods in use where they are to be applied.

It may be difficult to develop a single sedation policy that is equally relevant to the ICU, the emergency department (ED), the outpatient subspecialty procedure suite, the oncology clinic, the dental office, and the radiology suite; therefore, policies may differ slightly between facilities and departments. All, however, must comply with defined JCAHO standards. Policy developers should consider several factors (as noted below) when developing a sedation policy for their clinic, department, or facility.

Patients

Different patients have different levels of risk, depending on age, underlying disease, acute illness or injury, and fasting state. Children undergoing elective procedures in dental offices and outpatient clinics are generally healthy, with good physiologic reserve. Children presenting to emergency departments may be volume-depleted, hypoxic, head-injured, unfasted, or in acute pain when they require sedation and analgesia. Children referred to tertiary care units are more likely to be chronically ill or have underlying neurologic and cardiorespiratory disorders that place them at higher risk.

Procedures

Different procedures require different depths and durations of sedation and, therefore, have different sedation endpoints, depending on the degree of associated pain and anxiety. Undershooting the endpoint leads to inadequate sedation and analgesia. Overshooting the endpoint places the patient at unnecessary risk. Sedation policies must be flexible enough to take all these considerations into account.

Diagnostic imaging procedures may require only anxiolysis or light sedation. Many procedures, including foreign body removal and simple laceration repair, can be performed with no sedation or with light sedation if the child is frightened or uncooperative. Tongue, eyelid, and vermilion border lacerations demand high levels of cooperation, thus deeper levels of sedation. Some procedures, although painful (e.g., fracture reduction), last only seconds and require brief sedation, whereas other procedures (e.g., dental work) require prolonged sedation, placing children at higher risk of complications.

Planned procedures permit presedation fasting, but emergent procedures are necessary regardless of NPO (nothing by mouth) status. The nature and anatomic location of the procedure are also determinants of risk. Dental or nasal procedures may cause bleeding and aspiration, whereas endoscopy may compromise the upper airway. The exaggerated fetal position optimal for lumbar puncture predisposes a patient to hypoventilation.

Practitioners

Pediatric anesthesiologists possess the optimal combination of skills and experience for pediatric sedation; however, it is neither possible nor necessary to have a pediatric anesthesiologist attend every laceration repair, fracture reduction, CT scan, chest tube insertion, burn debridement, and bone marrow biopsy. Residency-trained emergency physicians, pediatric intensivists, and pediatric emergency physicians have pediatric expertise and are familiar with sedating drugs, potent opioids, and paralyzing agents and have resuscitation and airway management skills. Adult intensivists have similar skill sets but variable experience with children. General pediatricians have pediatric expertise but may have less comfort with "anesthetic" drugs, resuscitation, and airway management. Family physicians, dentists, general, orthopedists, plastic surgeons, and radiologists may have little experience with "anesthetic" drugs and limited critical care skills, yet find themselves dealing with sedated children. Within each field, wide ranges of ability and experience will exist. Sedation policies should take into account the skills of the physicians performing sedation.

Setting is a critical issue, and sedation policies should reflect geographic, regional, and departmental realities. Rural hospitals, which are less likely to have pediatric intensivists or trained emergency physicians, are often forced to deal with burns, fractures, and multiply traumatized children—difficult situations requiring procedural sedation skills. A recent survey showed that emergency physicians practicing in rural community hospitals use fewer pharmacologic interventions to manage acute procedural pain and anxiety in children. Ironically, physicians in tertiary referral settings, who are more likely to possess these skills, may be in less of a position to use them because of a high level of specialty back-up.

In some hospitals, ample OR time may make it logistically feasible to perform minor procedures in the OR. However, in many institutions, high volumes, limited OR availability, and cost-containment issues may make it preferable for both patient and institution to manage these procedures in the ED.

Within a hospital, some units (e.g., the ED and ICU) are staffed and equipped to manage emergencies, whereas others (endoscopy suites, diagnostic imaging, and orthopedic clinics) are not. Some areas are rich with critical care staff; others may have no one capable of managing an airway. Medical and dental offices also have varying levels of staffing and equipment to manage emergencies.

For the above reasons, different practitioners with different skills and experiences perform different procedures with differing risks on different patients in different settings. Policies must assure acceptable levels of patient safety, but also be relevant to the settings in which they are applied. Recognizing these issues, various specialty societies have developed their own sedation guidelines, which the reader is encouraged to review.

ESTABLISHING SEDATION GUIDELINES AND POLICIES

Every medical staff must be cautious when drafting sedation policies. A major consideration is when to expand beyond JCAHO mandates and when to keep things as simple as possible. Committees tend to introduce more complexity than necessary. A common strategy is to attempt to "impress" the JCAHO by exceeding basic standards; however, unduly complicated or lengthy policies may not be read, understood, or complied with, and overly restrictive policies will limit the appropriate and humane application of procedural sedation. Once a policy is established, the institution has set its standard and must document compliance or risk JCAHO censure.

Sedation policies should be tailored as much as possible to their target users, and should be developed with input from the practitioners who will be impacted by them. Policies that are developed from "the outside" without consultation may be rejected by the clinicians they are intended to help. "Consumers" must have confidence in both the recommendations and their developers, and policies may be embraced or rejected based strictly on who developed them.

The most appropriate way to develop a sedation policy is to review one or more of the specialty society guidelines referred to above and modify it according to specific local needs. Each of the guidelines has strengths and weaknesses and each has a slightly different focus. Of these, the ones that are most relevant to pediatric sedation include the AAP Guidelines, the ACEP Guidelines, and the ASA Guidelines. The ASA guidelines are global in scope and were written with the JCAHO in mind. Therefore, for the purpose of developing sedation policies in varied settings, these guidelines are probably the best starting point.

The specialty of the physician charged with developing the sedation policy is not stipulated by the JCAHO. However, an anesthesiologist should be integrally involved in the policy development process because anesthesiologists have a wealth of experience and perspective to offer. Because anesthesiologists may not be familiar with needs and sedation practices outside the OR, policies developed unilaterally by anesthetists may lack relevance to the specialists for which they are intended. Therefore, it is important to involve other specialists who perform procedural sedation.

IMPLEMENTATION OF GUIDELINES AND POLICIES

Implementation is the most crucial and difficult step. Ineffective implementation strategies diminish the potential of guidelines and policies to effect change. If the implementation process is ineffective, then months or years of planning, committee work, research, and writing will result in nothing.

Guideline publication alone will not lead to change. Information must be disseminated widely through journals and society publications and "marketed" by opinion leaders. Guidelines should be promoted regionally through provider associations and at a departmental and institutional level by committed individuals. Ideally, the adoption of guidelines is voluntary rather than compulsory, which means establishing a "buy-in" from physicians and health care providers at a grassroots level.

The most effective way to bring practitioners along is to encourage their participation in policy development, in which they have the opportunity to review and modify guidelines according to local and specialty needs. "Ownership" of process enhances the commitment to sustained practice change. Therefore, while some authors decry the proliferation of different sedation policies and guidelines, it is likely, in fact, that this apparent duplication represents widespread interest, which may translate into better guideline compliance and positive changes in clinical care.

Guidelines and policies should not be forgotten after implementation. Ongoing review and assessment is critical. Effectiveness should be assessed with a program that includes user feedback and outcome evaluation. Where guidelines and policies have cost and resource implications, processes for assigning resources to their implementation, evaluation, and revision should be established.

TRAINING AND CREDENTIALING

Practitioners who perform procedural sedation must be competent to use such techniques, to provide monitoring, and to recognize and manage the complications of sedation. They should be knowledgeable about the agents they are using and be familiar with relevant antagonists. These practitioners should be trained in pediatric basic life support and preferably advanced life support. They should be knowledgeable about all aspects of airway management, possess airway and vascular access skills, and have an understanding of drug interactions. If the practitioner performing the sedation does not have these skills, a person capable of airway management and advanced life support should be present during the procedure.

The JCAHO specifies that health care facilities establish mechanisms to assure that practitioners provide only services for which they have been determined to be competent. Consequently, some hospitals have instituted mandatory credentialing programs for procedural sedation. Physicians must apply for privileges and, in certain cases, be proctored before they may independently administer sedation. Currently, such credentialing methods are not required by the JCAHO.

Most anesthesia, emergency medicine, pediatric emergency medicine, and critical care residencies provide adequate training in procedural sedation, and the need for additional postgraduate training is generally unnecessary. However, in settings where practitioners with less training or experience perform procedural sedation, a specific training process or a policy restricting sedation privileges may be appropriate and necessary to assure optimal patient safety. Because of differences in patients, procedures, practitioner skills, and settings, every health care facility must determine the level of training and the process of credentialing for its own medical staff.

Increasingly, health practitioners are acknowledging that it is inhumane to perform painful procedures on children without taking steps to minimize the related pain and anxiety. As mentioned previously, health care reform (budget cutting) and managed care has limited access to health care facilities and specialists, thus increasing pressure to provide services on an outpatient basis. Therefore, procedural sedation and analgesia is a critical skill for many clinical settings. Skills, experience, and practices vary widely from specialty to specialty and between institutions. Well-designed sedation guidelines and policies will help assure optimal outcomes for both patients and practitioners.

SUGGESTED READING

The American Academy of Pediatric Dentistry. Guidelines for the elective use of pharmacologic conscious sedation and deep sedation in pediatric dental patients. Pediatr Dent 1993;15:297–301.

American Society of Anesthesiologists. Practice guidelines for sedation and analgesia by non-anesthesiologists. Anesthesiology 1996;84:459–471.

Bell GD, McCloy RF, Charlton JE, et al. Recommendations for standards of sedation and patient monitoring during gastrointestinal endoscopy. Gut 1991;32:823–827.

American Academy of Pediatrics, Committee on Drugs. Guidelines for monitoring and management of pediatric patients during and after sedation for diagnostic and therapeutic procedures. Pediatrics 1992;89(6):1110–1115.

Conroy M, Shannon W. Clinical guidelines: their implementation in general practice. Br J Gen Pract 1995;45:371–375.

Cook DJ, Greengold NL, Ellrodt AG, et al. The relation between systematic reviews and practice guidelines. Ann Intern Med 1997;127:210–216.

Cote CJ. Sedation protocols: why so many variations? Pediatrics 1994;94:281–283.

Department of Health Care and Promotion, Canadian Medical Association. Workshop on clinical practice guidelines: summary of proceedings. Can Med Assoc J 1993;148:1459–1462.

Graff KJ, Kennedy RM, Jaffe DM. Conscious sedation for pediatric orthopaedic emergencies. Pediatr Emerg Care 1996;12:31–35.

Hayward RSA. Clinical practice guidelines on trial. Can Med Assoc J 1997;156:1725–1727.

Innes GD, Murphy M, Nijssen-Jordan C, et al. Procedural sedation and analgesia in the emergency department: Canadian consensus guidelines. J Emerg Med 1998. In press.

Joint Commission on Accreditation of Healthcare Organizations (JCAHO): Accreditation Manual for Hospitals. Chicago, Illinois: JCAHO, 1993.Vol I:165–170. TX-15, LD-5, PE.1.7.1.

Sacchetti A, Schafermeyer R, Gerardi M, et al. Pediatric sedation and analgesia. Ann Emerg Med 1994;23:237–50.

U.S. Department of Health and Human Services, Public Health Service, Agency for Health Care Policy and Research, Acute Pain Management Guideline Panel. Clinical practice guideline, acute pain management: operative or medical procedures and trauma. February, 1992.

Chapter 17
Presedation Evaluation

Alejandro Mondolfi

Sedation and analgesia enhance patient cooperation and facilitate the successful completion of diagnostic or therapeutic procedures that cause stress and pain. Anxiety alleviation and amnesia are additional benefits particularly important for children, who may perceive even simple procedures as a terrifying experience. Procedural sedation and analgesia administered by nonanesthesiologists outside the operating room (ambulatory centers, diagnostic imaging suites, emergency departments, dental offices) has become a well-accepted practice. On the other hand, any sedation regimen, regardless of the agent and route of administration used, presents potential risks to the patient and may result in serious complications. Some patient-related risk factors associated with adverse outcomes during pediatric sedation/analgesia have been identified. Unfortunately, the majority of reported serious complications occur in previously healthy children and are secondary to inadequate monitoring for the level of sedation attained, medication overdose, or inadequate skills of the practitioners performing the sedation. Careful presedation preparation and compliance with published sedation guidelines allows the clinician to optimize the benefits of procedural sedation while minimizing risk to the patient.

PLANNING FOR PROCEDURAL SEDATION

The most important initial step is to decide if the benefits offered by procedural sedation to a particular patient for a given procedure outweigh the associated risks. Factors that may influence the decision include age and temperament of the patient, type of procedure, amount of pain involved, movement control required, and patient/parental anxiety level. Nonpharmacologic interventions such as parental presence, a nonthreatening and age-appropriate approach to the patient, distraction techniques, relaxation-imaginary techniques, and hypnosis may help direct the patient's attention away from the anxiety and pain associated with the procedure. Telling children, particularly toddlers and early school-age children, too much about a procedure may actually increase their anxiety level and decrease their pain threshold and sensitivity to stimuli. Nonpharmacologic interventions, combined with a local anesthetic when indicated, may obviate or greatly reduce the need for sedatives and/or analgesics. If pharmacologic intervention is indicated, the choice of drug(s) depends on desired effect (sedation, analgesia, amnesia, dissociation, agitation control, motion control); health status (American Society of Anesthesiologists [ASA] classification); recent medication use; time of the day; route of administration planned; patient's previous experience with sedative/analgesics; and practitioners skill and preference for certain agents. Failure to achieve an adequate level of sedation to successfully complete the procedure is a relatively common occurrence in the outpatient setting; therefore, it is important to have an alternative plan.

PRESEDATION EVALUATION

The presedation evaluation should be focused on recognizing patients at increased risk for sedation complications (Table 17.1). Patients with these conditions may benefit from consultation with an anesthesiologist before sedation and may require management in a more controlled environment such as the operating room. A screening history should inquire into medical and surgical history, allergies or

Table 17.1.   Patients at Increased Risk for Complications During Procedural Sedation

---

Age less than 5 years (especially younger than 1 year)
ASA class III or greater
History of prematurity with less than 60 weeks postconception age: increased risk for respiratory depression and apnea
Airway abnormalities (large tonsils or adenoids with signs of obstruction, obstructive sleep apnea, tracheomalacia or tracheal stenosis, previous airway instrumentation, congenital anomalies such as Pierre Robin syndrome, Treacher-Collins syndrome, Crouzon disease, trisomy 21): increased risk for upper airway obstruction
Pulmonary disorders (chronic lung disease, reactive airway disease, active respiratory infections): increased risk for hypoxia, bronchospasm, and laryngospasm
Cardiovascular disorders (heart failure, right-to-left shunt, rhythm disturbances): increased risk for hypotension and hypoxia
Neurologic/developmental/psychiatric disorders: level of sedation difficult to assess, paradoxical reactions to sedatives, increased metabolism of sedatives if taking anticonvulsants, drug interactions
Renal/hepatic disorders: altered metabolism of sedative/analgesics
History of sedation complications: increased risk for sedation failure, oversedation, and paradoxical reactions

---

ASA, American Society of Anesthesiologists.

previous drug reactions, medication use including prescription and over-the-counter drugs, time of last solid and fluid intake, administration of sedatives or opioids in the last 4 hours (that may potentiate the effect of the agents to be administered), recent consumption of alcohol or substances of abuse, and previous adverse experience to sedatives/analgesics. For emergency and nonelective sedations, the AMPLE (Allergies, Medications, Past medical problems, Last meal, Events) format is sufficient. Age, recent weight, and baseline vital signs, including room air oxygen saturation, should be documented. The physical examination should be directed at identifying patients with a difficult airway or cardiorespiratory instability. This examination should include evaluation of neck mobility, mouth opening, dentition and size of the tongue and mandible. If the tonsillar pillars and the uvula cannot be visualized, the patient may be difficult to ventilate and intubate. Assess hydration status and auscultate heart and lungs for equal normal ventilation and normal heart sounds and rhythm. Baseline mental status must be evaluated and documented. Presedation laboratory testing should be guided by the clinical situation; routine tests seldom, if ever, will change the sedation plan. Conditions such as active airway infections, dehydration, or fever may increase the risk of complications and should lead to cancellation of elective sedations and appropriate management before emergency sedations (enhanced monitoring, reduced level/depth of sedation, avoidance of agents that hypersensitize the laryngeal reflexes [ketamine], and use of intravenous titratable agents that can be reversed).

PRESEDATION DIETARY PRECAUTIONS

Sedation is considered a continuum in which light sedation may quickly and unpredictably progress to a deeper sedation with blunting of protective airway reflex and potential regurgitation and aspiration of gastric contents. Based on this premise, published guidelines suggest that presedation dietary precautions for *elective* procedures should be the same as for general anesthesia (Table 17.2). There is evidence that these guidelines are not strictly followed and that ample variations exist in local policies and institutional practice. Studies and clinical trials suggest that ingestion of clear fluids, defined as a liquid that one can see print through, up to 2 hours before sedation or general anesthesia does not significantly increase gas-

Table 17.2.   Recommended Presedation Dietary Precautions for Elective Procedures from American Academy of Pediatrics Section on Anesthesiology

Less than 5 months old: no milk or solids for 4 hours preprocedure
6–36 months old: no milk or solids for 6 hours preprocedure
More than 36 months old: no milk or solids for 8 hours preprocedure

Intake of clear fluids may continue up to 2 hours before sedation. Clear liquids include soft drinks, oral rehydration solutions, juices without pulp or water, but not juices with pulp or milk.

tric volumes or change gastric pH factors that may increase the risk of serious aspiration. Emergency patients usually have a history of recent oral intake and may have conditions (i.e., trauma, decreased level of consciousness) that may increase their risk of aspiration. The American College of Emergency Physicians does not consider lack of preprocedure fasting an absolute contraindication for nonelective and emergency sedation/analgesia. The decision to sedate a patient with a history of recent oral intake should be based on the benefits of sedation versus the risk of aspiration, taking into account the clinical situation, amount and type of ingestion, need for the procedure, and risk involved in deferring the procedure. Gastric emptying is unreliable for patients in pain, and delaying the procedure cannot always guarantee an empty stomach. For other situations, delaying the procedure to allow gastric emptying and administration of H_2-blockers and/or prokinetic/antiemetic drugs should be considered.

ASA CLASSIFICATION

The relationship between ASA physical status (Table 17.3) and the risk of adverse events related to general anesthesia has been established. Children with ASA physical status class III or IV experience adverse effects more often than children with ASA physical status class I or II and require more skilled personnel and intensive monitoring to ensure patient safety. Patients who are ASA class I or II are generally considered appropriate candidates for procedural sedation by nonanesthesiologists. Consultation with an anesthesiologist is recommended for ASA class III or IV patients.

PREPARATION FOR MONITORING AND RESUSCITATION

Even when appropriate precautions are taken and guidelines are followed, adverse reactions to sedation/analgesia may occur. Thinking through in advance the possible complications associated with the agent(s) used and preparing accordingly most likely will decrease the chance of serious complications. Enough time should be allowed to thoroughly set up and check the equipment and to calculate drug

Table 17.3.   American Society of Anesthesiologists Physical Status Classification

Class I:	A normally healthy patient
Class II:	A patient with mild systemic disease
Class III:	A patient with severe systemic disease
Class IV:	A patient with severe systemic disease that is a constant threat to life
Class V:	A moribund patient who is not expected to survive without the procedure
E:	Emergency procedure

doses, including reversal agents. The following are some relevant aspects to consider during presedation preparation.

Personnel

The person providing the sedation should understand the pharmacology of agents used for procedural sedation and be licensed to administer the agent(s) used (see Chapter 3). In addition, at least one designated individual should be present who is responsible for monitoring the level of sedation and physiologic parameters and in assisting resuscitation measures if needed. Training in pediatric basic life support is strongly encouraged, and staff trained in pediatric advanced life support and skilled in advanced airway management should be readily available.

Facilities

Regardless of the setting where procedural sedation is performed, the room should be well suited for the initial management of potential cardiorespiratory complications and to monitor the patient during recovery. If the patient requires transport before the sedation, check in advance if the setting and personnel are ready for the procedure. A plan to obtain emergency services back-up, such as more skilled personnel or transport to a facility with a more advanced level of care, should be in place, especially when sedation is performed in a nonhospital setting.

Consent

A practical explanation of the benefits and risks involved in the administration of sedation, the reasons for the sedation, and the expected behavioral changes during sedation should be provided to the patient and caretakers as appropriate. Written or verbal informed consent should be obtained and documented according to local policy (see Chapter 15).

Patient Safety

The patient should be positioned safely, with securing guardrails if necessary. A stretcher appropriate to transport sedated patients postprocedure should be available. A device for immobilization (i.e., papoose board) may be useful in certain patients to further control movements. The immobilization device should be checked frequently to assure that it does not compromise ventilation or limb perfusion.

Monitoring

Complications of procedural sedation can be avoided if adverse effects are detected early through adequate monitoring (see Chapter 3). The amount and type of monitoring required varies among published guidelines and among practitioners, depending on the level of sedation planned and interpretation of the guidelines. Adequate monitoring should include assessment of cardiovascular and respiratory function and evaluation of the level of sedation. The only practical way to monitor the level of sedation is by observing the type of response to verbal and physical stimulation, carefully selecting a time when the assessment will not disrupt the procedure. Cardiorespiratory function can be monitored by conventional physical examination and electronic monitoring. Visual assessment of chest movements and tissue color, measurements of respiratory rate and pulse and auscultation with a precordial stethoscope are useful but may not be sensitive for the detection of early hypoxia and respiratory depression. Monitoring through clinical evaluation may be sufficient for patients undergoing anxiety alleviation or simple analgesia; however, in patients undergoing sedation, a complement of electronic monitors should be used. A patient's uncooperative behavior may be exacerbated by monitoring devices such as blood pressure cuffs or finger probes; thus, it may be necessary to attach the probes after administration of the sedative has achieved some anxiety alleviation. In emergency situations, sedation/analgesia may be started using manual monitoring techniques until electronic devices can be applied.

Oxygen

A positive pressure oxygen delivery system must be available. If an oxygen tank is being used, check the amount available, turn on oxygen, and test bag-mask device before starting the procedure. Routine use of supplemental oxygen during sedation/analgesia may decrease the risk of hypoxemia but may also, by delaying the onset of hypoxemia, delay the detection of hypoventilation by means of pulse oximetry.

Airway Equipment

The most frequent complications of procedural sedation are airway related; therefore, readily available airway equipment that is suitable for all pediatric ages is mandatory (see Chapter 3). A bag-mask ventilation device with the appropriate size mask must be at the bedside, and the personnel should feel comfortable using the type of device available. Oropharyngeal and nasopharyngeal airways are useful to manage upper airway obstruction and to facilitate bag-mask ventilation in deeply sedated patients while the reversal takes place or the sedative agent wears off. A functioning laryngoscope with various sized blades, endotracheal tubes, and stylettes should be readily available.

Suction

At least one functioning suction device with large-bore suction catheters should be available at the bedside and should be turned on and tested before starting the procedure. A portable device should be available if the patient will be transported while still sedated.

Medications

An emergency kit with drugs and equipment for advanced resuscitation, as recommended by the American Academy of Pediatrics, that is suitable for all pediatric ages and checked periodically should be readily available. Establishing vascular access may increase patient safety, but in uncooperative children receiving sedation by other routes, starting an intravenous line may only serve to increase agitation and anxiety and defeat the purpose of the sedation. If administering intravenous sedation, enough saline flushes or running intravenous solution should be available. Sedatives/analgesics and reversal agents should be drawn up and placed close at hand in appropriately labeled syringes, allowing for titration of extra doses when indicated. Reversal agents do not need to be drawn into syringes; however, the drugs should be available in the room and proper doses in milligrams and milliliters should be calculated before the procedure. To decrease the chance of accidental medication errors, carefully calculate dosages, avoid abbreviations and decimal points in written orders (i.e., write 50 micrograms rather than 50 μg or 0.05 mg), and double-check the identity, doses, and volumes of drugs. Equipment for administration of nitrous oxide should not deliver a concentration of the agent higher than 60%, should provide an inspiratory fraction of oxygen of 100%, and should have a functioning gas scavenger.

SUGGESTED READING

American Academy of Pediatric Dentistry. Guidelines for the elective use of pharmacologic conscious sedation in pediatric dental patients. Pediatr Dent 1995;17:31–34.

American Academy of Pediatrics, Committee on Drugs. Guidelines for monitoring and management of pediatric patients during and after sedation for diagnostic and therapeutic procedures. Pediatrics 1992;89:1110–1114.

American Academy of Pediatrics, Section on Anesthesiology. Evaluation and preparation of pediatric patients undergoing anesthesia. Pediatrics 1996;98:502–508.

American Society of Anesthesiologists. Task force on sedation and analgesia by non-anesthesiologists. Practice guidelines for sedation and analgesia by non-anesthesiologists. Anesthesiology 1996;84:459–471.

Cote CJ. NPO after midnight for children: a reappraisal. Anesthesiology 1990;72:589–592.

Cote CJ, Alderfer RJ, Notterman DA, et al. Sedation disasters: adverse drug reports in pediatrics. Anesthesiology 1995;83:A1183.

Igebo KR, Rayhorn NJ, Hecht RM, et al. Sedation in children: adequacy of two-hour fasting. J Pediatr 1997;131:155–158.

Krauss BS, Shannon M, Damian FJ, et al, eds. Guidelines for pediatric sedation. American College of Emergency Physicians, 1995.

Malviya S, Voepel-Lewis T, Tait AR. Adverse events and risk factors associated with the sedation of children by non-anesthesiologists. Anesth Analg 1997;85:1207–1213.

Sacchetti A, Schafemeyer R, Gerardi M, et al. Pediatric analgesia and sedation. Ann Emerg Med 1994;23:237–250.

Wilson S. Review of monitors and monitoring during sedation with emphasis on clinical applications. Pediatr Dent 1995;17:413–418.

Chapter 18
Postsedation Evaluation

William Zempsky

The safe recovery and discharge of sedated patients is an essential component of outpatient sedation management. Patients continue to require close supervision during the immediate postprocedure period because this is a time when they are at high risk for complications. Continuous monitoring is therefore essential until the patient returns to baseline functioning or achieves predetermined criteria for a safe discharge.

It is not uncommon for health care workers to become less vigilant once a procedure is completed. However, a sedated patient can become particularly vulnerable in the postprocedure period. After the procedure is completed, patients receive less stimulation, allowing them to slip into a deeper level of sedation that can potentially lead to respiratory depression, airway compromise, or aspiration if vomiting occurs. The patient who was able to talk during the procedure can lapse into unconsciousness in the postprocedure period. Furthermore, medications given for sedation may outlast a brief procedure or peak after the procedure is finished. Children may also be transported away from the procedure area with inappropriate monitoring either to a recovery area or for postprocedure testing (e.g., postreduction films after fracture or dislocation reduction). This chapter discusses the mechanics of safe monitoring and time-efficient discharge of the sedated patient.

POSTSEDATION MONITORING

Whether a patient remains in the procedure room postsedation or is transported to a recovery area, proper monitoring must be maintained throughout this period (see chapters 3, 14, 16, and 17). The level of monitoring should not be different than that available during the procedure. The patient should remain on a pulse oximeter with cardiorespiratory monitoring as indicated and capnography as a useful adjunct. Oxygen should be available and administered when appropriate, especially during transport. Table 18.1 lists the equipment necessary for proper postsedation care. Only nurses, physicians, or physician extenders with advanced airway skills should be responsible for monitoring recovering patients. Nursing assistants should not be

Table 18.1.   Postsedation Care Equipment

Supplies
    Suction apparatus with Yankauer tip
    Oral/nasal airways
    Bag-valve-mask
    Laryngoscope/endotracheal tubes
    Oxygen tubing/masks
Monitors
    Cardiorespiratory monitor
    Pulse oximeter
    Capnograph
    Sphygmomanometer (manual or automated)
Medications
    Oxygen
    Epinephrine
    Atropine
    Lidocaine
    Naloxone
    Flumazenil
    Steroids
    Diphenhydramine

called on to transport or monitor the sedated patient. A single caregiver is adequate for most situations with assistance including physician backup close at hand.

If patients are transported to a recovery area, they should be placed in the lateral position or have the head of the bed elevated to prevent the aspiration of oral secretions. A warm blanket should be used to cover patients and to prevent hypothermia. Transported patients should have a clinician in attendance during the transport who is trained in advanced airway management. An appropriate size bag-valve-mask and airway equipment should be available. Intravenous tubing should be well secured to prevent loss of access during transport. Side rails should be secured to prevent the child from falling or escaping during transport. If a new clinician is assuming care of the patient during the postsedation period, a proper report should be given that includes relevant present and past history (including time of last meal and any history of allergies); type of procedure performed; baseline medications, medications given for sedation and analgesia; problems experienced during the procedure; and potential postsedation complications.

POSTSEDATION COMPLICATIONS

Postsedation problems are not uncommon in the pediatric patient (see Chapter 19). The clinician needs to be aware of the potential problems and how to recognize and treat them (Table 18.2).

Table 18.2. Postsedation Complications

Complication	Etiology
Pain	Procedural pain
Delayed awakening	Prolonged drug action
	Hypoxemia, hypercarbia, hypovolemia
Agitation	Pain, hypoxemia, hypercarbia, full bladder
	Paradoxical reactions
	Emergence reactions
Nausea and vomiting	Sedative agents
	Premature oral fluids
Cardiorespiratory events	
Tachycardia	Pain, hypovolemia, impaired ventilation
Bradycardia	Vagal stimulation, opioids, hypoxia
Hypoxia	Laryngospasm, airway obstruction, oversedation

Postprocedure Pain

Postprocedure pain depends on the type of procedure performed and the age of the patient. Persistent pain can cause tachycardia, nausea, vomiting, and agitation. Pain should be recognized (which can be difficult in infants and young children), the cause determined, and treated with the appropriate medications. Postsedation care may need to be prolonged in patients who require pain control with parenteral opioids, but this should not deter the appropriate treatment of pain.

Delayed Awakening

Delayed awakening can be the result of prolonged drug action (long half-life, decreased metabolism, slowed elimination), excessive sedative administration, hypoxemia, hypothermia, hypercarbia, hypovolemia, or electrolyte abnormalities. Patients with delayed arousal should be carefully evaluated. A trial of reversal agents, where appropriate, may be considered to determine if oversedation is the cause (see Chapter 12).

Emergence Agitation

Agitation on emergence can occur in up to 15% of children who receive sedation. Common causes include postprocedure pain, hypoxemia, hypercarbia, hypotension, and electrolyte abnormalities, as well as the effect of specific drugs such as ketamine (emergence reactions) or benzodiazepines (paradoxical reactions). Serious causes of agitation must be ruled out, and pain should be treated appropriately.

Nausea and Vomiting

Nausea and vomiting can occur anytime in the postsedation period. The cause is most commonly the medication(s) given during the procedure, but premature introduction of oral fluids is often a contributing factor. Children, where age appropriate, should express thirst or hunger before being offered fluids. This recommendation is often impractical for young toddlers (ages 1 to 3) who undergo sedation at a time past their normal bedtime and who rarely want to do anything except sleep postprocedure. If persistent vomiting occurs, the patient may be given an antiemetic (e.g., metoclopramide, ondansetron, droperidol, or diphenhydramine) once other causes for the vomiting have been ruled out.

Cardiorespiratory Events

Patients should be monitored closely for respiratory or cardiovascular events. Causes of inadequate ventilation include laryngospasm, upper airway obstruction from pooled secretions or soft tissue relaxation, and hypoventilation from oversedation. Laryngospasm itself can occur secondary to stimulation of the laryngeal reflexes by excessive secretions or bleeding from the mouth or pharynx. Bradycardia can result from vagal stimulation, opioid administration, or hypoxia. Tachycardia can result from pain, hypovolemia, a full bladder, or impaired ventilation. Other arrhythmias are rare but merit immediate attention.

POSTSEDATION ASSESSMENT

Patients require close observation and assessment after the completion of the procedure and should remain on a monitor until fully awake (Fig. 18.1) (see Chapter 14). Vital signs including heart rate, respiratory rate, blood pressure and pulse oximetry, and a full assessment of the patient should be done at regular intervals. Temperature should be recorded on admission to the recovery area at 60-minute intervals and at discharge. Assessment of the level of sedation should accompany vital sign evaluation. This can be done using one of several postanesthetic systems. The Steward Post-Anesthetic System uses three criteria: level of consciousness, airway, and movement (Table 18.3). The Aldrete score evaluates five criteria: activity, respiration, circulation, consciousness, and color. A modified sedation score based on the Aldrete score may be used for infants and children (Table 18.4). The frequency of assessment is determined by the level of sedation. For patients who are more deeply sedated (sedation score of 0–3), vital signs should be obtained at least every 5 minutes; for moderately sedated patient (sedation score 4–6) every 10 minutes; and for minimally sedated patients (sedation score >6) at least every 15–20 minutes.

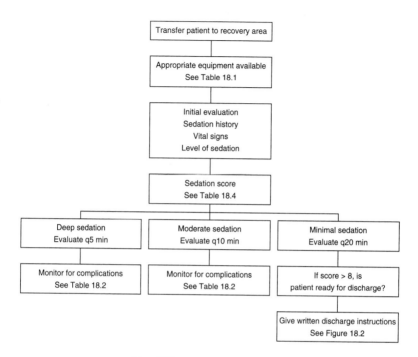

Figure 18.1. Postsedation flow chart.

Table 18.3.   Steward Postanesthetic Recovery Score

Consciousness
Awake	2
Responding to stimuli	1
Not responding	0

Airway
Coughing on command or crying	2
Maintaining good airway	1
Airway requires maintenance	0

Movement
Moving limbs purposefully	2
Nonpurposeful movements	1
Not moving	0

Table 18.4.   Sample Sedation Scoring System from Connecticut Children's Medical Center

Vital signs
Stable	1
Unstable	0

Respirations
Normal	2
Shallow respirations/tachypnea	1
Apnea	0

Level of consciousness
Alert, oriented/returned to pre-procedural level	2
Arousable, giddy, agitated	1
Unresponsive	0

Oxygen saturation
95–100% or preprocedural level	2
90–94%	1
<90%	0

Color
Pink/preprocedural color	2
Pale/dusky	1
Cyanotic	0

Activity
Moves on command/preprocedural level	2
Moves extremities/uncoordinated walking	1
No spontaneous movement	0

SEDATION SCORE	ACTION
>8	Consider discharge if no score = 0
7–8	Vital signs q 20 min
4–6	Vital signs q 10 min
0–3	Vital signs q 5 min—consider further evaluation if prolonged

DISCHARGE CRITERIA

The child who is ready for discharge should be alert and oriented or at his or her presedation state (taking into account the individual child's baseline at that hour of the day or night). The sedation score can be used as a guideline. For example, a total score of greater than or equal to 8 on the sedation scale in Table 18.4, or a score equal to the presedation score is necessary for discharge. There should be no score of zero in any category. Several other criteria also must be met. Oxygen saturation should be equal to preprocedural levels. The patient should be able to tolerate oral fluids without vomiting, although this premise has been challenged by some centers. Understandably, this may not be feasible if the procedure is completed at night after the child's bedtime. The child should also be able to sit unaided and walk with assistance if developmentally appro-

Your child has received the medications_____ to help his or her anxiety and to treat any pain experienced during the procedure today.

What to expect
Your child may remain drowsy or sleepy for the rest of the day. He or she may have difficulty walking or complain of dizziness. He or she may experience one or more episodes of nausea or vomiting. He or she may also be fussy or agitated. He or she may not want to eat or drink for a few hours.

Activity
Your child should be allowed to rest. Position your child on his or her side or stomach when sleeping. Your child should be woken up 2 hours after discharge even if it is nighttime. Watch your child closely when he or she is walking, crawling, or eating. Your child must avoid activities such as bike riding, swimming, or contact sports for at least 24 hours. Encourage "quiet" play.

Diet
Encourage your child to drink clear fluids (fluids you can see through). Your child can return to a normal diet when he or she is drinking well without vomiting.

Calling the doctor
Contact your doctor if you have concerns related to your child's sedation, or if your child experiences any breathing problems, prolonged sleeping, inability to be aroused from sleep, or frequent vomiting. You may contact Dr._____ at ___-___ .

I fully understand these instructions. If I have any problems or concerns, I will contact my doctor.

_____   _____
Parent/Guardian Signature   Date

_____
Nurse Signature

Figure 18.2. Sample discharge instructions. (Adapted from form used by Connecticut Children's Medical Center, Hartford, CT.)

priate. Before discharge, sufficient time, as much as 2 to 3 hours, should have passed since the last administration of reversal agents to ensure that resedation does not occur after discharge. Children should be discharged with a responsible adult who has been provided with written discharge instructions.

Discharge instructions should be clear, concise, and easily understood. They should include the following: instructions for diet, activity, sleep, and common problems that occur postsedation, and contact persons and phone numbers should a question or problem arise. A follow-up call should be considered in 24 to 48 hours to uncover any postsedation problems, improve patient and family satisfaction, and provide a mechanism for quality improvement. Sample discharge instructions are shown in Figure 18.2.

SUGGESTED READING

Aldrete JA, Kroulik D. A postanaesthetic recovery score. Anesth Analg 1970;49:924–934.

American Academy of Pediatrics, Committee on Drugs. Guidelines for monitoring and management of pediatric patients during and after sedation for diagnostic and therapeutic procedures. Pediatrics 1992;89:1110–1115.

Holzman RS, Cullen DJ, Eichhorn JH, et al. Guidelines for sedation by nonanesthesiologists during diagnostic and therapeutic procedures. J Clin Anesth 1994;6:265–275.

Practice guidelines for sedation and analgesia by non-anesthesiologists: a report by the American Society of Anesthesiologists. Anesthesiology 1996;84:459–471.

Sacchetti A, Schafermeyer R, Gerardi M, et al. Pediatric analgesia and sedation. Ann Emerg Med 1994;23:237–250.

Sievers TD, Yee JD, Foley ME, et al. Midazolam for conscious sedation during pediatric oncology procedures: safety and recovery parameters. Pediatrics 1991;88:1172–1179.

Steward DJ. A simplified scoring system for the post-operative recovery room. Canad Anaesth Soc J 1975;22:111–113.

Webster DE. The pediatric patient in the postanesthesia care unit. In: Rasch DK, Webster DE, eds. Clinical manual of pediatric anesthesia. New York: McGraw-Hill, 1994;8:126–144.

Yaster M. Recovery from sedation. In: Yaster M, Krane EJ, Kaplan RF, Cote CJ, Lappe DG. Pediatric pain management and sedation handbook. St. Louis: Mosby-Year Book 1997;22: 423–434.

Chapter 19
Management of Complications

Cheryl Vance

When a child cries out in fear or pain, the distress is both audible and infectious. The challenge to medical care providers is to supply prompt and effective relief without subjecting the patient to further harm.

In the last few years, a large variety of drugs have become available for use in the outpatient setting, some of which have previously been used only in the well-controlled environment of the operating room. Practitioners are often hesitant to use these drugs in their young patients for fear of potential complications. In this chapter, we will identify these complications, discuss their frequency, and determine how they can be quickly identified and managed to prevent serious sequelae.

Unfortunately, there are few good studies in the pediatric population on the use of these drugs for outpatient sedation and analgesia, and what is available presents a contradictory picture. On one hand, several studies suggest that complications are few, minor, and easily managed. A series of 2000 patients reported only three cases of respiratory depression requiring naloxone when IV fentanyl was used for analgesia. Another review of the use of ketamine in over 11,000 patients revealed an incidence of only 0.017% of laryngospasm. No cases of apnea were reported in this series. Serious complications with midazolam are also relatively uncommon, the most frequent being minor desaturations in 4.6% of patients. On the other hand, numerous case reports exist of significant adverse outcomes scattered throughout the literature. Fatal metabolic acidosis has been reported with the use of propofol, whereas cardiopulmonary arrest has occurred with the combination of midazolam and fentanyl. A review of sedation-related complications compiled from reports by the Food and Drug Administration, the United States Pharmacopoeia, and by individual physicians found 52 deaths and 6 permanent neurologic injuries reported since 1967. Although these complications could not be attributed to any specific drug or drug combination and occurred in many different practice settings, they demonstrate clearly that although uncommon, serious complications do occur in pediatric outpatient sedation and analgesia. The risk is not significant enough to prevent us from using these drugs but it is sufficient to increase our realization that with the opportunity for pain and anxiety intervention comes responsibility to manage potentially serious adverse events.

SPECIAL CONSIDERATIONS IN THE PEDIATRIC PATIENT

The pediatric patient requires special consideration when drugs are used for pain or anxiety relief. The basic anatomy of the child makes them more prone to respiratory compromise. The large occiput, proportionally large tongue, and soft larynx quickly cause airway obstruction when resting tone is decreased. Children sedated with midazolam are particularly vulnerable to this. The bronchi of the child are also smaller and more easily collapsible, and children have less pulmonary reserve. When respiratory drive is blunted by medication, there is rapid transition from adequate oxygenation to desaturation and hypoxia. If intervention is not quick and effective, full cardiopulmonary arrest will quickly follow.

The effects of medication are also less predictable in children. In infants less than 3 months of age, the opiates exhibit both decreased protein binding and decreased clearance compared with older children and adults. This allows for a greater than expected free fraction of the drug. Morphine, fentanyl, and meperidine must be given at lower doses in this age group and at less frequent intervals to avoid complications from excess drug availability. In older children, in whom drug metabolism is considered more predictable, dosing still requires careful titration to desired effect. Reduced effectiveness of drugs is commonly seen because of a child's heightened anxiety level in the frightening environment of the doctors office or emergency department.

PLANNING FOR COMPLICATIONS

Reports of adverse effects in children undergoing sedation and analgesia led the American Academy of Pediatrics (AAP) in 1985 and 1992 to issue guidelines to help assure high-quality care to pediatric patients undergoing outpatient procedures. These guidelines emphasize appropriate selection of patients, drugs, and dosages for sedation and analgesia and careful monitoring during the process. Two recent studies have looked at adverse effects after the implementation of a structured sedation program modeled after the guidelines proposed by the AAP. These studies suggest that with careful preparation, children can be safely sedated as outpatients with minimal adverse effects. Planning is the most critical step in both prevention and management of complications and in assuring a good outcome.

STEPS TO AVOID ADVERSE EVENTS

1. *Choose your patient:* Although some children will respond well to preprocedural preparation, local analgesia, and verbal support by parents and

caregivers, most children (especially in the toddler age group) will require some form of analgesia and/or sedation for outpatient procedures. The challenge is to correctly identify those patients who will benefit from the addition of drugs and those who may be at increased risk of adverse events. A good health history is an absolute prerequisite. Children with viral respiratory infections, obstructive airway disease, or history of psychosis or drug allergies need to be identified because they have an increased risk of complications with certain drugs. Children with severe systemic disease are also at increased risk and are probably better served by the anesthesiologist in the operating suite rather than attempting intervention in the outpatient setting.

2. *Know your drugs:* To avoid complications, it is essential to know the correct dose of the drug being used. The dosage should not only be weight dependent, but also age and disease dependent. It is also essential to be familiar with the pharmacokinetics of each drug, potential drug interactions, and the complications and side effects with different routes of administration. It is important to remember that medication requirements are not the same for all pediatric patients.

3. *Monitor patients carefully:* All patients should be monitored by continuous pulse oximetry by an independent observer who periodically records vital signs. This monitoring will assure early identification of problems and is the key to preventing adverse outcome. Monitoring should continue after the procedure until the patient has returned to baseline. Patients are particularly prone to develop respiratory complications at the completion of the procedure when the painful stimulus is removed. The use of capnography also should be considered because studies have shown that it can detect respiratory depression even earlier than pulse oximetry.

4. *Be prepared to intervene:* Quick intervention can often prevent the development of serious adverse events. For example, if mild hypoxia or hypercarbia is identified early, the patient will often respond to simple measures like gentle stimulation and the application of oxygen. If severe hypoxia or respiratory arrest occurs, age-appropriate resuscitative equipment, reversal agents, and persons skilled in advanced pediatric life support should be immediately available.

PREVENTION AND MANAGEMENT OF SPECIFIC COMPLICATIONS

Untoward reactions either to the procedure or to medication can occur at any time and can affect any body system. When the clinician is well informed and prepared, many of these can be prevented or easily managed (Table 19.1).

Table 19.1.   Drug Complications and Treatment

Medication	Complications	Treatment
Opioids Fentanyl Sufentanil Meperidine Morphine	**General** Respiratory depression	Stimulation; reposition head; oxygen; reversal agents; mechanical ventilation
	Vomiting	Antiemetic
	Pruritis	Antihistamine
Reversal agents Naloxone Nalmefene	**Drug specific** Fentanyl—chest wall rigidity	Avoid high-dose/rapid bolus; reversal agents; paralysis; intubation; mechanical ventilation
	Meperidine/morphine— hypotension	Fluid bolus
Benzodiazepines Diazepam Midazolam *Reversal agent* Flumazenil	**General** Respiratory depression	Stimulation; reposition head; oxygen; reversal agents; mechanical ventilation
	Paradoxical reactions (agitation)	Flumazenil
	Drug specific Diazepam—burning on injection	
Barbiturates Methohexital Pentobarbital	**General** Respiratory depression	Stimulation; reposition head; oxygen; mechanical ventilation
	Drug specific Methohexital—seizures	Avoid with known seizure disorder
Sedative/hypnotics Chloral hydrate Propofol	**General** Respiratory depression	Stimulation; reposition head; oxygen; mechanical ventilation
	Drug specific Propofol—cardiorespiratory depression	Avoid rapid infusion; assure euvolemia; stimulation; reposition head; oxygen; mechanical ventilation
	Propofol—burning on injection	Pretreat with lidocaine
Dissociative agents Ketamine	**General** Laryngospasm	Mechanical ventilation
	Increased secretions	Antisialogue
	Emergence reactions	Benzodiazepine
	$\uparrow$ICP	Avoid in patients with $\uparrow$ICP
Topical anesthetics TAC (cocaine-based)	**General** Systemic absorption	Avoid application to mucous membranes; avoid sniffing or ingestion

Respiratory Depression

The most common and concerning adverse effect of the drugs used for pediatric sedation and analgesia is respiratory depression. This is usually associated with use of the benzodiazepines and opiates and is most common in children less than 3 months of age or those with chronic lung disease. The potential of these drugs to cause respiratory depression increases when they are used in combination or when they are given with other central nervous system (CNS) depressants like the barbiturates or ethanol (ETOH). Respiratory depression also has been reported with ketamine, propofol, and chloral hydrate, and like the opiates and benzodiazepines, can be caused by too large a dose and/or rapid infusion. Careful patient selection, calculation of drug dosages, and appropriate administration is usually preventive. If respiratory depression occurs, initial treatment is gentle patient stimulation. Often, the patient will just need a "reminder" to breathe. Repositioning the head to open the airway, applying oxygen, administering positive pressure ventilation or intubation, and administering reversal agents may be required in those patients with persistent respiratory depression.

Increased Secretions

Ketamine can cause increased salivary and tracheobronchial secretions, which can interfere with respiratory effort. Premedication with an anticholinergic such as atropine or glycopyrrolate has been recommended when ketamine is used (see Chapter 7).

Laryngospasm

Upper airway obstruction from spasmodic closure of the larynx is a rare complication reported with the use of ketamine. Infants less than 3 months of age and children with viral upper respiratory tract infections are at increased risk, although the phenomena has also been reported in children with an easy "gag" or history of asthma. Excessive secretions may also be a precipitant. Initial management is repositioning the head and gentle suctioning of the airway. If laryngospasm persists, respiratory compromise will quickly follow, and the airway should be controlled by paralysis, intubation, and positive pressure ventilation. Ketamine should probably be avoided in those procedures that either stimulate the gag reflex or cause increased secretions.

Chest Wall and Glottic Rigidity

Rapid boluses of fentanyl cause "wooden chest syndrome," a complication in which the chest wall and glottis become rigid, making even manual ventilation difficult to impossible. Wooden chest syndrome is usually seen when fentanyl is used in doses of greater than 15 μg/kg but also has been associated with rapid infusion of smaller amounts of the drug. Chest wall rigidity has not been reported as a complication of procedural sedation in which low bolus doses (1–2 μg/kg) are given. This complication may only be partially reversed with naloxone, and treatment is usually a skeletal muscle relaxant and intubation with ventilatory support until effects of the drug have worn off.

Cardiovascular Complications

Propofol has no vagolytic activity and has been associated with reports of hypotension, bradycardia, and asystole. Volume loading before administration of propofol and continuous infusion rather than bolus doses is recommended to prevent these complications. The opiates, barbiturates, and benzodiazepines also can cause hypotension. Euvolemia should be assured before the administration of these drugs and patients should be monitored closely. The treatment algorithm is immediate discontinuation of the drug, fluid boluses, administration of reversal agents, and vasopressor therapy.

Emergence Phenomena

Dysphoric reactions, or "weird trips," are occasionally seen in the recovery phase of sedation with ketamine. The incidence is as high as 50% in adults but is relatively uncommon in children. Risk factors for emergence hallucinations include an age greater than 10 years, female gender, rapid IV administration, excessive environmental noise or stimulation during recovery, and a prior personality disorder. The use of ketamine in patients with any of these risk factors should be avoided. Premedication with a benzodiazepine may reduce psychic reactions in older children but will also prolong recovery time.

Seizure and Seizure-Like Activity

Seizures, although uncommon, have been reported with several of the drugs that are frequently used for pediatric sedation and analgesia. The topical anesthetic, TAC (tetracaine, epinephrine, cocaine), has been associated with seizures secondary to systemic absorption of cocaine. This medication should not be used for topical anesthesia of lacerations on or near mucous membranes, nor should it be used if there is a chance that the patient may sniff or swallow it. Methohexital can exacerbate seizures in patients with an underlying seizure disorder and its use should be avoided in these patients. Myoclonus, twitching, random movements, and hypertonicity can occur in patients sedated with ketamine or methohexital. These "pseudoseizures" self-resolve and rarely interfere with the performance of procedures.

Paradoxical Excitement, Hyperactivity, and Combativeness

Paradoxical excitement, hyperactivity, and combativeness are complications often associated with use of benzodiazepines. The etiology of these reactions is uncertain, but may be related to inadequate or excessive dosing, cerebral hypoxia, or may actually be a true paradoxical reaction. The benzodiazepine antagonist flumazenil will reverse these effects. Excitation reactions are also a complication seen with chloral hydrate and may be an age-specific phenomena because they are more common in older children.

Increased Intracranial Pressure

Ketamine causes increased intracranial pressure, and fentanyl has been associated with acute elevations of intracranial pressure in the head-injured child. Both of these agents should be avoided in patients with head trauma or in those in whom there is concern of an intracranial disorder.

Anaphylactic Reactions

Although anaphylactic reactions are uncommon, they may be life-threatening and can potentially occur with any of the agents used for sedation and analgesia. A careful history before administering any drug is essential. Most reports of anaphylaxis have occurred with propofol. Its use should be avoided in patients with a known reaction to muscle relaxants or in patients with several proven drug allergies. Should anaphylaxis occur, management includes discontinuing the drug; assuring a patent airway and applying oxygen; supporting blood pressure with fluid resuscitation; and administering drug therapy with epinephrine, antihistamines, bronchodilators, and steroids as indicated.

Nausea and Vomiting

Nausea and vomiting are reported with many of the agents used for sedation and analgesia including opioids, benzodiazepines, ketamine, chloral hydrate, and barbiturates. If airway-protective reflexes are lost because of a deep level of sedation, the patient is at risk for aspiration. Vomiting can be relieved with an antiemetic. Reversal agents can also be used. Readily available large bore suction will also assist in minimizing the potential complications from vomiting.

Pruritis

Itching is common side effect of the opiates and can be relieved with diphenhydramine. It is noted less with fentanyl because this opiate causes little to no histamine release.

Pain with Infusion

Intravenous infusion of propofol and diazepam can cause pain. Premedication with IV lidocaine (1 mL of a 1% solution), slow intravenous infusion of the drug, and avoidance of small veins all help to reduce the incidence of this complication.

SUGGESTED READING

Abramo TJ, Bates BA, Wiebe RA, et al. Noninvasive capnometry for monitoring during pediatric conscious sedation. SAEM Annual Meeting Abstracts 1994;#060.

Andrews J. Conscious sedation in the pediatric emergency department. Curr Opin Pediatr 1995;7:309–313.

Bailey PL, Pace NL, Ashburn MA, et al. Frequent hypoxemia and apnea after sedation with midazolam and fentanyl. Anesthesiology 1990;73(5):826–830.

Billmire DA, Neale HW, Gregory RO. Use of IV fentanyl in the outpatient treatment of pediatric facial trauma. J Trauma 1985;25(11):1079–1080.

Bloomfield EL, Masaryk TJ, Caplin A, et al. Intravenous sedation for MR imaging of the brain and spine in children: pentobarbital versus propofol. Pediatr Radiol 1993;186:93–97.

Cauldwell CB, Fisher DM. Sedating pediatric patients: is propofol a panacea? Radiology 1993;186:9–10.

Chuang E, Wenner WJ, Piccoli DA, et al. Intravenous sedation in pediatric upper gastrointestinal endoscopy. Gastrointest Endosc 1995;42(2):156–160.

Chudnofsky CR, Wright SW, Dronen SC, et al. The safety of fentanyl use in the emergency department. Ann Emerg Med 1989;18(6):635–639.

Committee on Drugs: guidelines for monitoring and management of pediatric patients during and after sedation for diagnostic and therapeutic procedures. Pediatrics 1992;89:1110–1115.

Correspondence. EMLA: Complications. British Journal of Anaesthesia 1990;295.

Correspondence. Norman J, Jones PL. Complications of the use of EMLA. Br J Anaesth 1990;64:403–406.

Cote CJ. Sedation for the pediatric patient. Pediatr Anesth 1994;41(1):31–58.

Council on Scientific Affairs, American Medical Association. The use of pulse oximetry during conscious sedation. JAMA, September 22/29, 1993;270(12):1463–1467.

Dailey RH. Fatality secondary to misuse of TAC solution. Ann Emerg Med 1988;17(2):159–160.

Damian FJ, Smith MF, Krauss BS. Conscious sedation roundtable: a collaborative practice model for problem solving in the emergency department. J Emerg Nurs 1997;23(2):153–155.

Daya MR, Burton BT, Schleiss MR, et al. Recurrent seizures following mucosal application of TAC. Ann of Emerg Med 1988;17(6):646–648.

Egelhoff JC, Ball WS, Koch BL, et al. Safety and efficacy of sedation in children using a structured sedation program. Am J Roentgenology 1997;168:1259–1262.

Goad RN, Webster D. Sedation, analgesia, and anesthesia issues in the pediatric patient. Clin Pediatr Med Surg 1997;14(1):131–148.

Graff KJ, Kennedy RM, Jaffe DM. Conscious sedation for pediatric orthopaedic emergencies. Pediatr Emerg Care 1996;12(1):31–35.

Green SM, Nakamura R, Johnson NE. Ketamine sedation for pediatric procedures: part 1, a prospective series. Ann Emerg Med 1990;19(9):1024–1032.

Green SM, Johnson NE. Ketamine sedation for pediatric procedures: part 2, review and implications. Ann Emerg Med 1990;19(9):1033–1043.

Green SM. Letters to the Editor. The safety of ketamine for emergency department pediatric sedation. J Oral Maxillofac Surg 1995;53:1232–1233.

Hart LS, Berns SD, Houck CS, et al. The value of end-tidal CO_2 monitoring when comparing three methods of conscious sedation for children undergoing painful procedures in the emergency department. Pediatr Emerg Care 1997;13(3):189–193.

Laxenaire MC, Mata-Bermejo E, Moneret-Vautrin DA, et al. Life-threatening anaphylactoid reactions to propofol (Diprivan). Anesthesiology 1992;77(2):275–279.

Liebelt EL. Reducing pain during procedures. Curr Opin Pediatr 1996;8:436–441.

Lipshitz M, Marino BL, Sanders, ST. Chloral hydrate side effects in young children: causes and management. Heart and Lung 1993;22(5):408–414.

Litman RS, Berkowitz RJ, Ward DS. Poster discussion—effects of anesthesia on ventilatory control. Anesthesiology 1995;83(3A).

Malviya S, Voepel-Lewis T, Tait A. Adverse events and risk factors associated with the sedation of children by nonanesthesiologists. Anesth Analg 1997;85:1207–1213.

Parker, RI, Mahan RA, Giugliano D, et al. Efficacy and safety of intravenous midazolam and ketamine as sedation for therapeutic and diagnostic procedures in children. Pediatrics 1997;99(3):427–431.

Pohlgeers AP, Friedland LR, Keegan-Jones L. Combination fentanyl and diazepam for pediatric conscious sedation. Acad Emerg Med 1995:2(10):879–883.

Policy Statements: American College of Emergency Physicians. Use of pediatric sedation and analgesia. Ann Emerg Med 1997;29:834–835.

Proudfoot J. Analgesia, anesthesia, and conscious sedation. Emerg Med Clin North Am 1995;13(2):357–379.

Proudfoot J, Petrack E. The six skills of highly effective pediatric sedation. Pediatr Emerg Med Rep 1997;2(8):79–90.

Sacchetti A, Schafermeyer R, Gerardi M, et al. Pediatric analgesia and sedation. Ann Emerg Med 1994;23(2):237–250.

Sievers TD, Yee JD, Foley ME, et al. Midazolam for conscious sedation during pediatric oncology procedures: safety and recovery parameters. Pediatrics 1991;88(6):1172–1179.

Smith JA, Santer LJ. Respiratory arrest following intramuscular ketamine injection in a 4-year-old child. Ann Emerg Med 1993;22(3):613–615.

Strickland RA, Murray MJ. Fatal metabolic acidosis in a pediatric patient receiving an infusion of propofol in the intensive care unit: is there a relationship? Crit Care Med 1995; 23(2):405–409.

Theroux MC, West DW, Corddry DH, et al. Efficacy of intranasal midazolam in facilitating suturing of lacerations in preschool children in the emergency department. Pediatrics 1993;91(3):624–627.

Tobias JD. Increased intracranial pressure after fentanyl administration in a child with closed head trauma. Pediatr Emerg Care 1994;10:89–90.

Trotter C, Serpell MG. Neurological sequelae in children after prolonged propofol infusion. Anaesthesia 1992;47:340–342.

Vade A, Sukhani R, Dolenga M, et al. Chloral hydrate sedation of children undergoing CT and MR imaging: safety as judged by American Academy of Pediatrics Guidelines. Am J Roentgenol 1995;165:905–909.

Woolard DJ, Terndrup TE. Sedative-analgesic agent administration in children: analysis of use and complications in the emergency department. J Emerg Med 1994;12(4):453–461.

Wright SW, Chudnofsky CR, Dronen SC, et al. Midazolam use in the emergency department. Am J Emerg Med 1990;8(2):97–100.

Yaster M, Nichols DG, Deshpande JK, et al. Midazolam-fentanyl intravenous sedation in children: case report of respiratory arrest. Pediatrics 1990;86(3):463–466.

Ziegler VL, Brown LE. Conscious sedation in the pediatric population. Crit Care Nurs Clin North Am 1997;9(3):381–394.

Chapter 20
Procedural Sedation
in the Emergency Department

Douglas Nelson

Sedation of children in the emergency department (ED) facilitates the wide range of medical procedures frequently performed in this setting including laceration repair, fracture and dislocation reduction, foreign body removal, and abscess drainage. The goals of ED sedation use include the following:

- Assuring the patient's safety
- Minimizing the pain and anxiety
- Minimizing the patient's motion
- Maximizing the chances of success for the procedure being performed
- Returning the patient to his or her presedated state as quickly as possible

Many agents and techniques are available to accomplish these goals, and several options are usually available for each patient in whom sedation is judged desirable. The ideal agent for ED use would have the following characteristics:

- Painless administration
- Wide therapeutic margin with no associated respiratory depression, emergence, or paradoxical reactions
- Effective duration of less than 30 minutes after which its effects would dissipate completely
- Low cost

No agent in use today satisfies these criteria.

The practice of procedural sedation and analgesia has evolved over the last 15 years to better attain the goals outlined above. Recent trends in the field include increased reliance on newer and shorter-acting medications, which are in some cases pharmacologically reversible. Traditional intramuscular cocktails, such as the mixture of meperidine, promethazine, and chlorpromazine (DPT), have fallen out of favor because of their high failure rate, delayed onset, prolonged duration of effect, possibility of serious adverse reactions, and lack of titratability. Another change is the increased desirability of nonparenteral routes of administration such as oral, transmucosal, intranasal, and rectal. Better monitoring, particularly the use of pulse oximetry and capnography, has allowed deeper levels of sedation to be attained without compromising patient safety.

The type of sedation performed in the ED is procedural sedation, which is defined as the use of sedative, analgesic, and dissociative agents to facilitate the performance of medically necessary procedures. This is different from conscious sedation, defined as a sedated state in which a patient is alert enough to follow commands. Any young child conscious enough to respond to verbal stimuli will not allow potentially painful medical procedures to be performed on him or her. Implicit in this description of procedural sedation is the knowledge that it is not being performed in an operating room, and that the drugs and doses given will allow the patient to maintain airway reflexes and respiratory drive.

SPECIAL CONSIDERATIONS

The emergency physician caring for the agitated child must first decide whether sedation is required at all. Table 20.1 lists factors known to decrease the need for sedation. Even if the need for sedation cannot totally be eliminated, awareness of these techniques will allow lower and therefore safer doses of medications to be

Table 20.1.   Factors Decreasing Sedation Needs

Environment
    Parental presence
    Distraction techniques
    Quiet environment
Systemic pain relief
    Ketorolac
    Ibuprofen
    Acetaminophen
Local pain relief
    TAC/LET
    Buffered lidocaine infiltration
    EMLA
    Vapocoolant spray (ethylene chloride)
Nonpainful wound repair
    Cyanoacrylate skin adhesive

Table 20.2.   Factors Affecting Sedation Decisions

Medical risks
    Respiratory depression/arrest
    Paradoxical reaction
    Nausea, vomiting, and aspiration
    Allergic reaction
Financial considerations
    Increased cost to family/insurance
    Increased length of outpatient stay
Potential benefits
    Calmer patient
    Impaired memory of upsetting medical interaction
    Improved parental satisfaction
    Better cosmesis (wound repair)
    Less stress for medical personnel
Characteristics of patient and family
    Patient baseline emotional state/degree of agitation and anxiety
    Parental preference
    History of oral intake (NPO status)
Medical factors
    Source of patient's distress (pain and anxiety)
    Presence of high-risk criteria
    Depth of sedation required
    Preferred duration of sedation
    Available access (IV)
Institutional factors
    Published hospital guidelines
    Availability of equipment and personnel
    Comfort level of emergency physicians—adult vs. pediatric facility

used. All the items listed reduce either pain or anxiety. Ketorolac is currently the only parenteral analgesic that does not produce sedation or potentiate respiratory depression. If sedation is desired, its depth, route of administration, and duration must be carefully chosen. The many factors to consider when making this decision are listed in Table 20.2.

The financial and temporal costs of sedation use are not trivial to most families and overcrowded emergency departments. A recent study examining the oral administration of midazolam in a pediatric emergency department showed an increase in combined nursing/hospital charges and total charges by $73 to $87, depending on laceration type. Physician charges did not increase with sedation administration but are expected because of the recent approval of CPT codes for sedation. Mean length of stay increased by 17 to 31 minutes as well.

The potential benefits of sedation are well known to any physician who has sutured a screaming child while anxious parents look on, convinced that the patient is experiencing excruciating pain. Accomplishing the goals of a medical procedure is easer in a calm patient: the physician is not rushing to finish the job and the affected body part requiring treatment is not moving. Parents will be calmer as well. The amnestic properties of newer medications such as midazolam may prevent the patient from remembering his or her upsetting experience, even if they cry uncontrollably throughout the procedure. These benefits of sedation will lower the stress level of the ED personnel involved, who usually do not lack for adrenal stimulation.

The emotional characteristics of the child being sedated, particularly the child's anxiety level, strongly influences the need for sedation. This degree of anxiety depends on a multitude of mutually interacting factors including baseline personality, parental anxiety level, past medical experiences, the current ED environment (especially noises and sights), demeanor of medical caregivers, length of wait, time of day, degree of pain, and size or type of injury. Despite the apparent complexity of anxiogenesis, discerning the total quantity of anxiety present is usually not difficult. Some children requiring laceration repair peel off their bandage proudly to show the physician, whereas others scream if caregivers approach within several feet of the wound. The latter type of child is sedated more often than the former. Some parents may express strong preferences regarding the use of sedation as well.

The final set of factors to consider when making sedation decisions depends on the medical facility at which the physician is practicing. Every institution where sedation is performed should have sedation guidelines detailing requirements for informed consent, vital sign charting, required equipment and personnel, and discharge criteria. In some cases, an ED may limit sedation to certain age ranges or prohibit the use of a particular agent; these regulations may also vary between general and exclusively pediatric EDs. These policies have been written for the protection of the patient and should be followed; if the practitioner consistently needs to deviate from them, efforts should be made to revise them (see Chapter 16).

Significant differences also exist between pediatric and general community hospital EDs in terms of frequency of sedation use and agents chosen. Recent studies have shown a higher rate of sedation administration and a preference for shorter-acting agents (such as fentanyl and ketamine) among children seen at a pediatric facility when compared with a general facility. Midazolam is currently the most frequently used sedative in either type of ED.

EQUIPMENT

The equipment required in the ED for safe administration of sedation and analgesia is discussed in chapters 3, 17 and 18. None of this equipment is used solely for purposes of insuring sedation safety. All of the airway equipment, monitoring devices, and medications are in widespread use for the treatment of respiratory difficulties and/or cardiopulmonary arrest and would normally be found in a well-equipped ED.

Nonmedical equipment has proven useful in the practice of procedural sedation because most agents are not specifically made in a pediatric preparation. Sugar syrups in which bitter medications such as crushed pills or the intravenous formulation of midazolam or ketamine (where an oral preparation is not available) may be mixed are helpful. Commercially available chocolate and strawberry syrups sold for topping desserts or flavoring milk work well. A source of soothing music such as a portable tape or compact disc player along with age-appropriate musical selections is helpful. Children may be calmed by being able to choose their medication flavor or background music tape. Photographs or cartoon posters on the ceiling over the bed where young patients are sutured provide distraction and can be the focus of a prolonged discussion with a young patient.

PERSONNEL

The physician supervising the care of the sedated child is responsible first and foremost for the safety of this patient. Despite the presence in the room of nurses, nursing assistants, child life workers, parents, and monitoring devices, nothing facilitates patient safety more than the bedside presence of a treating doctor who is familiar with the patient. Another physician responsibility is the obtaining of informed consent for sedation, which needs to be documented in writing. Depending on institutional guidelines, this may require completion of a dedicated form or a notation in the chart. Regardless of its format, it should include the information that indicates that the risks and benefits of sedation have been discussed. The two risks most worth discussing are respiratory depression and vomiting with the risk of aspiration. Although stylistic differences in obtaining consent exist, the form might also include a discussion of the financial and temporal costs incurred, especially for uninsured patients (see Chapter 15).

The role of the nursing staff in the care of a sedated patient is multifaceted (see Chapter 14). Administering the sedative agent may involve considerable cajoling skills and patience in the case of oral or intranasal medications and excellent intravenous placement skills for parenteral medications. Physical restraint, often needed in the lightly sedated child, is provided by a combination of a cloth and Velcro papoose and a nurse's arms. Once the patient is sedated and the physicians attention is directed toward completion of the medical procedure, the most important nursing role is the continuous monitoring of the patient's vital signs. At no point should one individual be responsible both for the performance of the medical procedure and patient monitoring.

Child Life Specialists

Some emergency departments are fortunate to have a child life worker, which is a nonmedical staff person whose role is to put children at ease. Through the use of gentle conversation, distraction techniques, and dolls who undergo mock procedures, less sedation may be needed, and may possibly be avoided altogether.

Parents

The role of the sedated child's parents has changed substantially in recent years. Once, it was common to usher parents out of the examination room while a procedure was performed. Parental presence at the bedside is now preferred, because this decreases patient (and parent) anxiety and therefore the need for sedation. Parents may need to be coached on where to sit, which hand to hold, and what to discuss with the patient; if successfully performed, this calming effect may be equivalent to several milligrams of midazolam. Despite the desirability of a calming parental presence, there are both parents and procedures for which this technique would not be advised.

PHARMACOPOEIA

The procedural sedation needs of most if not all patients in the emergency department may be met with midazolam, fentanyl, ketamine, and nitrous oxide (Table 20.3). These agents have in common a short duration of action. Two are reversible (midazolam and fentanyl), and two may be administered via a wide variety of

Table 20.3. Pharmacopoeia for Procedural Sedation in the Emergency Department

Anxiolytics (benzodiazapine)
   Midazolam[a]
   Diazepam
Sedative analgesics (opioids)
   Fentanyl[a]
   Sufentanil[a]
   Morphine
   Meperidine
Dissociative agents
   Ketamine[a]
Inhalational agents
   Nitrous oxide[a]
Reversal agents
   Naloxone
   Nalmefene
   Flumazenil
Pure sedatives
   Chloral hydrate
   Methohexital
   Pentobarbital

[a]Especially useful short-acting agents.

routes (midazolam and ketamine). As with the pharmacologic treatment of any condition, better results will be obtained if the practitioner uses one or two agents frequently and becomes experienced with their side effects, advantages, and disadvantages. Sedatives with a longer duration of action such as morphine, meperidine, and diazepam are no longer practical for ED use because they increase the duration of postprocedural monitoring and observation and therefore the time until discharge.

The most important factor affecting the choice of sedative is the physician's assessment of what will cause the patient's distress: pain or anxiety. Patients expected to be agitated because of severe pain are best sedated with fentanyl or ketamine. If mild to moderate pain and anxiety are anticipated, nitrous oxide is usually sufficient. If anxiety alone will be encountered, midazolam is the drug of choice. It is preferable (but not always possible) to use one drug class per patient to avoid potentiating respiratory depression. This occurs most commonly with the combination of benzodiazepines and opioids. Fortunately, drugs from both of these classes are reversible.

The extremely variable response of children to these agents ensures that the task of providing effective procedural sedation will always involve equal parts of art and science. Fortunately, newer agents and monitoring equipment have made procedural sedation in the ED safe and more reliable than in the past. Clinicians performing procedures on injured children should be acquainted with the use of several common agents to minimize the pain and anxiety of their young patients.

SUGGESTED READING

AAP Committee on Drugs. Guidelines for monitoring and management of pediatric patients during and after sedation for diagnostic and therapeutic procedures. Pediatrics 1992;89:1110–1115.

AAP Committee on Drugs. Reappraisal of lytic cocktail/Demerol, Phenergan, Thorazine (DPT) for the sedation of children. Pediatrics 1995;95:598–601.

Bates B, Schutzman S, Fleisher G. A comparison of intranasal sufentanil and midazolam to meperidine, promethazine, and chlorpromazine for conscious sedation in children. Ann Emerg Med 1994;24:646–51.

Billmire DA, Neale HW, Gregory RO. Use of IV fentanyl in the outpatient treatment of pediatric facial trauma. J Trauma 1985;25:1079–1080.

Cote, CJ. Sedation for the pediatric patient. Pediatr Clin North Am 1994:41;31–58.

Green SM, Johnson NE. Ketamine sedation for pediatric procedures: part 2, review and implications. Ann Emerg Med 1990;19:1033–1046.

Green SM, Nakamura R, Johnson NE. Ketamine sedation for pediatric procedures: part 1, a prospective series. Ann Emerg Med 1990;19:1024–1032.

Hennes HM, et al. The effect of oral midazolam on anxiety of preschool children during laceration repair. Ann Emerg Med 1990;19:1006–1009.

Hoagland JR, Nelson DS. The Costs of Sedation Using Oral Midazolam: Money, Time, and Parental Attitudes. Presented at American Academy of Pediatrics, November 1997, New Orleans, Louisiana.

Krauss B, Shannon M, Damian F, et al. Guidelines for pediatric sedation. American College of Emergency Physicians, 1995.

Krauss B, Zurakowski D. Sedation patterns in pediatric and general community hospital emergency departments. Pediatr Emerg Care 1998;14:99–103.

Menegazzi J, Paris P, et al. A randomized, controlled trial of the use of music during laceration repair. Ann Emerg Med 1991;20:348–50.

Sacchetti A, Schafermeyer R, et al. Pediatric analgesia and sedation. Ann Emerg Med 1994;23:237–250.

Schutzman S, Burg J, et al. Oral transmucosal fentanyl citrate for premedication of children undergoing laceration repair. Ann Emerg Med 1994;24:1059–1064.

Yealy DM, et al. Intranasal Midazolam as a sedative for children during laceration repair. Am J Emerg Med 1992;10:584–587.

Chapter 21
Sedation for Radiologic Imaging

Carl Chudnofsky

Advances in imaging technology have revolutionized the evaluation of a wide variety of acute and chronic pediatric disorders. Advanced imaging procedures (i.e., computed tomography [CT], magnetic resonance imaging [MRI]) generally require children to remain motionless for the duration of the scan. Thus, the ability to provide safe and effective sedation in the radiology suite has become a necessity for many providers of pediatric health care.

The need to prevent children from moving requires the use of sedation for most infants and toddlers. In the appropriate setting (i.e., scheduled elective scan), adjunctive measures such as sleep deprivation can also be helpful. In older children, verbal reassurance may be sufficient. In addition, simulation is an effective alternative to sedation for elective MRI in children greater than 6 years of age.

The Joint Commission on Accreditation of Healthcare Organizations mandates that sedation practices be uniform throughout any one institution. Therefore, hospitals performing imaging procedures on children must establish policies and procedures governing the use of sedation in the radiology suite. To assure institutional uniformity, these policies and procedures should be made in conjunction with the anesthesia department and should address issues such as patient selection, personnel, equipment, monitoring, drug selection and administration, recovery, disposition, and management of emergency situations (see Chapter 16). Many institutions have found that implementing a structured sedation program for the radiology department increases the safety, efficiency, and success rates for imaging procedures.

SPECIAL CONSIDERATIONS

Sedating children for radiologic imaging posses some unique problems not encountered in other outpatient settings. These include the need to keep the child motionless during the imaging procedure and the difficulty associated with monitoring and resuscitating children in the radiology suite.

Slight movement during a painful or invasive procedure (e.g., laceration repair, fracture reduction) is usually of little consequence. However, for advanced imaging procedures, even small movements can prevent satisfactory interpretation. Therefore, the agent or agents chosen to sedate a child for radiologic imaging must also render the child motionless.

Children sedated for radiologic imaging require the same level and type of monitoring required for other outpatient settings (see Chapter 3). However, observing children from the CT or MRI control room through a glass window is much more difficult than direct observation at the bedside and increases the practitioner's reliance on monitoring devices. Monitoring is further complicated during MRI because the scanner generates strong static, radio frequency, and time-varied magnetic fields. A static magnetic field within the bore of the scanner is roughly 15,000 times greater than the magnetic field of the earth's surface. This can cause ferromagnetic devices to become airborne, damaging the equipment or scanner or injuring the patient. In addition, radio frequency and time-varied magnetic fields can interfere with the operation of standard ferromagnetic monitoring devices. Conversely, without specific radio frequency shielding, standard monitoring devices and cables may induce artifactual radio frequency current, which degrades the magnetic resonance image. It has also been reported that heat generated by the increased magnetic fields has resulted in serious burns when standard cables were looped around a patient's extremity.

Many of these problems have been eliminated by the use of new nonferromagnetic monitors and cables made specifically to be safe and reliable within the scanning suite. Standard ferromagnetic monitors can also be used but must be placed outside the magnetic field. If standard ferromagnetic cables are used, they should be wrapped in aluminum foil to decrease radio frequency interference. Finally, oximeter probes should be placed as far from the magnetic bore as possible (e.g., on a toe), and care should be taken to avoid looping the cable around the patient's extremity to prevent burns.

The radiology suite also can be a hostile environment for managing children with apnea or cardiac arrest. Poor lighting, limited space, and inadequate patient access and lack of appropriate support staff, supplies, and equipment are all potential obstacles to successful resuscitation. Therefore, a resuscitation plan specific to the radiology department should be developed before sedation (see Chapter 17).

EQUIPMENT

Monitoring devices described in Part One of this book are also required when sedating children for radiologic imaging (see chapters 3, 14, 17, and 18). If the radiology suite is not equipped with wall outlets for oxygen and suction, portable oxygen tanks and suction apparatus should be available. Also, a crash cart with resuscitation drugs and reversal agents, a defibrillator, and age- and size-appropriate equipment for oxygen administration to establish a patent airway, positive pressure ventilation, and intubation must be immediately available. It should also be remembered that for MRI, all monitoring devices and equipment must be nonferromagnetic, or carefully shielded and/or placed outside the static magnetic field of the scanner.

PERSONNEL

Personnel requirements for sedating children in the radiology suite are also similar to other outpatient settings (see chapters 3, 14, 17, and 18). One individual, other than the technician performing the scan, must be assigned to monitor the patient. This person should be adept at recognizing hemodynamic and respiratory compromise and must be able to establish a patent airway and provide positive pressure ventilation. In the emergency department setting, this individual is usually an emergency department nurse experienced or credentialed in procedural sedation. For outpatient scans, a designated sedation nurse with special training or experience in pediatric sedation usually fills this role. A physician should be present during drug administration but does not need to remain in the control room unless using an agent, such as propofol, that is administered by constant infusion. However, a physician who is trained in pediatric advanced life support and capable of performing endotracheal intubation must be immediately available. Therefore, if the scanner is not readily accessible from the emergency department for emergency department patients, the emergency physician may be required to remain with the child during the scan. In the outpatient setting, if the radiologist does not have the necessary training and skills, an anesthesiologist or other physician with training in pediatric advanced life support and advanced airway skills must be present.

PHARMACOLOGY

When choosing an agent to sedate a child for an imaging procedure, the clinician must consider the child's age, weight, acute and chronic medical problems, and the type of scan being performed. In addition, the need for intravenous (IV) contrast and the difficulty associated with obtaining IV accesses will impact the choice of the sedating agent and the route of administration (Table 21.1).

OPIOIDS

Opioids should be avoided for painless imaging procedures because they increase the risk of adverse effects, particularly respiratory depression. When opioid analgesia is desired (i.e., interventional radiologic procedure or when a reversal agent is needed), intravenous fentanyl is recommended because of its rapid onset and short duration of action, ease of titration, and established safety record in the

Table 21.1. Agents for Radiologic Imaging

Agent	Class	Route	Usual Total Dose[a]	Onset	Duration[b]	Comments
Fentanyl (Sublimase)	Opioid	IV	2–4 µg/kg	1–2 min	20–30 min	Use only when analgesia required.
Midazolam (Versed)	Benzodiazepine	IV	0.05–0.15 mg/kg	1–2 min	30 min	Bezodiazepines do not consistently prevent movement; therefore, they are not recommended as first line agents for radiologic imaging. They may be used as an adjunct to other sedation strategies.
		IM	0.05–0.15 mg/kg	2–5 min	30–40 min	
		PO	0.5–0.75 mg/kg	15–20 min	45–60 min	
		PR	0.5–0.75 mg/kg	10–15 min	45 min	
		IN	0.2–0.5 mg/kg	10–15 min	45 min	
Methohexital (Brevital)	Barbiturate	IV	0.75–1.0 mg/kg	<1 min	5–10 min	Disadvantage of the IM route is pain at the injection site. The PR route may decrease risk of cardiorespiratory complications associated with rapid IV administration. To reduce sedation failures (20 mg/kg) and adverse effects (30 mg/kg), the author recommends 25 mg/kg.
		IM	10 mg/kg	3–5 min	85 min	
		PR	20–30 mg/kg	5–10 min	60 min	
Pentobarbital	Barbiturate	IV	1–6 mg/kg	3–5 min	15–30 min	The IV route has shorter induction times and higher success rates than IM or PR routes. Given in increments of 1–2 mg/kg/dose.
Thiopental	Barbiturate	PR	25–50 mg/kg	12–30 min	90 min	Level of sedation is deeper than with rectal methohexital.

Drug	Class	Route	Dose[a]	Onset[b]	Duration[b]	Comments
Chloral hydrate	Nonbarbiturate sedative-hypnotic	PO	25–100 mg/kg	20–30 min	60 min	Prolonged sedation in up to 11% of children. Sedation failures are more common in older (3–4 years of age) and heavier (> 15 kg) children, and in those with underlying neurologic disease.
Ketamine (Ketalar)	Phencyclidine derivative	IV IM	1–1.5 mg/kg 4 mg/kg	1 min 5 min	15 min 15–30 min	Limited use for radiologic imaging because it is contraindicated in conditions that may be associated with increased intracranial pressure. Combination analgesia and sedation is an advantage for painful interventional procedures.
Propofol (Diprivan)	Alkylphenol derivative	IV	1.5 mg/kg, followed by continuous infusion at 25–125 µg/kg/min	< 1 min	1–10 min	Limited data on use by nonanesthesiologists.

[a]Doses provided are usual total doses.
[b]Times are approximate and may vary with dose.

outpatient setting. The recommended total dose of intravenous fentanyl is 2 to 4 μg/kg. However, the ultimate dose will depend on the child's pain threshold and level of anxiety, the procedure being performed, the concomitant use of other agents, and the presence of underlying medical problems. Achieving adequate analgesia without adverse effects should dictate the dose of fentanyl.

BENZODIAZEPINES

Benzodiazepines exhibit sedative, hypnotic, anxiolytic, amnestic, anticonvulsant, and muscle relaxant properties. In addition, they may be administered by multiple routes and are reversible. As a result, they are among the most widely used agents for sedating both children and adults for a variety of outpatient procedures. However, because they do not consistently prevent the child from moving, benzodiazepines alone are not recommended as first line agents for imaging procedures. In many institutions, benzodiazepines serve as a backup or adjunct when other agents have failed or when a reversible agent is needed.

BARBITURATES

Pentobarbital, methohexital, and thiopental are the most widely used barbiturates to sedate children for imaging procedures. However, long induction times (intramuscular [IM] route) and prolonged sleep have resulted in the diminished use of pentobarbital. Nevertheless, when prolonged sedation is required (i.e., multiple scans), pentobarbital may be an alternative to other agents. In these cases, the IV route is recommended because it has significantly shorter induction times and higher success rates.

In contrast, rapid onset of sleep with a low incidence of prolonged sedation, high success rates, and an excellent safety record have made methohexital a popular agent for imaging procedures. Because of its brief duration of action (approximately 10 minutes), the IV route of methohexital is best suited for short imaging studies such as cranial CT. The recommended dose of IV methohexital is 0.75 to 1.0 mg/kg. When a longer period of sedation is required, or IV access is either not possible or not required, methohexital may be given rectally. The rectal route offers high success rates, ease of administration, and high patient and parent acceptance. In addition, slower absorption helps circumvent the potential cardiorespiratory complications associated with the rapid IV administration of barbiturates. The dose of rectal methohexital ranges from 20 to 30 mg/kg. However, because the 20 mg/kg dose is associated with higher failure rates, and using 30 mg/kg increases the risk of adverse effects, the author recommends using 25 mg/kg. Intramuscular administration of methohexital (10 mg/kg) is also associated with a high success rate and a low incidence of adverse effects and is a good alternative when rectal administration is not possible. The major drawback to IM administration is pain at the injection site.

Thiopental has also been used to sedate children for radiologic imaging and is most often given rectally because the IV route frequently causes a profound dose-dependent respiratory depression. When given rectally, thiopental has an onset and duration of action longer than rectal methohexital. Thiopental also produces a deeper level of sedation, which may be an advantage when sedating children for MRI in which a deeper level of sedation might prevent awakening from associated scanner noise. The usual dose of rectal thiopental is 25 mg/kg; however, when needed, up to 50 mg/kg has been used.

OTHER SEDATIVE HYPNOTICS

Chloral Hydrate

Years of experience, ease of administration, and an excellent safety record have made chloral hydrate the most widely used sedative for children undergoing radiologic imaging. For years, the recommended dose of chloral hydrate for imaging procedures was 30 to 50 mg/kg. Although safe, these doses are associated with an unacceptably high failure rate. Recent studies using 70 to 100 mg/kg have demonstrated success rates in excess of 90% without significantly increasing adverse effects. However, at these higher doses, prolonged sedation (i.e., >2 hours) has been reported in as many as 11% of children. In addition, regardless of the dose, sedation failures are more common in older (more than 3 to 4 years of age) and heavier (more than 15 kg) children and in those with underlying neurologic disorders, particularly white matter disease. Therefore, the use of chloral hydrate should be avoided in these children. Long induction times (20 to 30 minutes) and prolonged sedation make chloral hydrate less desirable than other nonparenteral agents (i.e., rectal methohexital) for outpatient use.

Propofol

A rapid onset, short duration of action, and lack of prolonged or residual sedation suggest that IV propofol would be an ideal agent for sedating children during radiologic imaging. This has been supported by several studies, which have demonstrated that propofol provides effective sedation with a low incidence of adverse effects and extremely rapid recovery. However, the total number of patients enrolled in these studies was small (141 children), making it difficult to draw any firm conclusions regarding the safety and efficacy of propofol in this setting.

Most radiologists do not have the necessary training, skills, or experience to manage a child who requires endotracheal intubation or resuscitation. As a result, the use of propofol by radiologists to sedate children for imaging procedures has been called into question. In the studies previously described, propofol was administered by an anesthesiologist in all but 16 patients. Hence, it is unclear whether the results of these studies can be extrapolated to other physicians, particularly those unfamiliar with its use. Therefore, larger studies conducted by nonanesthesiologists are needed before propofol can be recommended for widespread use during radiologic imaging. However, if shown to be safe, propofol will undoubtedly become a popular agent, particularly among emergency physicians.

For radiologic imaging, the author recommends an initial bolus dose of 1.0 to 1.5 mg/kg, followed by additional doses of 0.5 mg/kg every 30 seconds until loss of consciousness occurs. Sedation is maintained by constant infusion at 25 μg/kg per minute. If the child moves, the infusion can be increased in 25 μg/kg/per minute increments as needed. Doses in excess of 125 μg/kg/per minute are seldom required.

DISSOCIATIVE AGENTS

Ketamine

Ketamine is a safe and effective agent for pediatric outpatient sedation and analgesia. Ketamine can be given by multiple routes and is one of only a few agents that are extremely predictable when administered intramuscularly. Furthermore, unlike benzodiazepines, barbiturates, and sedative/hypnotic agents, ketamine is a cardiovascular stimulant and seldom causes respiratory depression. For radiologic imaging, however, these favorable properties are often overshadowed by the fact that ketamine elevates intracranial pressure (ICP). This makes ketamine contraindicated in conditions that may be associated with elevated ICP, such as head trauma, hydrocephalus, and intracerebral masses. Unfortunately, these are common indications for imaging studies and, therefore, limit the use of ketamine in this setting. However, in the appropriate child, ketamine is a safe and effective agent for radiologic imaging. Because ketamine also provides excellent analgesia, it is especially useful for painful interventional imaging procedures.

Demerol, Promethazine, Chlorpromazine (DPT)

The combination of meperidine (Demerol), promethazine (Phenergan), and chlorpromazine (Thorazine), also know as DPT, or the "lytic" cocktail, has been popular as an analgesic and sedative to facilitate a variety of painful or anxiety-provoking procedures in children. However, for painless diagnostic imaging, meperidine is unnecessary and increases the risk of respiratory depression. Moreover, unacceptable rates of sedation failure, prolonged sedation times, and the possibility of dystonic reactions (from the combination of phenothiazines) argue against the use of DPT in any setting.

SUGGESTED READING

Accreditation Manual for Hospitals, Vol 1, 1998. Joint Commission on Accreditation of Healthcare Organizations. Oakbrook Terrace: Illinois, 1997.

Beekman RP, Hoorntje TM, Beek FJA, et al. Sedation for children undergoing magnetic resonance imaging: efficacy and safety of rectal thiopental. Eur J Pediatr 1996;155:820–822.

Bell C, Conte AH. Monitoring oxygenation and ventilation during magnetic resonance imaging: a pictorial essay. J Clin Monitoring 1996;12:71–74.

Billmire DA, Neale HW, Gregory RO. Use of IV fentanyl in the outpatient treatment of pediatric facial trauma. J Trauma 1985;25:1079.

Bloomfield EL, Masaryk TJ, Caplin A, et al. Intravenous sedation for MR imaging of the brain and spine in children: pentobarbital versus propofol. Radiology 1993;186:93–97.

Breedy R, Spear R, Fisher B, et al. Propofol infusion: dose-response for CT scans in children (abstract). Anesth Analg 1992;74:S36.

Cauldwell CB, Fisher DM. Sedating pediatric patients: is propofol a panacea? Radiology 1993;186:9–10.

Chudnofsky CR, Lozon M. Sedation and analgesia for procedures. In: Rosen P, et al, eds. Emergency Medicine: Concepts and Clinical Practice. 4th ed. St. Louis: Mosby Year Book, 1998:301–313.

Chudnofsky CR, Pomeranz ES, Lozon MM, et al. Rectal methohexital sedation for CT imaging of pediatric patients in the ED (abstract). Acad Emerg Med 1997;4:383.

Cote CJ. Sedation for the pediatric patient. Pediatr Clin North Am 1994;41:31–57.

Cotsen MR, Donaldson JS, Uejima T, et al. Efficacy of ketamine hydrochloride sedation in children for interventional radiologic procedures. AJR 1997;169:1019–1022.

Coventry DM, Martin CS, Burke AM. Sedation for paediatric computerized tomography-a double-blind assessment of rectal midazolam. Eur J Anaesth 1991;8:29–32.

Egelhoff JC, Ball WS Jr, Koch BL, et al. Safety and efficacy of sedation in children using a structured sedation program. AJR 1997;168:1259–1262.

Glasier CM, Stark JE, Brown R, et al. Rectal thiopental sodium for sedation of pediatric patients undergoing MR and other imaging studies. Am J Neuroradiol 1995;16:111–114.

Green R. Clearer images in pediatric MRI. Canadian Nurse 1995;91:47–48.

Green SM, Johnson NE. Ketamine sedation for pediatric procedures: part 2, review and implications. Ann of Emerg Med 1990;19:1033–1046.

Green SM, Nakamura R, Johnson NE. Ketamine sedation for pediatric procedures: part 1, a prospective series. Ann Emerg Med 1990;19:1024–1032.

Greenberg SB, Faerber EN, Aspinall CL. High dose chloral hydrate sedation for children undergoing CT. J of Comput Assist Tomogr 1991;15:467–469.

Greenberg SB, Faerber EN, Aspinall CL, et al. High-dose chloral hydrate sedation for children undergoing MR imaging: safety and efficacy in relation to age. AJR 1993;161:639–641.

Griswold JD, Liu LMP. Rectal methohexital in children undergoing computerized cranial tomography and magnetic resonance imaging scans (abstract). Anesthesiology 1987;67:A494.

Hollman GA, Elderbrook MK, VanDenLangenberg B. Results of a pediatric sedation program on head MRI scan success rates and procedure duration times. Clin Pediatr 1995; 34:300–305.

Holshouser BA, Hinshaw DB Jr, Shellock FG. Sedation, anesthesia, and physiologic monitoring during MR imaging: evaluation of procedures and equipment. JMRI 1993;3:553–558.

Hubbard AM, Markowitz RI, Kimmel B, et al. Sedation for pediatric patients undergoing CT and MRI. J Comput Assist Tomogr 1992;16:3–6.

Keeter S, Benator RM, Weinberg SM, et al. Sedation in pediatric CT: national survey of current practice. Radiology 1990;175:745–752.

Lefever EB, Potter PS, Seeley NR. Propofol sedation for pediatric MRI. Anesth Analg 1993;76:919–920.

Malis DJ, Burton DM. Safe pediatric outpatient sedation: the chloral hydrate debate revisited. Otolaryngol Head Neck Surg 1997;116:53–57.

Manuli MA, Davies L. Rectal methohexital for sedation of children during imaging procedures. AJR 1993;160:577–582.

Marti-Bonmati L, Ronchera-Oms CL, Casillas C, et al. Randomised double-blind clinical trial of intermediate- versus high-dose chloral hydrate for neuroimaging of children. Neuroradiology 1995;37:687–691.

Mitchell AA, Louik C, Lacouture P, et al. Risks to children from computed tomographic scan premedication. JAMA 1982;247:2385–2388.

Pereira JK, Burrows PE, Richards HM, et al. Comparison of sedation regimens for pediatric outpatient CT. Pediatr Radiol 1993;23:341–344.

Petrack EM, Marx CM, Wright MS. Intramuscular ketamine is superior to meperidine, promethazine, and chlorpromazine for pediatric emergency department sedation. Arch Pediatr Adolesc Med 1996;150:676–681.

Pruitt JW, Goldwasser MS, Sabol SR, et al. Intramuscular ketamine, midazolam, and glycopyrrolate for pediatric sedation in the emergency department. J Oral Maxillofac Surg 1995;53:13–17.

Ronchera-Oms CL, Casillas C, Marti-Bonmati L, et al. Oral chloral hydrate provides effective and safe sedation in paediatric magnetic resonance imaging. J Clin Pharm Ther 1994;19:239–243.

Rosenberg DR, Sweeney JA, Gillen JS, et al. Magnetic resonance imaging of children without sedation: preparation with simulation. J Am Acad Child Adolesc Psychiatry 1997;36:853–859.

Rumm PD, Takao RT, Fox DJ, et al. Efficacy of sedation of children with chloral hydrate. South Med J 1990;83:1040–1043.

Sacchetti A, Schafermeyer R, Gerardi M, et al. Pediatric analgesia and sedation. Ann Emerg Med 1994;23:237–250.

Slovis TL, Parks C, Reneau D, et al. Pediatric sedation: short-term effects. Pediatr Radiol 1993;23:345–348.

Terndrup TE, Dire DJ, Madden CM, et al. A prospective analysis of intramuscular meperidine, promethazine, and chlorpromazine in pediatric emergency department patients. Ann Emerg Med 1991;20:31–35.

Valtonen M. Anaesthesia for computerised tomography of the brain in children: a comparison of propofol and thiopentone. Acta Anaesthesiol Scand 1989;33:170–173.

Vangerven M, Wouters P, Vandermeersch E, et al. Total intravenous anesthesia with propofol and without intubation for magnetic resonance imaging (MRI) in pediatric patients (abstract). Anesthesiology 1990;73:A1239.

Varner PD, Ebert JP, McKay RD, et al. Methohexital sedation of children undergoing CT scan. Anesth Analg 1985;64:643–645.

Weir MR, Segapeli JH, Tremper LJ. Sedation for pediatric procedures. Mil Med 1986;151:181–184.

Chapter 22
Sedation and Analgesia in Dental Office Practice

Annie Pham-Cheng, Howard Needleman

The specialty of pediatric dentistry has long been concerned with managing the pain and anxiety of children and adolescents requiring dental treatment. In the late 1970s, the American Academy of Pediatric Dentistry (AAPD) recognized the need to develop guidelines for the use of sedation and analgesia. The first of these guidelines was published in 1985 and lead to the development of similar guidelines in anesthesia and pediatrics. Currently, the AAPD sedation/analgesia guidelines closely mirror the American Society of Anesthesiologists (ASA) guidelines. In addition to these guidelines, the AAPD has developed a template of new definitions and characteristics for the levels of sedation to help dentists evaluate and monitor the sedated patient (Table 22.1).

SPECIAL CONSIDERATIONS

Indications for Systemic Sedation and Analgesia

Nonpharmacologic techniques are the primary interventions used to manage children receiving dental care. Pharmacologic interventions are used by pediatric dentists to treat difficult and/or young patients requiring extensive or complex dental procedures. As many as 10% of the children brought into the dental office of pediatric dentists are not successfully managed by standard behavioral techniques and require sedation or analgesia.

The majority of children over 4 years old can be managed in the dental office using behavioral techniques such as tell/show/do, modeling, and positive reinforcement. Conversely, many children under the age of 4 require pharmacologic management for restorative or surgical dental procedures, in addition to the application of either block or infiltrative local anesthesia. Similarly, the child with special needs whose emotional, cognitive, or physical status is compromised often requires more than standard behavioral techniques to accept invasive dental

Table 22.1. Definitions and Characteristics of Levels of Sedation

Functional Level of Sedation	Anxiolysis Mild Sedation	Interactive	Noninteractive/Arousable with Mild/Moderate Stimulus	Noninteractive/Nonarousable Except with Intense Stimulus
Goal	Decrease anxiety; facilitate coping skills	Decrease or eliminate anxiety; facilitate coping skills	Decrease or eliminate anxiety; facilitate coping skills; promote sleep	Eliminate anxiety; coping skills over-ridden
Responsiveness	Uninterrupted interactive ability; totally awake	Minimally depressed level of consciousness; eyes open or temporarily closed; responds appropriately to verbal commands	Moderately depressed level of consciousness; mimics physiologic sleep (vitals not different from that of sleep); eyes closed most of the time; may or may not respond to verbal prompts alone; responds to mild/moderate stimuli (e.g., repeated trapezius pinching or needle insertion in oral tissues elicits reflex withdrawal and appropriate verbalization [complaint, moan, crying]); airway only occasionally may require readjustment via chin thrust	Deeply depressed level of consciousness; sleeplike state, but vitals may be slightly depressed compared with physiologic sleep; eyes closed; does not respond to verbal prompts alone; reflex withdrawal with no verbalization when intense stimuli occurs (e.g., repeated prolonged and intense pinching of the trapezius); airway expected to require constant monitoring and frequent management

Personnel	2	2	2	3
Monitoring Equipment	Clinical observation	PO$_x$; precordial recommended[a]	PO$_x$; precordial; BP; CA desirable[a]	PO$_x$; CA; precordial; BP; ECG Defibrillator desirable
Monitoring information	None	HR, RR, O$_2$ presedation; during (q 15 min); post as needed	Continuous HR, RR, O$_2$, BP, [CO$_2$] if available presedation; during (q 10 min); post until stable/discharge criteria	Continuous HR, RR, O$_2$, [CO$_2$], BP presedation; during (q 5 min); post until stable/discharge criteria

BP, blood pressure cuff; CA, capnography; ECG, electrocardiograph; HR, heart rate; PO$_x$, pulse oximetry; precordial, precordial stethescope; RR, respiratory rate.

[a]"Recommended" and "desirable" imply use as an adjunct in assessing patient status, not a necessity.

Adapted from AAPD.

Table 22.2.   Selection Criteria for Pharmacologic Intervention

Age
- Younger than 4 years
- Any age for noxious or invasive intra-oral procedures

Behavior
- Separation anxiety
- Short attention span
- Inability to understand simple commands or follow directions

Special needs
- Language barrier
- Learning disability

Medical status
- ASA Class I or II

Extent of dental work
- Operative time 45 minutes or less per session
- Requires less than the maximum dose of local anesthesia

Noxious and/or extensive dental procedures
- Extensive restorative procedures, e.g., crowns, root canals
- Traumatic dental injuries, e.g., crown fractures, displacements, avulsions
- Incision and drainage of dentoalveolar infections
- Oral and maxillofacial surgery, e.g., removal or exposure of impacted teeth, frenectomy, suturing of traumatic lacerations

Table 22.3.   Contraindications to Sedation/Analgesia in Pediatric Dental Patients

- ASA Class > II (anesthesia consult recommended)
- Extensive restorative needs
- Upper respiratory infection; nasal congestion; cough; severe pulmonary disease
- Psychoses
- Nasal congestion; mouth breathing habit
- Increased risk for pulmonary aspiration of gastric contents (gastroesophageal reflux, extreme obesity)

procedures. Pediatric dentists also use pharmacologic interventions on some healthy older children when the procedure itself is particularly noxious or frightening, such as exposure or removal of an impacted tooth. Table 22.2 lists the criteria used to select pediatric dental patients for pharmacologic intervention. The contraindications to sedation/analgesia in the pediatric dental patient are listed in Table 22.3.

Airway Management

Because the operative site for dental care is the oral cavity, consideration must be given to airway maintenance and patency. Special attention must be paid to preventing occlusion of the airway by manipulating the neck and retruding the tongue during the dental procedure. In addition, special care must be provided to prevent foreign objects such as dental materials, tooth fragments, and small dental devices from falling into the oropharynx during the procedure. The dental rubber dam greatly reduces this risk of aspiration.

Topical and Local Anesthetics

Local anesthetics remain the key to painless intra-oral hard and soft tissue dental procedures. Topical anesthetics such as benzocaine (5 or 20% gel) and the innovative Dentipatch® system (46.1 mg of lidocaine on a 2 cm² adhesive patch) are frequently used by dentists before local injection of lidocaine. Current investigation into the use of EMLA cream for mucosal analgesia may eventually provide a more powerful topical anesthetic for dentists. The emulsion droplet concentration of lidocaine and prilocaine in EMLA is approximately 80%, compared with the 20% maximum of a topical containing lidocaine alone.

Although their systemic absorption is rapid, topical anesthetics rarely are used alone for painful dental procedures because of their slower rate of onset, shorter duration, and poor penetration into the dental pulp. Local injection or block injection of anesthetics such as lidocaine are still required to provide complete dental anesthesia. When used in conjunction with sedative drugs, especially when sedative agents are used in combination, local anesthetics have been correlated with an increase in intra-operative morbidity and mortality. Therefore, it is especially important that the amount of local anesthetic administered not exceed the recommended dosage based on the child's weight (see Chapter 8).

PHARMACOPOEIA

Tables 22.4 and 22.5 list the common sedative/analgesic agents, dosages, and combinations currently used in pediatric dentistry. It is important to note that drug combinations are mainly used in hospital-based pediatric dental programs and less used in private practices. The selection of the individual or combination drugs to be used is primarily determined by the dental practitioner. Previous pediatric dentistry training, familiarity with the sedatives, perceived success and safety of the regimen as reported in the literature, and confidence in managing adverse effects are several of the factors affecting drug selection. In addition to the combination of oral sedatives, nitrous oxide is frequently used as an adjunct. Nitrous oxide can be easily titrated depending on the noxious level of the dental procedures (e.g., local injection, rubber dam clamp placement).

Although dental procedures are limited in number and are similar in nature (i.e., local anesthetics followed by tooth preparation and restoration, or local anesthetic followed by extraction), there are a few different combinations of sedative drugs (Table 22.5). The ideal combination of agents, which provides sufficient working time (30–60 minutes), easy administration and titration, and relative safety that does not require the support of anesthesiology or nursing staff, has not been found. Combinations involving opioids or neuroleptics may provide longer working time

Table 22.4. Drugs Commonly Used for Sedation/Analgesia in Pediatric Dentistry

Agents	Route/Dose
Antihistamines	
Diphenhydramine	PO: 1.25 mg/kg
Hydroxyzine	PO: 1–2 mg/kg
	IM: 0.6 mg/kg
Barbiturates	
Pentobarbital	PO: 2 mg/kg
Benzodiazepines	
Diazepam	PO: 0.3–0.5 mg/kg
	IV: 0.2 mg/kg
Midazolam	PO: 0.3–0.7 mg/kg
	IM: 0.04–0.1 mg/kg
Dissociative agents	
Ketamine	IV: 1–2 mg/kg (for 10–15 min working time)
Local anesthetics	
Lidocaine	2% with 1:100,000 epinephrine (maximum: 4 mg/kg)
Neuroleptics	
Chlorpromazine	PO/IM: 0.25–0.5 mg/kg
	PR: 0.5–1 mg/kg
	IV: 0.5–2 mg
Promethazine	PO: 1–2 mg/kg
	IM: 1 mg/kg
Nitrous oxide	40–60% N_2O/O_2
Opioids	
Fentanyl	IV: 1–4 µg/kg
Meperidine	PO: 1–3 mg/kg
	IM: 1–1.5 mg/kg
	IV: 1–2 mg/kg
Sedative/Hypnotic	
Chloral hydrate	PO: 50–55 mg/kg (maximum: 1 gm)

Table 22.5.   Indications for Common Drug Combinations Used in Pediatric Dental Practice

Procedures	Combinations	Route/Dose
Age: < 3 y Treatment: < 30 min Behavior: moderately difficult to approach Weight: < 20 kg	Chloral hydrate Hydroxyzine	PO/PR: 55 mg/kg PO: 2 mg/kg
Age: > 2 years Treatment: < 30 min Behavior: difficult to approach	Meperidine Promethazine	IM: 1.1 mg/kg IM: 1.1 mg/kg
Age: > 3 y Treatment: 30–60 min Behavior: moderate to very difficult; disruptive Weight: > 20 kg	Chloral hydrate Meperidine Hydroxyzine	PO: 30–50 mg/kg PO: 1 mg/kg PO: 25 mg

Age: > 6 y
Treatment: < 30 min
 	
Behavior: moderate anxiety; special needs
   (e.g., cerebral palsy)
	Diazepam
	Fentanyl
		PO: 0.25 mg/kg
		SL: 4 μg/kg 1 h after
		   diazepam

SL, sublingual.

and predictability but carry more liability. Hypnotic/antihistamine combinations are usually safer, although less predictable in terms of success.

Nitrous Oxide

The majority of private pediatric dental offices limit sedation/analgesia to the inhalation route using a mixture of nitrous oxide and oxygen. In a 1993 survey of all active and fellow AAPD members in the United States and Canada, nitrous oxide was reported to be the most popular (89%) sedation/analgesia regimen. Nitrous oxide analgesia alone was employed more than five times per week by a majority of pediatric dentists. The AAPD also reported that 20% or less of their patients required either nitrous oxide alone or a combination of nitrous oxide with other sedative agents. Sedative agents in combination with nitrous oxide were used less often than nitrous oxide alone, which was similar to findings of a 1991 survey.

Nitrous oxide in combination with oxygen is the most popular agent used because of its relative safety and reliability in controlling a patient's behavior. This combination has several advantages such as its rapid induction and emergence rates and ease of titration. Nitrous oxide with oxygen is also relatively safe, universally accepted, nonthreatening, and inexpensive. Children receiving an appropriate mixture of nitrous oxide (40–60%) and oxygen (40–60%) remain awake, responsive to verbal commands, and mildly insensitive to pain. Although a useful adjunct to behavioral intervention, nitrous oxide can only be effective if the child accepts the placement of the nasal inhaler and understands basic commands. Children less than 3 years of age and those who are extremely apprehensive seldom accept the nasal mask. In these cases, the use of oral or rectal sedation/analgesia in addition to, or instead of, nitrous oxide is indicated.

Enteral Agents

Enteral (oral or rectal) sedation in combination with nitrous oxide is used both in private offices and hospital-based clinics to manage the difficult pediatric dental patients for whom nitrous oxide alone proves insufficient. A common regimen to promote sleep includes the use of chloral hydrate, hydroxyzine, and nitrous oxide.

If the child refuses oral administration of a sedative, the rectal route can be used. Routinely, this route is used only if patient compliance, gagging, and vomiting preclude the patient from taking medication orally. Drug effect tends to be erratic with rectal administration because of the variable rate and amount of absorption.

Parenteral Agents

The parenteral route is not commonly used in private pediatric dental offices because of documented dangers and the lack of training received in pediatric dental training programs. Although didactics in pharmacology and a rotation in anesthesiology are required during their training, pediatric dentists usually do not gain sufficient training and experience in parenteral sedation to make them comfortable using this route in their office practice. In addition, dental office staff may not be trained sufficiently to monitor and assist during a parenteral sedation. When the parenteral route is used, pediatric dentists usually involve an anesthesiologist to medically screen the patients, deliver the sedative agents, and monitor the patients during and after the procedure.

Guidelines

Since the introduction of the AAPD sedation guidelines, many pediatric dentists have discontinued the use of enteral and parenteral agents in their private offices. Similarly, the overall use of analgesia/sedation has decreased in pediatric dental training programs, with a large decrease in the use of the parenteral routes, and a modest increase in the oral route and the use of general anesthesia. These changes are primarily because of changes in state legislation of sedation, rising professional liability malpractice insurance premiums, and adoption of sedation guidelines requiring additional monitoring equipment, personnel, recording, and documentation.

Although clear monitoring guidelines exist within the AAPD sedation guidelines, specific recommendations differ from those guidelines established by other organizations such as the American Academy of Pediatrics. The most obvious differences exist in the explicit or implicit requirements for the monitoring of patients when nitrous oxide is used alone. In the 1993 survey of AAPD members, 74% did *not* use any monitoring when using nitrous oxide alone, whereas 90% did use monitoring when using nitrous oxide in combination with other agents. The pulse oximeter was the single most commonly used monitoring device, and the most frequent combination of monitors was the pulse oximeter, blood pressure cuff, and precordial stethoscope.

Most recently, the guidelines for monitoring sedated patients has been revised by the AAPD. The new guidelines highlight the sedative state as a continuum and clearly state the minimum recommendations in monitoring to ensure patient safety and minimize the dentist's liability. The minimum recommended monitoring devices include the precordial stethoscope and pulse oximeter (Table 22.1). Once the patient is sedated, if the possibility of a minimally depressed level of consciousness exists, blood pressure and capnography should be added to pulse oximetry and precordial stethoscope. Continuous monitoring and frequent visual examinations are recommended, requiring at least an operator and an additional trained person to read the monitors.

SUGGESTED READING

Acs G, Musson CA, Burke MJ. Current teaching of restraint and sedation in pediatric dentistry: a survey of program directors. Pediatr Dent 1990;12:364–367.

de Jong RH. Physiology and Pharmacology of Local Anesthetics. Springfield: Charles C Thomas, 1970.

Goodson JM, Moore PA. Life-threatening reactions after pedodontic sedation: an assessment of narcotic, local anesthetic, and antiemetic drug interaction. J Am Dent Assoc 1983;107: 239–245.

Guidelines for the elective use of pharmacologic conscious sedation and deep sedation in pediatric dentistry. Pediatr Dent 1997;19:48–52 (Special issue: Reference Manual).

Lu D. The use of hypnosis for smooth sedation induction and reduction of postoperative violent emergencies from anesthesia in pediatric dental patients. ASDC J Dent Child 1994; 61:182–185.

Needleman HL, Joshi A, Griffith DG. Conscious sedation of pediatric dental patients using chloral hydrate, hydroxyzine, and nitrous oxide—a retrospective study of 382 sedations. Pediatr Dent 1995;17:424–431.

Wilson S. Patient monitoring in the conscious sedation of children for dental care. Curr Opin Dent 1991;1:570–575.

Wilson S, Creedon RL, George M, et al. A history of sedation guidelines: where we are heading. Pediatr Dent 1996;18:194–199.

Wilson S. A survey of the American Academy of Pediatric Dentistry membership: nitrous oxide and sedation. Pediatr Dent 1996;18:287–293.

Chapter 23
Procedural Sedation for Patients with Special Health Needs

Alfred Sacchetti, Michael Gerardi

*Editor's note: Consultation with an anesthesiologist is
recommended for ASA class III and IV patients.*

The sedation of a child with special health needs should be approached no differently than the sedation of any other child. The selection of an appropriate sedation agent is determined by the indications for sedation, the child's acute problem, the outpatient facility's capabilities, and the child's underlying medical or psychiatric conditions. There exists a temptation to limit pharmacologic interventions in children with special health care needs to avoid disrupting a perceived fragile medical or mental baseline. In fact, a well-designed pharmacologic approach is safer than forcibly attempting a procedure or avoiding a study altogether. This chapter will review the approach to sedation and control of children with special health care needs.

BEHAVIORAL, DEVELOPMENTAL, AND PSYCHIATRIC PATIENTS

Management Principles

Patients with behavioral, developmental, or psychiatric disorders (BDP) may perceive the outpatient facility or emergency department differently than other age-appropriate children. Benign conditions may be threatening, minor procedures may be intolerable, and simple actions by personnel may precipitate dramatic and unexpected responses. This immature reaction may persist into adolescence and adulthood, leading to an uncooperative patient who is physically incapable of being forcibly immobilized as is often done with an infant or toddler.

Making an early commitment to use pharmacologic management is important in dealing with children with BDP disorders. A failed attempt at a procedure may sensitize a child and make any further interactions much more difficult. However, appropriate use of sedatives in behaviorally challenged children will increase the probability of successful completion of the procedure with a minimum of anxiety or discomfort to the patient.

Selection of sedative analgesic agents for children with BDP disorders should depend on both the underlying problem and the indications for the sedation. Many children with BDP disorders may already be on medications with sedative/hypnotic properties as part of their daily treatment regimen. In these children, it may be possible to simply increase the dose of one of these agents to produce an increased degree of sedation. A careful interview with the caretaker may identify those patients who would be candidates for this approach. If the child demonstrates increased drowsiness after the normal dose of the sedative agent, then simply providing a larger dose of the medication may provide adequate procedural sedation. The advantage of this approach is that it limits the problems encountered with combining agents with similar adverse actions. A similar effect can be produced by sleep depriving children who generally take a nap and scheduling the diagnostic study during the nap time.

If the parent or caretaker relates no discernible effects with administration of the child's medications, then that child may have developed a tolerance to the sedative properties of the agent. In these instances, sedation may be best accomplished by picking a drug with a different mechanism of action or different metabolic pathway. For example, a child on chronic barbiturate therapy may not be sensitive to drugs that work through the gamma-aminobutyric acid (GABA) receptor such as barbiturates or benzodiazepines. Sedation of these children may require large doses of these drugs. Drugs that operate through a different mechanism, such as propofol or chloral hydrate, might be considered as an alternative. A heightened sensitivity should be kept for the possibility of additive adverse effects when combining different agents.

The appropriate dosing is especially important in patients with BDP disorders. Just as with any child, a suboptimal dose of any sedating agent may only disinhibit the child and produce uncontrolled agitated behavior. In children with limited impulse control such a loss of any emotional or behavioral restraint can be troublesome. Again, this may be compounded with stronger older children.

Children with behavioral or developmental problems may not be able to articulate complaints of pain well and are at risk for oligoanalgesia. In many instances, a change from a stable behavioral pattern may be the only means by which such a child can communicate the presence of pain. As a general rule, any condition that would prompt the use of an opioid in an adult should prompt the same pain management in a child with BDP disorders. Analgesia for extremely painful conditions, such as postfracture care, is best provided by an opioid. Unlike the sedatives, these agents do not tend to disinhibit children and have no special restrictions in children with BDP disorders. For less painful conditions, acetaminophen or a nonsteroidal anti-inflammatory agent (e.g., ibuprofen, ketorolac) is appropriate.

OPTIONS FOR DRUG DELIVERY

Intravenous

The route of drug administration in children with BDP disorders is a deciding factor in selecting an appropriate agent(s). The intravenous (IV) route permits titration, rapid administration, the ability to combine different agents, and an easy means to add supplemental doses if the procedure exceeds the expected treatment time. Although, securing the access site may be extremely difficult in this population. In infants and small children, restraint of an extremity by an assistant is adequate to obtain IV access. Older, stronger children may require multiple assistants to obtain enough control to complete the procedure. The greater strength of these children may be offset by their relatively larger, more easily cannulated veins. Pretreatment with a topical anesthetic such as EMLA cream may permit easier IV placement in conjunction with distraction of the patient.

Intramuscular

Intramuscular (IM) injections are an alternative means of delivering parenteral medications in patients with BDP disorders. The advantage of this route is that the injection need not be as precisely placed as with an intravenous attempt, allowing a more rapid puncture in a struggling child or adolescent. The IM route also permits a child to be distracted and the needle introduced with no prior visualization or lead in. One disadvantage to this route is that the injection will still leave the child agitated, requiring physical restraint or comforting until the medication takes effect. Additionally, if an ineffective dose was delivered, the child will need to undergo a second injection while still excited. The child will also be more suspicious with a second injection, limiting the usefulness of distraction or deception maneuvers. These problems may be greatly amplified if the initial injection produces a disinhibited state.

Enteral

Enteral medications have the advantage of providing a nonthreatening delivery route while avoiding the use of "frightening" needles. However, both oral and rectal medications exhibit erratic absorption, variable efficacy, and prolonged onset times. In instances in which an extended lead time is present, such as with a scheduled outpatient diagnostic study, an oral preparation may be the optimum route of delivery. If an agent with a reliable dose response profile is selected, then a dose may be administered at a set time before the study, allowing for adequate preparation of the child.

Inhalational

The inhalation agent nitrous oxide has a number of advantages in children who are able to cooperate with the delivery systems. The safest inhalation systems are those that employ some form of self-delivery system (e.g., demand valve mask). Unfortunately, the nature of some children with behavioral or developmental problems may preclude their ability to use inhalation masks or nasal cannula.

Nonpharmacologic Interventions

Behavior modification, hypnosis, diversions, and distractions are of some value in the management of most patients with BDP disorders, depending on patients' attention spans and abilities to cooperate. These techniques have been documented as effective in children with behavioral problems undergoing dental procedures, but the time requirements involved in these applications may make them impractical in outpatient settings such as the emergency department.

SELECTING THE APPROPRIATE AGENT

Ketamine

Agents with overt psychological actions or those with unreliable actions should be avoided in patients with BDP disorders. Ketamine is one agent that should be used with caution in children with psychiatric problems. The hallucinogenic properties of this drug and its potential for emergence reactions limit its application in this population. In circumstances in which ketamine must be used, a benzodiazepine should be added to depress awareness until the effects of ketamine have dissipated.

For nonpainful diagnostic procedures, short-acting sedatives may be the best treatment option. Agents to consider in this class include barbiturates, benzodiazepines, propofol, and chloral hydrate.

Pentobarbital

The barbiturate pentobarbital, which has a reliable therapeutic profile, rapid onset time and short duration of action, is an excellent agent for these patients in the IM or IV routes.

Propofol

Propofol may prove to be an excellent option for short-term sedation of patients with BDP disorders, although currently no data exist on its use for children undergoing procedural sedation in the emergency department. The ability of propofol to be carefully titrated in conjunction with a short half-life allows precise control of sedation for procedures.

Benzodiazepines

The benzodiazepines possess pure sedative properties similar to those of the barbiturates. One major limitation of the benzodiazepines in patients with BDP disorders is the large therapeutic window associated with this class of agents. As noted earlier, doses at the low end of the therapeutic range produce disinhibition and exaggeration of excited behavior. If a benzodiazepine is selected, an adequate dose should be used to ensure the desired effect.

Chloral Hydrate

Given enough lead time, chloral hydrate may be used effectively in children with BDP disorders who are undergoing painless diagnostic procedures, especially radiologic imaging.

Transmucosal Fentanyl

Transmucosal fentanyl ("lollipops") has been successful as a nonparenteral agent but its high rate of emesis limits it effectiveness in these patients. The combination of droperidol with transmucosal fentanyl does limit emesis and provides an effective sedative analgesic combination.

CHILDREN WITH SPECIAL HEALTH NEEDS

As with children with BDP disorders, patients with physical or medical conditions may require special considerations in their sedation and analgesia management. Table 23.1 summarizes the physiologic effects of the different sedative and analgesic agents used to treat children with special health care needs.

The approach to children with special health needs begins with an appreciation of both the presenting condition and the child's underlying problem. Caretakers should be questioned concerning allergies and adverse reactions to medications in the past. The use of the term allergies is useful because many parents will classify any untoward reaction to a medication as an allergic reaction. Parents may also be able to provide information on what sedative or analgesics have worked successfully in prior situations. Ideally, these children will be identified with some form

Table 23.1. Physiologic Effects of Sedative and Analgesic Agents

Medication	Systemic Vascular Resistance	Cardiac Output	Anticonvulsant Activity	Analgesic	Sedative	Respiratory Depressant	Specific Contraindications
Benzodiazepines							
Midazolam	<	0	>>	0	>>>	>>	
Diazepam	<	0	>>	0	>>	>	
Lorazepam	<	0	>>	0	>	>	
Barbiturates							Caution with porphyria
Pentobarbital	0	0	>	0	>>	>>	
Thiopental	0	<	>>	½>	>>>	>>>	
Methohexital	0	<	>	½>	>>>	>>	
Opioids							
Morphine	<	0	0	>>	>	>>	
Fentanyl	0	0	0	>>>	>	>>	
Meperidine	<	0	0	>>	>	>	Accumulation of metabolites
Other							
Propofol	<	<	>	>	>>	>>	
Chloral hydrate	0	0	>	0	>>	>	
Ketamine	>	>	0	>>>	>>>	0	Increased intracranial pressure

>, increases; <, decreases.

of medical identification jewelry relating to an accessible data repository on the child. The child's present medications must also be examined for possible interactions. As with children with BDP disorders, if a child is already on a sedative medication, the safest approach may be to use this medication in an increased dose to provide sedation for the required procedure.

Consideration must be given to the fact that the agent(s) chosen for procedural sedation may change the metabolism of a child's maintenance medications. Single-dose therapy with a sedative or analgesic agent is unlikely to significantly alter a stable medication regimen; however, caution must be used with any agent that is prescribed for more extended use. Barbiturates are notorious for inducing hepatic enzymes, displacing protein-bound drugs, and altering the half-lives of multiple agents.

METABOLIC AND ENDOCRINE PATIENTS

The patient history is especially important in children with endocrine or metabolic abnormalities. Drugs may be metabolized differently, or unusually high levels of metabolic intermediaries may produce unexpected interactions in these patients. Children with enzymatic deficiencies and liver abnormalities are at particular risk for these types of problems. Almost all of the benzodiazepines, barbiturates, and opioids are metabolized to some extent through the liver. Most of the standard sedative and analgesic agents can be used in patients with liver abnormalities, but delayed metabolism and an extended duration of action should be expected and thus lower initial doses should be used. Propofol is unique among the sedatives in that although it is metabolized in the liver, its duration of action is not prolonged in patients with chronic hepatic or renal failure.

Children with inborn errors of metabolism are relatively unique and generally possess a specific metabolic pathway abnormality. Unlike patients with generalized liver problems, metabolic patients do not appear to have an increased risk from barbiturates, benzodiazepines, or opioids unless the patients have a specific defect in pathways that metabolizes these drugs. Children with porphyria are probably the best known example of children at risk for this type of reaction. These patients can develop hemolysis if administered barbiturates.

NEUROLOGIC ABNORMALITIES

Many patients with neurologic problems will also have some form of behavioral or developmental abnormalities. Other neurologic conditions that may appear in children requiring sedation and analgesia include seizure disorders, increased intracranial pressure, and shunts or other conditions requiring intracranial devices.

Most of the sedative agents used for procedural purposes have antiseizure properties and are safe to use in these patients. Barbiturates and propofol also possess intracranial pressure (ICP) lowering properties, which make them particularly useful for procedures in children with indwelling shunts. However, benzodiazepines have a relatively neutral effect on ICP in children; fentanyl has been shown to have variable effects on patients with elevated ICPs; and ketamine has been proven to elevate intracranial pressure. All three of these agents should be avoided in children in whom a suspicion of elevated ICP exists. In patients in whom a ventricular shunt is present and functioning, there is no real contraindication to the use of morphine, pentobarbital, or propofol.

Clinicians must be cautious not to oversedate these children when using agents possessing an accumulative action with their native medications. Oversedation with any drug can lead to hypoventilation resulting in hypercarbia, worsening ICP. Some anti-seizure medications have intrinsic sedative properties and the addition of a new sedative is probably best performed through intravenous titration.

Some form of sedative combined with a local anesthetic is strongly recommended to facilitate performance of a lumbar puncture in these children. The use of either a barbiturate or a benzodiazepine before beginning these procedures will enhance cooperation with positioning, especially in a child who has undergone multiple lumbar punctures. Ketamine has also been used successfully in performing lumbar punctures, although it is contraindicated for procedural sedation in patients with increased intracranial pressure.

CARDIOVASCULAR PROBLEMS

Patients with cardiovascular abnormalities may be divided into two groups: those with anatomic problems and those with myocardial problems. Pediatric cardiac patients with anatomic problems may be further subclassified into those having undergone a definitive repair and those with some form of temporizing or palliative procedure. Children who have received a definitive correction of their anatomic problem will generally have separate pulmonary and systemic circulations with relatively good oxygenation, if not near normal exercise tolerance. Unless an associated myocardial problem exists, these children will have few if any sedation or analgesic limitations. Drugs with potential cardiovascular depressant actions such as thiopental or propofol are not contraindicated but should be delivered slowly to allow the systemic vasculature to adjust gradually to any vasodilating properties. All other agents such as the benzodiazepines, opioids, barbiturates, benzodiazepines, chloral hydrate, and ketamine can be used relatively safely in this group. As with any child, hypovolemic or dehydrated cardiac patients should receive some form of intravenous rehydration before initiation of any drug with the potential to produce vasodilation andhypotension.

Pediatric cardiac patients with palliative procedures frequently have parallel pulmonary and systemic circulations. In these patients, admixing of blood occurs from the two circulations, which results in chronic hypoxia, polycythemia, and a physiologic univentricular heart equivalent. These patients require careful assessment and consultation with their cardiologist and an anesthesiologist as part of the presedation evaluation.

Children with myocardial problems, such as cardiomyopathy or myocarditis, are best managed with sedatives with minimal direct cardiovascular actions. Any of the pure sedatives have the potential to depress the myocardium or precipitously drop the systemic vascular resistance, thus stressing the pumping capacity of the heart. Fentanyl has little or no cardiovascular depressant actions and is an excellent sedative analgesic choice for these types of patients. Ketamine can also be used in these patients because its inherent sympathomimetic actions tend to negate any myocardial depressant actions of the drug. Children with myocardial problems are also more prone to congestive heart failure and passive liver dysfunction. Therefore, those patients should receive decreased doses of any sedative agent to guard against any prolonged actions from these agents.

RENAL PROBLEMS

Children with chronic renal failure generally do not present a major sedation or analgesia problem. Most of the sedative agents used in these patients are metabolized by the liver to inactive or less active forms that are excreted by the kidneys. Initial doses of medications will produce a minimal accumulation of metabolites, which will be cleared with the next course of peritoneal or hemodialysis. Repeated doses of sedative or analgesic agents may lead to symptomatic levels of metabolites, and any child receiving extended treatments should be monitored closely for signs of over accumulations.

Patients with hypertension are not considered a problem with the use of pure sedative or analgesic agents. Ketamine should be used with caution in these patients because it stimulates the release of catecholamines and may produce an increase in systemic blood pressure.

PULMONARY PROBLEMS

Oxygenation is the major concern in patients with underlying lung problems. Any of the sedatives have the potential to depress respirations and should be used with caution in these patients. Chronic lung problems should not be considered a contraindication to sedation, but only an indication that careful monitoring be maintained during and after the sedation. Ketamine, because of its bronchodilatory properties and rare respiratory depression, may be the ideal agent for use in these patients. Problems with increased secretions can be managed with either glycopyrrolate or atropine. Excessive drying and inspissation of mucus is not a problem with single-time use of these agents.

CHILDREN WITH CHRONIC PAIN CONDITIONS

Patients with medical conditions that render them susceptible to recurrent painful conditions frequently present to the emergency department during acute crises. Children with sickle cell disease, cancer, and any number of chronic debilitating diseases are at risk for painful events that cannot be managed with standard oral or outpatient medications. Unfortunately, many of these patients, especially older patients, may develop antagonistic relationships with medical staff secondary to frequent emergency department visits and suspicions of drug abuse. Because of the large emotional components involved in the care of these children, an objective, protocol-driven treatment plan is the safest and most humane approach to acute pain management in this population.

Children presenting with acute painful episodes should be examined quickly and carefully for a medical cause to their pain. Patients with sickle cell should be investigated for signs of infection, end organ ischemia, or infarction. Baseline hematologic parameters should be obtained including a complete blood and reticulocyte count. Patients with cancer also should be investigated for evidence of sepsis or hypoperfusion. In children with autoimmune disorders, evidence of early arthritis or inflammation may be sought with erythrocyte sedimentation rates or C-reactive protein levels. Children with long-standing abdominal problems including inflammatory bowel diseases, chronic obstructions, pancreatitis, and recurrent renal calculi should all be investigated for evidence of perforation or infection with serial abdominal examinations, diagnostic imaging, and laboratory studies as needed. The presence of abdominal pain does not preclude the use of opioids. The notion that opioids will mask significant intra-abdominal problems has never been proven, and a number of recent studies in adults have clearly shown this concept to be unfounded.

Measures to address a child's pain should begin simultaneously with any investigation of a relevant cause of the child's immediate problem. If possible, these children should have a preset analgesic regimen established in conjunction with their primary or subspecialty physician to address acute painful scenarios. These protocols should center on titratable regimens, preferably intravenous, with escalating doses depending on the child's response. Visual analog scales should be used whenever possible to quantify the child's pain status and progress. Older children may use patient-controlled analgesia pumps and devices to titrate their own level of comfort. The use of such protocols relieves the physician of having to wrestle with any emotional concerns that he or she is being manipulated by a patient with chronic pain. Private physicians should be encouraged to complete Emergency Data Sets detailing the analgesic management of their patients in the event a child presents to a department unfamiliar with the child's condition. It is more helpful for a patient to present a formal document with an analgesic regimen than to have the patient relay the information verbally. Many clinicians become suspicious and withhold medications when patients describe pain regimens involving opioids.

For new patients, a safe approach is to begin the child with a standard dose of morphine while the diagnostic studies are being completed. Demerol should be avoided in these children because of the risk of accumulation of the metabolite normeperidine with extended use of this agent.

Children with special health needs require as much or more sedation or analgesia than children without such problems. More liberal use of these agents results not only in more comfortable treatment but also safer treatment of these patients.

SUGGESTED READING

Bezold LI, Ayres NA. Sedation and monitoring during cardiac diagnostic procedures. In: Garson A, Bricker JT, Fisher DJ, et al, eds. The Science and Practice of Pediatric Cardiology. Baltimore: Williams & Wilkins 1998:1065–1080.

Egelhoff JC, Ball WS Jr, Koch BL, et al. Safety and efficacy of sedation in children using a structured sedation program. Am J Roentgenol 1997;68:1259–1262.

EMSC Task Force on Children with Special Health Care Needs. EMS for children: recommendations for coordinating care for children with special health care needs. Ann Emerg Med 1997;30:274–280.

LoVecchio F, Oster N, Sturmann K, et al. The use of analgesics in patients with acute abdominal pain. J Emerg Med 1997;15:775–779.

Malis DJ, Burton DM. Safe pediatric outpatient sedation: the chloral hydrate debate revisited. Otolaryngol Head Neck Surg 1997;116:53–57.

Pace S, Burke TF. Intravenous morphine for early pain relief in patients with acute abdominal pain. Acad Emerg Med 1996;3:1086–1092.

Sacchetti AD, Gerardi M, Barkin R, et al. Emergency data set for children with special needs. Ann Emerg Med 1996;28:324–327.

Sacchetti AD, Schafermeyer R, Gerardi M, et al. Pediatric analgesia and sedation. Ann Emerg Med 1994;23:237–250.

Silen W. Cope's early diagnosis of the acute abdomen. 19th ed. New York: Oxford University Press, 1996:5–6.

Chapter 24

Sedation and Analgesia for Trauma Patients

John Burton

A rational, evidence-based approach toward analgesia and sedation for acquired injuries and procedural pain in the trauma patient is a subject that has largely been ignored throughout trauma literature, education, and teaching. This observation is true for both the adult and pediatric trauma populations. The current standard of certification for assessment and management of the trauma patient, the American College of Surgeon's Advanced Trauma Life Support (ATLS) course, devotes little attention toward providing analgesia and sedation. Trauma patient management has historically emphasized rapid diagnosis and stabilization as the critical factors in trauma patients. Amidst the intense focus on assessment and stabilization, patient comfort frequently becomes lost in this paradigm.

Over the last 10 years, concern has increased for the needs of patients in acute pain and discomfort. This interest has prompted the development of clinical practice guidelines by the Department of Health and Human Services. Despite increased attention, studies continue to document the inadequate and untimely administration of analgesics to acutely injured patients.

Multiple studies have shown that pediatric patients are less likely to receive adequate pain control in comparison with adults. Pediatric trauma patients may also selectively suffer from increased neglect of pain and discomfort. If such a bias does exist, the causes likely include inaccurate perceptions by caregivers and parents of pediatric patients' pain; an inability or unwillingness of pediatric patients to request analgesia; and health professionals' fear of complications and inexperience in administering meaningful analgesia to children in the setting of acute trauma.

Despite these issues, comfort in the form of analgesics and sedatives (including the use of regional anesthesia) can be safely and meaningfully administered to acutely injured pediatric patients. A heightened attention toward safely relieving suffering in the acute trauma-care setting must be accompanied by a thorough knowledge of current analgesic and sedative agents, potential complications, and monitoring principles. Established treatment protocols specifically directed toward

Table 24.1.   Sedation and Analgesia Assessment in the Trauma Patient

1. Is the patient in pain?
2. What is the etiology/etiologies of the pain?
3. Is the patient hemodynamically stable?
4. What form of pain control is appropriate (regional, systemic, both)?
5. Would the patient benefit from anxiolysis?
6. What form of anxiolysis is appropriate (benzodiazepine, neuroleptic, both)?

relief of pain and suffering may further prompt the appropriate implementation of comfort-directed therapies (Table 24.1).

SPECIAL CONSIDERATIONS

The multitude and severity of potential injuries in any trauma patient mandates the need for a careful and thorough assessment before administering medications for relief of pain and anxiety. This directive assumes that the patient is alert and cooperative. Trauma patients with altered mental status or other injuries placing the patency and function of the airway at risk are considered unstable and thus are not candidates for systemic analgesia. These patients most likely require endotracheal intubation, with the choice of a sedative induction agent and neuromuscular blockade depending on the nature of the injuries the degree of hemodynamic stability. Patients who present with altered mental status secondary to intoxication or substance abuse (in contradistinction to altered mental status as a consequence of head injury, hypoxemia, or hypoperfusion) may also require preemptive sedation or chemical restraint to facilitate injury assessment and stabilization. The following examples are demonstrative of these situations and are meant to provide suggestions for commonly encountered difficult scenarios in the management and assessment of these patients. Review of drugs, profiles of agents, and comments regarding their use are not intended to be exhaustive or complete but rather to provide an overview of common medications and concerns. A general approach to the assessment and pharmacologic management of the trauma patient is illustrated in Figure 24.1 and Table 24.2.

MANAGEMENT OF PAIN IN THE HEMODYNAMICALLY UNSTABLE TRAUMA PATIENT (FIG. 24.2)

The hemodynamically unstable trauma patient presents a critical challenge to the clinician. The initial emphasis must be placed on attempts to diagnose the cause and extent of the patient's compromising injuries. Once this injury or injuries have been diagnosed, the emphasis must then focus on stabilization of the patient's con-

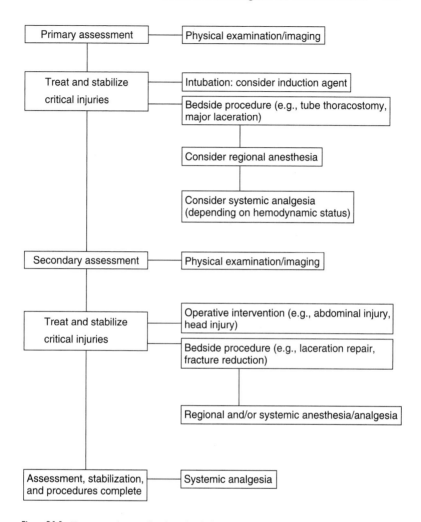

Figure 24.1. Trauma patient analgesic and sedative management in the emergency department.

dition and definitive procedures to correct the cause of instability. An example in this setting would be the diagnosis of compromising intra-abdominal injuries followed by rapid transfer to the operating room for definitive exploration and stabilization of identified injuries.

Once identification and stabilization of injuries has occurred, then the focus may shift toward analgesia and sedation. The absence of attempts to provide analgesia in this setting is justified by the immediate, life-threatening potential of an unstable trauma patient. Further, the implementation of systemic analgesic or sedative agents might predictably compromise the assessment and stability of the pa-

Table 24.2.   Drug Considerations in the Trauma Patient

Agent	Advantages	Disadvantages
Regional anesthesia		
Lidocaine	Minimal complications	Relatively short-acting (1–2 h)
Lidocaine with epinephrine	Hemostasis at site; epinephrine prolongs duration of lidocaine's effects	Contraindicated in areas at risk for ischemic injury
Bupivacaine	Long-acting	Relative longer onset of action (5–10 min)
Systemic analgesic		
Ketorolac	No significant cardiovascular/ neurologic effects	Expensive; mild analgesic effects; ↑ bleeding time
Fentanyl	Rapid onset; short-acting; easily titratable	Short-acting; chest wall rigidity (rare)
Morphine	Long duration (2–4 h)	↓ Central venous return; vasodilatation; ↓ BP
Meperidine	Long duration (2–4 h)	Toxic metabolites—normeperidine (seizures)
Ketamine	Analgesic/sedative effects; short-acting	Hypersalivation; emergence reactions; laryngospasm
Nitrous oxide	Analgesic and sedative effects; no significant cardiovascular effects; short-acting	Variable analgesic/sedative effects; requires apparatus
Systemic sedative		
Midazolam	Rapid onset; short-acting; easily titratable	Respiratory depression potentiated with other agents
Diazepam	Long-acting	Long-acting metabolites
Thiopental	Rapid onset; short-acting; neuroprotective	↓ Central venous return; ↓ BP
Methohexital	Rapid onset; short-acting	↓ Central venous return; ↓ BP
Ketamine	Analgesic/sedative effects; short-acting	Hypersalivation; emergence reactions; laryngospasm
Nitrous oxide	Analgesic and sedative effects; no significant cardiovascular effects; short-acting	Variable analgesic/sedative effects; requires apparatus

tient's condition. This belief, however, should not be a directive against appropriate use of regional anesthesia for selected injuries or induction agents when the decision to intubate an unstable patient is made.

Intravenous fentanyl or midazolam offers attractive hemodynamic profiles for the sedation of unstable patients after or apart from induction for endotracheal intubation. Both drugs have short onset times and short half-lives, with the added benefit of available reversal agents. Caution should be used with the common practice

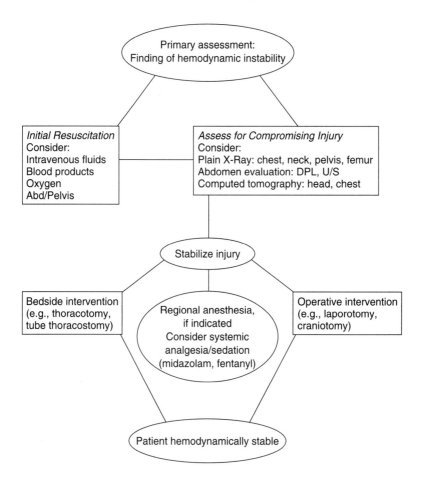

Figure 24.2. Management of pain in the hemodynamically unstable trauma patient.

of combining these drugs, which is often done in stable patients requiring analgesia and sedation for brief procedures. The combination of these drugs will frequently cause deterioration in the hemodynamic stability of the tenuous trauma patient because of enhanced negative inotropic function and decreased venous return.

MANAGEMENT OF PAIN IN THE TRAUMA PATIENT WITH ALTERED MENTAL STATUS (FIG. 24.3)

The possible etiologies of altered mental status in the trauma patient include the following: head injury, hypoxia from inadequate oxygenation, hypoxemia from

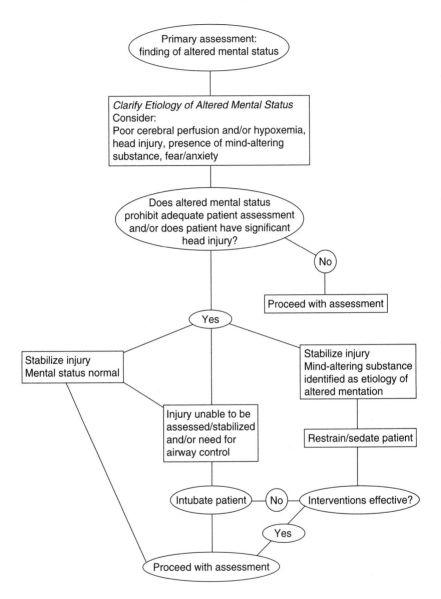

Figure 24.3. Management of pain in the trauma patient with altered mental status.

poor cerebral circulation, and mental status-altering substances (alcohol, cocaine, marijuana, etc.). The management of pain in the trauma patient with altered mental status is best undertaken once the etiology of the mental status changes is clarified. Initial efforts should therefore focus on identifying the etiology of the altered mental status as a prerequisite to analgesia or sedation. However, altered mental status can preclude an adequate assessment of the patient. When this occurs, the worst case scenario (typically intracranial head injury or hypoxemia) are the safest working diagnoses and may require endotracheal intubation to enhance oxygenation, protect the airway, and facilitate assessment of the patient's injuries.

MANAGEMENT OF PAIN IN THE COMBATIVE, INTOXICATED TRAUMA PATIENT (FIG. 24.4)

Intoxicated patients with traumatic injuries are frequently seen in the emergent setting. Unfortunately, many of these patients will become violent and threatening

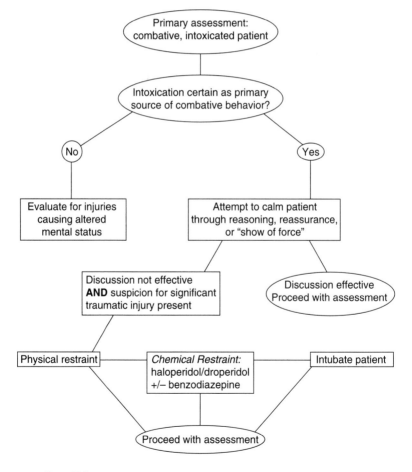

Figure 24.4. Management of pain in the combative, intoxicated trauma patient.

toward caregivers. Each physician must have a strategy for dealing with these difficult patients.

Considerations in formulating a management strategy for traumatic injuries (head injury, hypoxemia) resulting in combative behavior include the following: the nature of the injury, substances used by the patient, the physician's legal responsibility to the intoxicated patient, and the danger these patients represent to themselves and the medical staff. In this setting, aggressive attempts to intervene with chemical or physical restraints may ultimately be in the best interest of the patient. A reluctance to intervene, or a delay in intervention, can result in the physician missing significant traumatic and often life-threatening pathology.

Approaches to chemical or physical restraint to facilitate the trauma assessment vary. Intramuscular (IM) or intravenous (IV) neuroleptic agents (primarily the butyrophenones) are frequently employed after calm reasoning, reassurance, or shows of force fail to convince the patient to cooperate with medical treatment. Haloperidol (5–10 mg IM/IV) or droperidol (2.5–5 mg IM/IV) offer the advantages of minimal cardiovascular compromise and mild sedation in addition to antipsychotic effects. Many providers will use one or two doses of these agents in an attempt to calm or sedate the patient. Intramuscular lorazepam (1–2 mg IM/IV) may be used as a sedative adjunct to butyrophenones. Neuroleptics can also be combined with opioids for combative patients who require analgesia.

If all else fails, the final step in controlling the combative, intoxicated trauma patient is rapid sequence intubation. Choice of induction agents should account for hemodynamically compromising injuries or head injuries with an additional emphasis on rapid onset of induction and paralysis. This step, once employed, removes the combative altered mental status that poses a formidable obstacle to rapid assessment and stabilization of the trauma patient.

Once assessment and stabilization are complete, appropriate analgesia or sedation directed toward identified injuries may be considered. Ongoing sedation is probably best achieved by liberal use of benzodiazepines. In this setting, benzodiazepines offer the benefit of titratable sedation in addition to providing early treatment for withdrawal and central nervous system depression and raising the seizure threshold.

SUGGESTED READING

Acute Pain Management Guideline Panel. Acute pain management: operative and medical procedures and trauma. Clinical practice guidelines. AHCPR Pub. No. 92–0032. Rockville, MD: Agency for Health Care Policy and Research, Public Health Service. US Department of Health and Human Services, February 1992.

Algren JT, Algren CL. Sedation and analgesia for minor pediatric procedures. Ped Emerg Care 1996;12:435–441.

American College of Surgeons. Advanced Trauma Life Support. Course for Physicians. 5th ed. Chicago: American College of Surgeons, 1993.

Friedland LR, Kulick RM. Emergency department analgesic use in pediatric trauma victims with fractures. Ann Emerg Med 1994;23:203–207.

Friedland LR, Pancioli AM, Duncan KM. Pediatric emergency department analgesic practice. Pediatr Emerg Care 1997;13:103–106.

Gerardi MJ, Sacchetti AD, Cantor RM, et al. Rapid-sequence intubation of the pediatric patient. Ann Emerg Med 1996;28:55–74.

Goodacre SW, Roden RK. A protocol to improve analgesia use in the accident and emergency department. J Accid Emerg Med 1996;13:177–179.

Henretig FM, King C. Textbook of Pediatric Emergency Procedures. Baltimore: Williams & Wilkins, 1997.

Jylli L, Olsson GL. Procedural pain in a paediatric surgical emergency unit. Acta Paed 1995;84:1403–1408

Chapter 25
Sedation and Analgesia for Transport

George Woodward, Joel Fein

Pediatric transport can be divided into three general categories: prehospital (often performed by emergency medical services [EMS] personnel), interfacility, and intrafacility transport. The management of pain and anxiety is important in all three categories, but perhaps most relevant for the inter- and intrahospital settings. To maximize the usefulness and minimize the risks of sedation and analgesia during transport, one must be familiar with the transport environment, the patient's specific disease process, and the available options for sedation. Patients who require sedation or analgesia during transport may fall along the entire continuum of illness or injury. Interhospital transport of a child with relatively minor trauma may suggest the need for one particular type of sedation or analgesia, whereas the intrahospital transport of a child on extracorporeal membrane oxygenation (ECMO) will require an entirely differentapproach.

Patients are transported for myriad of reasons. Interfacility transport can occur for second opinions, continuation or augmentation of initial care, or for specialized services or personnel not available at the referring institution. Intrafacility transport is often undertaken to attain studies, for preoperative or postoperative transfer, or simply for a location change. Primary goals of the transport are to maintain stability of the patient, react efficiently to predictable and unpredictable changes, prevent iatrogenic deterioration, and ensure transport team safety. Sophisticated pediatric transport systems will also offer pediatric-specific diagnosis and intervention capabilities.

INDICATIONS

In addition to providing medical support, the transport clinician should concentrate on alleviating the pain or anxiety that the child is experiencing, as well as anticipating the child's needs during and after the transport (Table 25.1). Importantly, once the decision has been made to intervene pharmacologically, the team must discern whether the child is suffering from pain, anxiety, or both, and choose the medication(s) most appropriate for the situation. The relative indications and

Table 25.1.   Sedation and Analgesia Issues to Consider In a Child Undergoing Transport

- Is the child suffering pain, anxiety, or both?
- Is the child demonstrating significant stress of leaving a family? Does he or she feel abandoned?
- Can nonpharmacologic interventions be used to control pain and anxiety?
- Will the sedation plan be in the patient's best interest during the pretransport, transport, and posttransport periods?
- Will pharmacologic means compromise the further evaluation and management?
- What are the risks and benefits of the medications chosen for this particular patient?

contraindications to using the various sedatives and analgesics are reviewed elsewhere in this text.

Characteristics of ideal sedative and analgesic agents for transport include the following:

1. Wide therapeutic range
2. Reversible effects
3. Short duration of action to allow frequent reevaluation when necessary

To provide the optimal care, the transport team needs to be aware of the actions, interactions with other medications, side effects, onset and duration of the medications used for analgesia and sedation (see Chapter 26). Consideration of analgesic or sedative use can originate from the transport team, referring physician, medical control physician, patient, and parents. The overall goal is for the patient to arrive at the receiving hospital in as good or better medical condition than when he or she left the referring institution. Additionally, the patient should be maintained as comfortably as possible during the transport without the addition of any new problems. The transport team also must be mindful of the potential need for further evaluation and the management considerations of health care providers at the receiving hospital. One should avoid overzealous administration of sedative medications if the ensuing examination is critical in the decision process for the patient's care. Examples include the patient with a potential surgical abdomen or the patient with altered mental status.

Situations in which a child will require sedation or analgesia on transport can be divided into three general categories:

1. The child with a stable medical process requiring no altered needs for sedation/analgesia.
   —This patient will most likely have a continued need for sedation/analgesia during and after the transport. Examples include the child with sickle cell disease, the child with a long bone fracture, and the postoperative patient.

2. The child with an evolving medical process that alters the sedation/analgesic requirements.
   —The child who is intubated just before or during transport will require sedation in addition to chemical paralysis. Likewise, the trauma patient who has deteriorated and requires insertion of a chest tube or one whose mental status has improved enough to allow him or her to feel the pain of the chest tube may require more analgesia than previously administered.
3. The child with a stable medical process in which the transport itself may increase pain or anxiety sufficiently to warrant additional analgesia or sedation.
   —The child with a long bone fracture or peritonitis may be comfortable while on a stationary hospital gurney but in severe pain during a bumpy ambulance journey.

The transport process may involve several transfers between location (hospital, ambulance, helicopter, and plane), each of which can add additional stress or pain. The transport environment is loud (especially in a helicopter) with significant vibration and temperature fluctuations. One will see pathophysiologic changes as the patient reacts to these environmental stresses. If necessary, the level of sedation and analgesia should be titrated in response to these environmental issues.

Nonpharmacologic Interventions

Interfacility transport involves placing the patient in a foreign environment with unfamiliar caretakers. The stress of leaving a family and the concept of abandonment are often major issues for the child undergoing interfacility transport. The transport team should be aware of nonpharmacologic methods of pain and anxiety management, such as calming and distraction techniques, positioning and immobilization, and play therapy. These techniques can be instituted after a quick evaluation of the patient and family. For example, the parent who responds hysterically to the child's distress calls may not be the ideal candidate to help with immobilization, yet may best be assigned the job of singing favorite songs or telling a favorite story. The family should also be informed of what to expect during and after the transport. Because the parents know the child well, they can be of assistance in the important role of preparing the child for the ambulance journey and any procedures or diagnostic tests that will be performed at the receiving institution. Accompaniment of a family member during the transport can help the patient transition into the new environment, and perhaps lessen the need for pharmacologic intervention.

TRANSPORT ENVIRONMENT

Personnel

The level of sophistication of personnel in a transport environment can vary greatly. The providers can include volunteers, emergency medical technicians

Table 25.2.   Ambulance Terminology and Participant Level

- No medical capabilities
    Volunteer
- Basic life support (BLS)
    Emergency Medical Technician (EMT)
- Advance life support (ALS)
    Paramedics
- Critical care ambulance
    Paramedics
    Critical care nurse
    +/− Respiratory therapist
- Specialized pediatric critical care transports
    Pediatric critical care transport nurse(s)
    +/− Physicians, respiratory therapists, paramedics

Table 25.3.   General Skill Levels of Transport Personnel

- Volunteer
    Lack of formal medical education
- Emergency medical technician (EMT)
    Basic CPR, extrication, and stabilization
- Paramedic (EMT-P)
    ALS capabilities—advanced airway, breathing, and circulatory management; use of medications and interventions; minimal pediatric training, and often limited pediatric experience
- Critical care nurse
    Similar skills as paramedic with advanced knowledge secondary to previous nursing education and experience; pediatric expertise directly related to previous experience
- Pediatric critical care transport nurse
    Same skills as critical care nurse with the addition of significant pediatric critical care nursing experience. Levels of advanced skills can include intubation, surgical airway, thoracostomy, and central venous access.
- Physicians
    Variable skills and cognitive knowledge
    Levels include resident, fellow, house, and attending physicians
    Most transport physicians, outside of the residency group, come from intensive care, neonatology, or emergency medicine. They can also include subspecialists (anesthesiologists, otolaryngologists, ECMO surgeons, etc.) as dictated by the patient's needs.

(EMT), paramedics (EMT-P), respiratory therapists, critical care nurses, pediatric critical care transport nurses, and physicians. Knowledge of the cognitive and skill levels of the transport personnel is imperative (Tables 25.2 and 25.3).

The sense of urgency surrounding an acutely ill patient in need of transport can lead one to opt for the transport service that can arrive the fastest. It is important to remember that a rapid response does not guarantee qualified care. While both can and do coexist, a potential pitfall in pediatric transport is responding to the urge to "get the child out of here as soon as possible." This is especially relevant for the community hospital setting where personnel may be uncomfortable managing a critically ill child. This approach can be dangerous for the patient and increase liability for the physician. A better approach is to consider "how do I obtain the best, most appropriate care for this patient as expediently as possible." Another important perspective is whether the patient needs transport to a pediatric care center, or whether specialized pediatric care needs to come to the child. With a sophisticated pediatric critical care transport service, the initial phone call to the medical control physician allows specialized pediatric care to begin immediately.

When selecting a transport service for interfacility transport, one should choose the team with the highest level of expertise required by the patient being transported. If the patient is a pediatric patient, ideally a pediatric critical care transport team should be chosen. A pediatric critical care transport team will include pediatric-specific transport equipment, personnel with expertise and experience in pediatrics, and pediatric medical control physicians. Choosing a general transport system may be efficient and appropriate in some circumstances; however, one should be careful not to assume that the team will provide specific pediatric diagnosis, intervention, or management capabilities. Although generic transport systems will usually have skilled personnel at the paramedic or critical care nurse level, the lack of specific pediatric training and expertise can be a significant liability. The potential exists for extrapolation from adult medicine to pediatric management and intervention, which might not be in the patient's best interest. Certification in pediatric advanced life support (PALS or APLS) is useful, but cannot replace specific pediatric experience. One of these certifications should be required for all members of a service that transports children.

Transport Time

Transport time is another issue to consider. The total transport time includes many steps as follows:

1. Time from injury or illness to initial care
2. Decision to transport
3. Transport service contact
4. Information flow
5. Transport acceptance
6. Team preparation and assembly
7. Transport service arrival
8. Time at the scene or referring hospital
9. Conveyance of the patient to receiving hospital

These times can be minimized by the following:

1. Anticipation of the need for transport
2. Predetermined transport team referral plans
3. Transport agreements
4. Concise patient presentations
5. Available and copied patient records and studies
6. Optimal stabilization of the patient before arrival of the transport team
7. Efficient transfer of care

Having the patient as stable as possible is helpful before the transport process unless a specific situation such as ongoing CPR dictates rapid transport to a more appropriate stabilization location. The time spent preparing a patient for transport is crucial and should not be discounted. This includes a review of previous and on-going therapy, the securing of catheters, lines, and tubes, verifying proper medication infusions and rates, and preparing equipment for potential use. If those procedures and interventions can be accomplished before the arrival of the transport team, the transition of care will be more efficient and will result in a more predictable patient outcome.

Roles and Responsibilities

It is important to assign tasks during transport, especially with a sedated patient. Although most interfacility transports will include at least two attendants, if the attendants have different skill sets, the patient may actually be receiving less than one-to-one care. For example, in a transport environment with a critical care transport nurse and a moonlighting physician, the nurse is often responsible for the patient's acute management and monitoring, as well as knowledge of the transport environment, documentation, and communication with the receiving facility. The physician may have been used as a participant in the transport for "physician" skills such as airway management, surgical intervention, or disease process evaluation, but may be unaware of the idiosyncrasies of the transport environment. The ideal transport team will have members who are all literate with the transport environment and have complementary skills. Those complementary skills allow the patient to be adequately managed, observed, and monitored while the issues of the transport environment are simultaneously addressed. Familiarity with the transport environment can lead to more efficient, directed, and appropriate medical care for the transported patient.

One may be confronted with issues regarding paralysis and the level of sedation during the transport process. The capabilities of the transport personnel should be considered when deciding on the use of paralytics for the transported patient. Paralysis, with appropriate sedation, may ease the transport for both the caretakers and the patient. However, loss of the artificial airway or inability to oxygenate and ventilate effectively can be disastrous if not promptly recognized and expertly managed. If advanced airway capabilities are not available with the chosen transport service and a more appropriate transport service is not available, not paralyzing the patient may add a margin of safety to the transport process. An alternate choice is to increase the level of sedation and be prepared to reverse the medications if the airway becomes compromised.

Communication

Communication is an important part of the transport process. Communication with the referring hospital personnel at the time of referral and with the patient, family, and personnel throughout the transport process is extremely important. The emotional pain a family member feels surrounding a transport can be lessened by honest, direct, and caring communication. One important aspect of communication is to avoid criticizing the management of other medical personnel. Recognizing that there are multiple options available for adequate sedation and analgesia and being cognizant of pretransport issues will help maintain collegial relationships. It is probably the exception rather than the rule that sedation and analgesic guidelines and therapies will be identical between hospitals or even services within a single hospital. The knowledge bases, comfort levels, and medication availability can be significantly diverse in those environments; therefore, one should expect the delivered care to vary. It is imperative, therefore, to be specific when communicating information regarding current or planned sedation or analgesia. This should include specific drugs and dosages for the particular patient as well as a review of potential issues or side effects with the selected medications. This type of communication can be especially important if a medication is chosen with which a transport team is relatively inexperienced.

DIFFICULTIES DURING TRANSPORT

Difficulties in transport can result from an unstable patient, altered monitoring capabilities, and logistical issues. Preparation for expected, unexpected, and iatrogenic issues surrounding sedation and transport are imperative. The transport environment is self-contained and must include all personnel, equipment, and medications that a particular patient can be reasonably expected to require (Table 25.4). The transport environment should mirror a hospital intensive care area. The patient should be monitored as closely as possible with direct visualization and monitoring tools such as automated blood pressure machines, cardiorespiratory, oxygen, and carbon dioxide monitors when appropriate. Measurement of arterial blood gases during the transport process with portable analyzers can be useful for monitoring respiratory status. Portable, handheld capnographs have become available to measure expired carbon dioxide in nonintubated patients. Performance of capnog-

Table 25.4.   Checklist for Transport of Sedated Patient

- ❏ Safety ensured for patient and transport personnel
    - ❏ Sophisticated transport system
    - ❏ Skilled personnel (assessment, diagnosis, intervention, communication)
    - ❏ Appropriate mode of transport
    - ❏ Disease progression and adverse events anticipated and prepared for
    - ❏ Appropriate receiving personnel and location (available and notified)
    - ❏ Alternate transport and intervention plans available if necessary
- ❏ Consent obtained
- ❏ All pertinent patient information communicated and copied
    - ❏ Acute medical information
        - ❏ History of present illness
        - ❏ Physical examination
    - ❏ Pertinent medical history
        - ❏ Communicable disease exposure
    - ❏ Interventions and responses
    - ❏ Working diagnosis
    - ❏ Laboratory and radiographic results
- ❏ Appropriate medical equipment available and functioning
    - ❏ Pediatric airway
        - ❏ Nasal and oral airway
        - ❏ Bag and valve devices
        - ❏ Masks
        - ❏ Laryngoscopes
        - ❏ Pediatric endotracheal tubes
        - ❏ Ventilator if appropriate (pressure and/or volume)
    - ❏ Intravenous and interosseous
    - ❏ Surgical airway
    - ❏ Monitors
        - ❏ Cardiorespiratory
        - ❏ Blood pressure
        - ❏ Pulse oximetry
        - ❏ Capnography
        - ❏ Invasive if required
    - ❏ Point of care testing
- ❏ Appropriate medications available (and understood)
    - ❏ Medication references and guidelines
    - ❏ Routine medications
    - ❏ Resuscitation medications
    - ❏ Disease-specific medications
    - ❏ Sedation and reversal agents
    - ❏ Intravenous fluids
    - ❏ Oxygen, medical gases
    - ❏ Complete documentation of process

raphy in these types of patients will be useful in the transport environment. The transport process should not proceed until all the necessary equipment has been checked and all personnel are available. Regardless of length of transport, inadequate preparation, personnel, equipment, or medications can lead to an unfavorable outcome. The child transported without incident from another hospital but who has a respiratory arrest while in the elevator without proper supplies and personnel, can still have a disastrous outcome. One must, as in other professions, prepare for the worst and hope for the best.

Given potential limitations in monitoring a patient during transport and the lack of an ideal, controlled environment for airway management, the transport team must anticipate the potential for adverse occurrences during analgesia and sedation. One of the principal rules of transport medicine is that the transport team knows all of the therapies that were administered to the patient at the referral institution. Specific medications and routes of administration can result in delayed effects that can manifest during the transport. For example, drugs administered intramuscularly may be erratically absorbed and can produce effects 30 to 90 minutes into the transport. When opioids and benzodiazepines are used together, they offer the advantage of providing analgesia and sedation using lower doses of opioids than if used alone. However, this synergy applies to adverse effects as well, occasionally resulting in neurologic, respiratory, or cardiovascular depression. Similarly, the combination of medications such as Vistaril (hydroxyzine) and opioids can result in delayed potentiation of opioid effects.

Transport also offers the potential for educational intervention. Although it is usually not appropriate to "educate" referring personnel at the time of transport, the case may spark interest in a review of specific disease processes or larger issues such as sedation and preparation for transport. This can become an invaluable tool for improving one's medical referral environment.

Intrafacility and interfacility transport should be considered an extension of hospital-based care. An understanding of the reasons and options for using sedation and analgesia on transport is imperative. In general, health care providers should use therapies with which they are familiar and confident. Three characteristics of ideal sedative and analgesic agents for transport are 1) wide therapeutic range; 2) reversible effects; and 3) short duration of action to allow frequent reevaluation when necessary. Medications such as midazolam, morphine, and fentanyl are therefore appropriate candidates for inclusion in a protocol. Conversely, medications with a narrow therapeutic window such as propofol, those with irreversible effects such as ketamine, and those with prolonged sedation effects such as phenobarbital should be administered only in consultation with all medical parties involved. The medical control physician at the receiving hospital, as well as critical care consultants, will be helpful in determining the need to "step out" of a protocol when one of these agents is required. Certain limitations exist to the transport environment potentially including the number and pertinent experience of personnel, equipment, medications, and protocols. However, the transport environment should be able to offer excellent, safe, controlled transfer of almost all pediatric patients. If a safe, knowledgeable transport cannot be guaranteed, the decision to transport the patient using that particular team or service should be revisited.

SUGGESTED READING

Aoki BY, McCloskey K. Evaluation, Stabilization, and Transport of the Critically Ill Child. St. Louis: Mosby Year Book, 1992.

Bauchner H, Vinci R, Bak S, Pearson C, Corwin MJ. Parents and procedures: a randomized controlled trial. Pediatrics 1996;98:861–867.

Cote CJ. Sedation for the pediatric patient. Pediatr Clin North Am 1994;41:31–58.

Edge WE, Kanter RK, et al. Reduction of morbidity in interhospital transport by specialized pediatric staff. Crit Care Med 1994;22(7):1186–1191.

Fein JA. Pain. In: Schwartz MW, ed. Pediatric Primary Care: A Problem Oriented Approach. 3rd ed. Philadelphia: Mosby Year Book, 1997.

Jaimovich DG, Vidyasagar D. Handbook of Pediatric and Neonatal Transport Medicine. Philadelphia: Hanley and Belfus, Inc., 1996.

Macnab AJ. Optimal escort for interhospital transport of pediatric emergencies. J Trauma 1991;31(2):205–209.

McCloskey K, Orr R. Pediatric Transport Medicine. St. Louis: Mosby Year Book, 1995.

McDonald TB, Berkowitz RA. Airway management and sedation for pediatric transport. Pediatr Clin North Am 1993;40(2):381–407.

Notcutt WG. Transporting patients with overwhelming pain. Anesthesia 1994;49:145–147.

Pace S, Burke TF. Intravenous morphine for early pain relief in patients with acute abdominal pain. Acad Emerg Med 1996;3(12):1086–92.

Rubenstein JS, Gomez MA, et al. Can the need for a physician as part of the pediatric transport team be predicted? A prospective study. Crit Care Med 1992;20(12):1657–1661.

Schecter NL. Pain and pain control in children. Curr Prob Pediatr 1985;15:1–67.

Szem JW, Hydo LJ, et al. High-risk intrahospital transport of critically ill patients: safety and outcome of the necessary "road trip." Crit Care Med 1995;23(10):1660–1666.

Part Three

Nonelective Procedures

Chapter 26

Practical Aspects of Procedural Sedation and Analgesia

Baruch Krauss

Sedation and analgesia in children can be used to relieve anxiety, control pain, decrease mobility, and enhance patient cooperation. Choosing the appropriate type of sedation or analgesia depends on the nature of the procedure and the type of intervention required, i.e. anxiolysis, sedation, dissociation, and local and/or systemic analgesia. Laceration repair in the toddler may require anxiolysis/sedation but minimal to no systemic analgesia, whereas abscess incision and drainage may require liberal use of systemic analgesia but only minimal sedation. When drugs are used in combination, the nature of the procedure performed will determine the appropriate ratio of analgesia to sedation. In each case, drugs with the appropriate analgesic or sedative properties should be carefully chosen. Sedative/hypnotics (barbiturates, benzodiazepines, chloral hydrate, propofol) have no analgesic properties and must be used with opioids or topical/local analgesia for procedures requiring both analgesia and sedation.

For the clinician who is just beginning to use procedural sedation, it is prudent to become thoroughly familiar with one or two agents. Although many choices are acceptable, fentanyl and midazolam provide much flexibility. Both agents are short-acting, easily titratable, and rapidly reversible. Midazolam can be used by various routes of administration, making it useful for a wide range of applications. Used appropriately, these two agents, alone or in combination, can provide sufficient sedation and analgesia for the majority of outpatient procedures.

Clinicians should perform a risk-benefit analysis before using procedural sedation. In children, a complex set of variables must be assessed to determine the need for sedation and analgesia (these variables will be discussed in depth in chapters 27 through 38). The benefits of reducing anxiety and controlling pain should be carefully weighed against the risks of respiratory depression and airway compromise.

This chapter presents an overview of the practical aspects of administration of the most commonly used agents for procedural sedation and analgesia. The following chapters should be referred to for in-depth discussions of and suggested readings for the pharmacology of these agents:

- Local analgesia—Chapter 8
- Topical analgesia—Chapter 9
- Midazolam—Chapter 4
- Ketamine—Chapter 7
- Fentanyl/sufentanil—Chapter 10
- Nitrous oxide—Chapter 11

TOPICAL AND LOCAL ANALGESIA

Topical Analgesia

- Topical anesthetics are available in aqueous and viscous preparations in varying strengths. These preparations are prepared by each hospital pharmacy. The viscous form is more adherent to the wound site and tends to drip less (an important consideration for lacerations in the orbital area).
- Available preparations include: tetracaine, epinephrine, cocaine (TAC), and tetracaine, epinephrine, lidocaine (LET).
- Apply LET or TAC for 20 to 30 minutes for optimal vasoconstriction and topical anesthesia.
- A cotton ball saturated with topical anesthetic provides better surface-to-wound contact than a gauze pad. The first application may be done with a Q-tip followed by saturating a cotton ball with the remainder of the medication. The cotton ball can then be taped to the patient's wound or the parents can hold the cotton ball. The use of tape allows children to play and remain active and mobile for 20 to 30 minutes and can free up the procedure room during that time.
- Studies have demonstrated equal efficacy in pain control and hemostasis between TAC and LET.
- The major indication for a topical anesthetic is in facial lacerations.

Local Anesthesia

Every effort should be made to provide painless administration of local anesthesia. It is well documented that a few simple maneuvers can significantly reduce the pain associated with infiltration of local anesthesia. These maneuvers include the following: choosing the smallest needle size (preferably a No. 27 or No. 30

gauge); buffering the local anesthetic with sodium bicarbonate in a ratio of 10:1 before injection; warming the local anesthetic; and infiltrating at a slow steady rate (because it is the rate of anesthetic injection that can be painful, in addition to the puncture itself).

Combined Topical and Local Anesthesia

Combined use of topical and local anesthesia is indicated for any deep wound that requires a two-layer closure. Topical anesthesia alone will not anesthetize the deeper skin layers and should be augmented with local anesthesia.

ORAL DRUG OPTIONS FOR PROCEDURAL SEDATION (TABLE 26.1)

Midazolam

1. Dosing range
   - Maximum recommended oral dose is 10 to 12 mg.
   - Doses greater than 0.5 mg/kg prolong recovery time, with minimal increase in anxiolytic effect, especially when administered in the evening to young children.
   - Use the 5 mg/mL intravenous preparation for oral administration.
2. Preparation
   Midazolam is only available in the intravenous preparation. Because

Table 26.1.   Oral Drug Options

	Midazolam	Ketamine
Dosing range	0.5–0.75 mg/kg	5–10 mg/kg
Preparation	1, 5 mg/mL	10 mg/mL
Advantages	1. Painless administration	1. Painless administration
	2. High safety profile	2. Mild analgesia, sedation, anxiolysis, dissociation
	3. Anxiolysis with minimal to mild sedation	
Disadvantages	1. Nontitratable	1. Nontitratable
	2. Limited sedative effect	2. Multiple contraindications
	3. Variable responses (first pass hepatic metabolism)	
	4. Paradoxical reactions (hyperactivity, excitation, dysphoria)	
	5. No analgesia	

there is currently no oral form of the drug, the intravenous preparation must be used for oral administration. Use the most concentrated preparation (5 mg/mL) to minimize the amount of liquid the child must drink. Mix the intravenous preparation, which is bitter tasting because of the preservative benzyl alcohol, in a sweet vehicle (e.g., fruit syrup, Tylenol, ibuprofen, or sugar). Deliver to the child in a syringe or cup depending child's age. If the child is drinking from a cup, make sure that the mixture is swallowed in one gulp because it tends to have a bitter aftertaste and the child will be reluctant to sip it again after an initial unpleasant experience. Adding ice to the mixture also may help decrease the bitterness.

3. Advantages
   - Midazolam produces effective anxiolysis with minimal to mild sedation.
   - This drug is particularly useful for fearful school-aged children (ages 4 to 7) who are so anxious that they are unable to focus their attention or follow instructions. Once anxiolysis is established, these children can usually be talked through the procedure.
   - The safety profile is high with no reported cases of apnea or respiratory arrest when administered orally.
4. Disadvantages
   - Onset is slow (15 to 30 minutes).
   - Utility is restricted to anxiolysis (because Midazolam does not produce reliable sedation).
   - First pass hepatic metabolism results in oral bioavailability of 10 to 15%, and gastrointestinal absorption can be variable. These factors may lead to unpredictable results after oral midazolam, with some children responding well and others showing minimal to no response.
   - Paradoxical reactions can occur, which are best treated by withholding further drug administration. It is important not to mistake a paradoxical reaction for undersedation.

Ketamine

1. Dosing range
   Studies assessing the appropriate oral dosing have shown that doses greater than 5 mg/kg reliably produce sedation with doses up to 10 mg/kg producing none of the adverse effects associated with the intramuscular or intravenous routes of administration (hypersalivation, emergence phenomena, laryngospasm).
2. Preparation
   - Use same instructions as with oral midazolam except the most concentrated preparation is 100 mg/mL and the preservative is benzethonium chloride.

- Because no serious adverse effects are associated with the oral form of ketamine, concomitant administration of atropine, glycopyrrolate, or midazolam is not required.

3. Advantages

    Even though oral bioavailability is approximately 16%, oral ketamine produces a more reliable sedative state than oral midazolam because of the enhanced effect of its active metabolite norketamine.

4. Disadvantages

- Onset is slow (15 to 30 minutes).
- Recovery time can be prolonged (up to 2 hours in some children).
- Ketamine has multiple contraindications (see section on intravenous ketamine).

INTRANASAL DRUG OPTIONS FOR PROCEDURAL SEDATION (TABLE 26.2)

Midazolam

1. Dosing range

- When used in combination with sufentanil, the low-end dose (0.2 mg/kg) should be used.
- This drug is most useful in children 5 years old or younger because the volume of drug instilled in the nose should not exceed about 1 mL. For example, an average 5-year-old weighs approximately 20 kg. Using the most concentrated preparation (5 mg/mL) and dosing at 0.3 mg/kg yields slightly more than 1 mL of solution.
- An active upper respiratory infection with nasal congestion is not a contraindication to the use of intranasal medications, although it may decrease the degree of drug absorption.

Table 26.2. Intranasal Drug Options

	Midazolam	Sufentanil
Dosing range	0.2–0.5 mg/kg	0.7–1.0 μg/kg
Preparation	5 mg/mL	50 μg/mL
Advantages	1. No IV required	1. No IV required
	2. High safety profile	2. Potent analgesia
	3. Short duration of action	3. Reversible
	4. Reversible	
Disadvantages	1. Nontitratable	1. Nontitratable
	2. Noxious administration	2. Noxious administration
	3. No analgesia	

Recommendation: Proper administration is crucial for maximal nasal mucosal absorption. The child must be supine with the head held in the neutral position, looking straight up. The solution is placed in a 1-mL syringe and instilled slowly, drop-by-drop, into the child's nostrils, alternating as one proceeds. If the child receives a drop and immediately swallows, then the solution bypassed the nasal mucosa and will be absorbed orally. Likewise, if the child coughs and gags after a drop then the solution has bypassed the nasal mucosa and irritated the glottic region. Time each instillation with the child's swallowing pattern, ideally instilling the solution immediately after the child swallows. Crying is helpful in creating back pressure to keep the solution out of the posterior pharynx. Most children will begin to cry after the first instillation.

Note: It is important to inform parents that even though the administration is noxious, once the drug has taken effect, children tend not to focus on the administration but rather on the comfortable and happy feelings produced by the drug.

2. Preparation
   - Use the undiluted intravenous form in the most concentrated preparation (5 mg/mL).
   - Use a 1-mL tuberculin syringe for controlled administration.
3. Advantages
   - As with oral midazolam, the safety profile is high with no reported cases of apnea or respiratory arrest attributed to this route of administration.
   - Onset is relatively rapid (10 to 15 minutes) and duration is brief (45 to 60 minutes).
   - Midazolam is reversible with flumazenil.
4. Disadvantages
   - Intranasal administration is noxious to children for three reasons:
   - The solution stings when instilled (a combination of the low pH and the presence of the preservative benzyl alcohol). Buffering the solution does not decrease the burning.
   - Toddlers do not like liquids placed in their noses.
   - Toddlers do not like to be held in a supine position.
   Note: The degree of absorption, and therefore effectiveness of the drug, is operator-dependent (see above discussion on proper administration technique).

Sufentanil

1. Dosing range
   When used in combination with midazolam, the low-end dose (0.7 μg/kg) should be used.
   Caution: Sufentanil is dosed in μg/kg unlike midazolam, which is given

in mg/kg. A tenfold error (overdose) will usually cause a respiratory arrest.

2. Preparation

No oral preparation is available and, therefore, the undiluted intravenous preparation must be administered, preferably in a 1-mL syringe for controlled delivery.

3. Advantages
- Currently, sufentanil is the only available opioid that has been studied for intranasal administration.
- Sufentanil provides systemic analgesia.
- This drug potentiates the effects of midazolam when used in combination.
- Sufentanil is reversible with naloxone.

4. Disadvantages
- Sufentanil is not practical in children over 5 years old (too large a volume to deliver in the nose—see discussion on intranasal midazolam).
- This drug has minimal sedative effects at normal dosing range.
- The combination of intranasal sufentanil and midazolam can prolong the recovery period for up to 2 hours.
- The safety profile is decreased when used in combination with midazolam (increased incidence of respiratory depression and apnea, especially if both drugs are dosed at the high end of the dosing range).

    Note: Degree of absorption depends on the operator administration technique (see discussion on intranasal midazolam).

INTRAMUSCULAR DRUG OPTIONS FOR PROCEDURAL SEDATION (TABLE 26.3)

Ketamine

1. Dosing range

Although the dosing range is 3 to 6 mg/kg, 4 mg/kg is needed to produce reliable dissociation.

2. Preparation
- Ketamine is a sialagogue and should be administered with atropine (0.15 to 0.5 mg at 0.02 mg/kg) or glycopyrrolate (0.005 mg/kg, max 0.25 mg).
- Ketamine can be administered with midazolam (0.025 mg/kg) and atropine in children under 8 years old to decrease hypertonicity. This small dose is usually sufficient to decrease hypertonicity without prolonging recovery time.
- All three drugs (ketamine, atropine or glycopyrrolate, and midazolam) are compatible in the same syringe.

Table 26.3.   Intramuscular Drug Options

Ketamine	
Dosing range	3–6 mg/kg
Preparation	10, 50, 100 mg/mL
Advantages	1. No IV required
	2. Reliable dissociative anesthesia
	3. Rapid onset
	4. Immobility
Disadvantages	1. Multiple contraindications
	2. Sialogogue
	3. Emergence reactions

- Use the most concentrated preparations of each drug (ketamine 100 mg/mL, atropine 0.4mg/mL, midazolam 5 mg/mL) to minimize the volume of injection.

3. Advantages
   - Onset is extremely rapid (2 to 10 minutes) for intramuscular administration.
   - Be set up and ready to go with the procedure before administering the drug.
   - No respiratory depression or loss of airway reflexes occurs.
   - Ketamine has a short duration of maximum anesthesia (30 minutes) with recovery time in 60 to 90 minutes.
   - Ketamine provides adequate systemic and local analgesia in most cases obviating the need for local anesthesia.
   - Emergence reactions are rare in children younger than 8 years old.

4. Disadvantages
   - Ketamine has multiple contraindications (see section on intravenous ketamine).
   - Ketamine requires an injection (although patients tend not to remember the injection).

INTRAVENOUS DRUG OPTIONS FOR PROCEDURAL SEDATION (TABLE 26.4)

Fentanyl

1. Dosing range

   Most procedures require dosing in the range of 2 to 5 μg/kg. An initial bolus of 5 μg/kg is considered an induction dose and should be avoided for outpatient procedures. Chest wall rigidity, a complication of the short-acting opioids, is a phenomenon restricted to rapid intravenous bolus administration of induction doses of fentanyl. This complication has not been reported in procedural sedation in which lower doses are used.

Note: Although the initial bolus should not exceed 1 to 2 µg/kg, the maximal endpoint of titration over a period often will exceed a total of 5 µg/kg. The maximum titrated dose depends on the clinical response of the patient.

- Dosing range per bolus for children who weigh 50 kg (adult dosing) is 50 to 100 µg (see comment No. 3).

2. Preparation

Fentanyl is only available as 50 µg/mL.

3. Initial and secondary dosing

Start with an initial bolus of 1 to 2 µg/kg, to a maximum of 50 to 100 µg, given over 15 to 30 seconds. Secondary dosing can continue with aliquots of 1 µg/dose, to a maximum of 50 µg/dose, titrated to desired effect.

Note: Exceptions to this dosing are individuals with high drug tolerance (chronic opioid users and abusers and individuals with large physical habitus and muscle mass) who should be titrated to effect rather than an absolute dosing range.

Table 26.4.   Intravenous Drug Options

	Fentanyl	Ketamine	Midazolam
Dosing range[a]	1–5 µg/kg	0.5–1.5 mg/kg	0.05–0.2 mg/kg
Preparation	50 µg/mL	10, 50, 100 mg/mL	1, 5 mg/mL
Initial dose	1–2 µg/kg Adults: 50-100 µg	0.5–1.5 mg/kg	0.05–0.1 mg/kg Adults: 1–2 mg
Secondary dose	1 µg/kg/dose Adults: 50 µg/dose	0.5–1 mg/kg	0.05 mg/kg/dose Adults: 1 mg/dose
Advantages	1. Titratable 2. Reversible 3. Rapid onset 4. Short duration	1. Titratable 2. Rapid onset 3. Brief duration 4. Dissociative anesthesia (analgesia, sedation, amnesia, dissociation)	1. Titratable 2. Reversible 3. Rapid onset 4. Short duration
Disadvantages	1. Requires IV 2. Minimal sedation	1. Requires IV 2. Multiple contraindications 3. Sialogogue 4. Emergence reactions	1. Requires IV 2. No analgesia

[a]Because these agents are titratable, higher cumulative doses may be given over time.

4. Advantages

Fentanyl is a potent short-acting analgesic agent (100 times more potent than morphine) with minimal histamine related side effects (nausea/vomiting, pruritus, hypotension). Its rapid onset (2 to 3 minutes) and reversibility make it extremely titratable and safe in experienced hands.

5. Disadvantages

Fentanyl provides potent analgesia but minimal to no sedation at the recommended dosing range for procedural procedures. Sedative effects can be obtained from higher dosing ranges, but the increased risk of respiratory depression with these doses make fentanyl an impractical agent for pure sedation. When performing procedures requiring both analgesia and sedation, fentanyl may be combined with a short-acting benzodiazepine (midazolam).

It is important to note that the risks of hypoxemia and apnea are significantly greater when opioids and benzodiazepines are used in combination than when either drug is given alone.

Recommendation: Although fentanyl causes minimal histamine release, children receiving the drug tend to experience pruritus restricted to the nasal area. It is therefore important to restrain patients' hands during facial laceration repair when fentanyl is administered.

Midazolam

1. Dosing range
   - The dosing range for midazolam is 0.05 to 0.1 mg/kg with a maximum dose of 4 mg. A bolus of 0.2 mg/kg is considered an induction dose and should be avoided for procedural sedation.
   - The dosing range for children who weigh 50 kg (adult dosing) is 1 to 4 mg.

   Individual sensitivities and responses to midazolam vary by age. A 0.1-mg/kg bolus in a 1-year-old weighing 10 kg (1 mg) may provide mild to moderate sedation, whereas the same 0.1-mg/kg bolus in an 8-year-old weighing 30 kg (3 mg) may result in a deep level of sedation.

   It should be noted, for completeness' sake, that the geriatric population is especially sensitive to the effects of midazolam, and the same 1-mg bolus given safely to the 10 kg 1-year-old may produce respiratory depression and apnea in a 70-year-old.

2. Preparation
   - Available as 1 mg/mL and 5mg/mL.

   Note: The concentration of midazolam should always be checked before administration because a 1-mL bolus of the higher concentration (5 mg/mL) will produce apnea and respiratory arrest in most patients.

3. Initial and secondary dosing

   Start with an initial bolus of 0.05 to 0.1 mg/kg, to a maximum of 3 mg, given over 15 to 30 seconds. Secondary dosing can continue with aliquots of 0.05 mg/dose, to a maximum of 1 mg/dose, titrated to desired effect.

Recommendation: For those who are first learning to use midazolam in the intravenous form in children, it is advisable to start with a test dose of 0.05 mg/kg or 1 mg in patients weighing over 10 kg until one is thoroughly familiar with the varied effects of midazolam on different age groups. This can be accomplished by administering the initial dose as a 1-mg bolus, waiting 2 to 3 minutes to determine the effect of this dose on the patient, then proceeding with the appropriate secondary dosing based on the response of the patient to the initial 1-mg bolus.

4. Advantages

   Midazolam is a reversible short-acting sedative/hypnotic with a rapid onset (2 to 3 minutes) and brief duration (45 to 60 minutes).

5. Disadvantages

   Midazolam is a pure sedative/hypnotic with no analgesic properties. It must be combined with an opioid to provide both analgesia and sedation.

   Paradoxical reactions to midazolam are characterized by excitation, agitation, and restlessness, and occur most commonly in younger children (younger than 5 years).

Ketamine

1. Dosing range

   The dosing range of ketamine is 0.5 to 1.5 mg/kg, although maximal cumulative doses may exceed this range, especially if repeated doses are given or if the procedure is extended beyond 10 to 15 minutes.

2. Preparation
   - Ketamine is available as 10, 50, and 100 mg/mL.
   - Dosing should be checked before administration because the 10-mg/mL vial can be mistaken for the 100-mg/mL vial.

3. Initial and secondary dosing
   - Start with an initial bolus of 0.5 to 1.5 mg/kg given slowly over 1 to 2 minutes. No secondary dosing is required if used for brief procedures. For longer procedures, dosing may be repeated at 0.5 to 1 mg/kg/dose.
   - The onset of ketamine is extremely rapid because it has a "one arm brain" circulation time (30 to 60 seconds) and its duration is brief (5 to 10 minutes). The duration of action of ketamine may be prolonged (up to 10 to 20 minutes) with the addition of midazolam.
   - Avoid rapid administration ("IV push") because respiratory depression and apnea have been reported.
   - Midazolam decreases ketamine-induced hypertonicity, blunts emergence reactions in older children, augments ketamine effect, and can prolong recovery time.

- Give ketamine with an antisialagogue (atropine or glycopyrrolate).

  Recommendation: The use of midazolam, soft voice tones, parental touching, and low lighting decrease the risk of emergence reactions in children, especially those older than 8 years.

  Note: Emergence reactions, or adverse reactions to ketamine in general, should not be misinterpreted as undersedation. The correct management in these circumstances is not to increase the dosing of ketamine but rather to withhold further administration of ketamine and treat as needed with a benzodiazepine.

4. Indications
   - Use for brief procedures (15 minutes).
5. Advantages

   Ketamine is a useful drug for brief procedures in which dissociation, analgesia, sedation, and potent agitation control are needed.
6. Disadvantages
   - Ketamine has a brief duration.
   - Emergence reactions occur. (Reactions occur in approximately one-third of adults [older than 15 years] but are rare in children younger than 8 years old. These reactions may be partially or completely blunted by benzodiazepines.)
   - Multiple contraindications exist.
     - Active upper or lower respiratory infection
     - History of asthma
     - History of hypertension
     - History of psychosis
     - Oral procedures with increased secretions or bleeding, especially procedures involving the posterior pharynx
     - Increased intracranial pressure states (including head trauma)

     Note: Active upper or lower respiratory infections or a history of asthma increase the risk of laryngospasm with ketamine and are contraindications to its use. Intravenous ketamine in conjunction with skeletal muscle relaxants is the drug of choice for intubation of the severe asthmatic. In this circumstance, the risk of laryngospasm is controlled by paralysis of the vocal cords.

INHALATIONAL DRUG OPTIONS FOR PROCEDURAL SEDATION (TABLE 26.5)

Nitrous Oxide

1. Dosing range

   Nitrous oxide is delivered in a fixed preset mixture of nitrous oxide and

Table 26.5. Inhalational Drug Options

Nitrous Oxide (N$_2$O)	
Preparation	Preset mixture of O$_2$ and N$_2$O delivered by demand valve mask
Advantages	1. Rapid onset
	2. Controlled delivery
	3. Controlled duration
	4. Brief recovery period
	5. No IV required
Disadvantages	1. Not useful for children under 3–5 y
	2. Relatively contraindicated when opioids or other sedating drugs have been given within 4 h
	3. Provides only mild analgesia and sedation

oxygen through a demand valve mask, which requires the patient to inspire to release the gas. Various mixtures have been used, ranging from 15% N$_2$O/85% O$_2$ to 70% N$_2$O/30% O$_2$, with the most common being 50/50. Nitrous oxide in a preset 50/50 mixture is extremely safe when the machinery is used properly. There is no time limit for the duration of sedation with nitrous oxide in this formulation. The onset is within 5 minutes (5 minutes of nitrous oxide inhalation is required before starting a procedure), and the duration is controlled by the length of time the patient is breathing the gas mixture. At the conclusion of the procedure, a 5-minute period of 100% oxygen is required to wash out residual nitrous oxide and prevent diffuse hypoxia.

2. Preparation
   - Nitrous oxide is available commercially as a Nitronox machine that includes nitrous oxide and oxygen tanks, a scavenger unit, and a demand valve mask setup. The flow of gas is only triggered when the patient takes a breath.
   - Nitrous oxide is available in metal cylinders or from a gas outlet in the wall.
   - The procedure room should have an appropriate scavenging system for the nitrous oxide.
3. Advantages
   - Nitrous oxide has a high safety profile when used properly.
   - Nitrous oxide has a rapid onset and controlled duration.
4. Disadvantages
   - The use of nitrous oxide is limited to children over the age of 4 to 5 years who are able to understand the use of the demand valve mask and cooperate with it. Some centers have modified this setup to allow

for free-flowing gas (as a nitrous-oxygen mixture) and have been successful in administering nitrous oxide to children 2 years and older.

- Nitrous oxide provides only mild analgesia and sedation and is only appropriate for selected procedures.
- Nitrous oxide is contraindicated during pregnancy.
- Avoid nitrous oxide if the patient is nauseous or vomiting.
- Nitrous oxide is relatively contraindicated when opioids or other sedating drugs have been given within 4 hours because the combination can blunt airway reflexes.

Recommendation: Medical personnel who are pregnant should avoid administering nitrous oxide because residual gas may be present in the procedure room. Some reports suggest low-level teratogenicity from chronic exposure on operating room personnel.

Chapter 27
Indirect and Fiber-Optic Laryngoscopy

Alfred Sacchetti, William Levin

Laryngoscopy for foreign body removal from the posterior pharynx and upper airway is a common procedure in school-aged children and adolescents. The fact that laryngoscopy is being performed on these patients indicates the potential for a possible airway compromise. Any techniques used to facilitate this procedure must not only render the patients cooperative, but also permit patients to maintain their airway. In selecting a pharmacologic approach, consideration should also be given to the fact that the laryngoscopy procedure itself may precipitate loss of the patient's airway; therefore, any technique chosen must not interfere with emergency airway procedures if needed. In addition, any child undergoing diagnostic laryngoscopy should be evaluated for the need for immediate endotracheal intubation. This is not always possible because the laryngoscopy itself may be the diagnostic procedure needed to determine the need for endotracheal intubation.

NONPHARMACOLOGIC MANAGEMENT

A laryngoscopy can only be performed with a cooperative patient. An awake, alert, calm child who can understand the procedure as explained may not require any sedation. In many instances, it is possible to examine older children and adolescents with no supplemental sedation. Younger children and those who are too apprehensive will require some degree of sedation to facilitate the examination.

As with all children, the response to the initial physical examination can set the tone for any further diagnostic maneuvers. Anxiety may be produced in an otherwise calm child by an unexpected, overly aggressive examination of the posterior pharynx with a tongue blade. If there is any question that a laryngoscopy may be required as part of the examination, the clinician should take great efforts to minimize any discomfort in the preliminary examination of this area.

PHARMACOLOGIC MANAGEMENT

Propofol, etomidate, midazolam, fentanyl, and ketamine have all been used successfully to sedate children for these types of examinations. Any sedative for a laryngoscopy is intended only to calm the child, not to produce deeper levels of sedation. In this respect, sedation is an adjunct to local anesthetic maneuvers. In any patient in whom an emergency airway maneuver is a possibility, secure intravenous access is important, and all medications should be titrated via this route. Figure 27.1 contains a flow chart for the preparation of a child for a laryngoscopy.

INDIRECT LARYNGOSCOPY

Topical Agents

Indirect laryngoscopy requires suppression of the posterior pharyngeal sensations either through topical anesthetics or regional nerve block. Choices for topi-

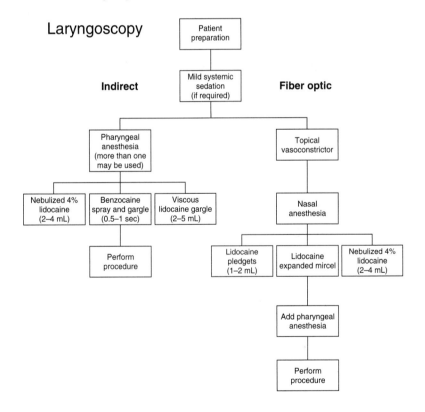

Figure 27.1. Pharmacologic approach to laryngoscopy.

cal agents include spray preparations of lidocaine, tetracaine, and benzocaine. Commercial preparations of each of these agents are available in either pressurized containers or pump delivery devices. When dealing with children, the taste of the anesthetic may be a major compliance issue. Benzocaine preparations (Cetacaine® [14%], Hurricaine® [20%]) are flavored, making them more palatable to children. Caution must be exercised with any benzocaine preparation because systemic absorption with creation of methemoglobin has been reported from topical application of this agent. Always using the lowest possible volume of solution is best when anesthetizing a child. Pressurized administration systems deliver approximately 200 mg per second, making a spraying duration of 0.5 to 1 second more than sufficient for even large adolescents. For pump systems, one pump for small children and two pumps for adolescents will deliver the appropriate amount of anesthetic.

An alternative anesthetic method for older children and adolescents involves having the patient gargle with a topical anesthetic solution. Benzocaine, lidocaine, and tetracaine have all been used in this manner to produce topical anesthesia. Again, the unpleasant taste of these agents may limit their applicability in children. Flavored preparations of these solutions may be prepared by adding powdered drink crystals to the solutions.

Viscous preparations of topical anesthetics can also be used to decrease posterior pharyngeal sensation. This preparation is made by adding some type of a flavored solution (i.e., an antacid) with 10 to 20 mL of viscous lidocaine (2 to 4%). The patient is again asked to gargle or slowly swallow the solution to produce posterior anesthesia.

A universally applicable mucosal anesthetic technique is nebulization of a concentrated anesthetic solution. Most commonly performed with 4% lidocaine, any mucosal anesthetic solution may be nebulized for this purpose. The standard nebulization set used in the delivery of albuterol is usually used to nebulize 3 to 5 mL of the anesthetic solution. In patients too young to cooperate with a mouthpiece, a mask may be used to deliver the vaporized solution.

Because of the open nature of these delivery systems, any personnel getting too close to the nebulized mist may experience numbness to their tongue and lips. Once again, the taste of the topical agents may limit patient cooperation. Because these agents will be inhaled, flavoring additives cannot be used. If a child will not cooperate with the nebulization technique, a sedative may be employed first and the mask with aerosol applied after the child becomes less defiant.

The maximum safe dose of systemic lidocaine is 3 mg/kg. A 4% solution of lidocaine will contain 40 mg of lidocaine for every milliliter of solution, meaning that only 1.5 mL of such a solution would contain enough lidocaine to produce toxic effects in a child weighing 20 kg. Also having the same potential is 3 mL of a 2% preparation. Transmucosal absorption is never 100%, so an inherent safety margin is built in, limiting the applied dose of lidocaine preparations to 3 mg/kg. Because the lidocaine is applied topically, it is the concentration and not the volume of the mixture that is important. When inducing posterior pharyngeal anesthesia, a smaller volume of a higher concentration solution (4%) will be more effective than a larger volume of a more dilute solution.

Once adequate topical anesthesia is obtained, indirect laryngoscopy can be performed. Covering the patient's eyes during performance of this procedure is often helpful. Although the posterior pharynx may be completely anesthetized, the patient may still withdraw if he or she observes the physician approaching with any type of instrument. Having a parent hold the tongue and instructing the child to pant like a puppy will help limit any gagging during the procedure.

In addition to benzocaine, any of the topical anesthetics (especially prilocaine in EMLA) have the potential to produce methemoglobinemia if absorbed in sufficient quantities. To protect against such problems, the lowest possible dose of a topical anesthetic agent should be used.

FLEXIBLE FIBER-OPTIC LARYNGOSCOPY

Flexible fiber-optic nasopharyngoscopes have supplanted indirect laryngoscopy as the visualization technique of choice in performing laryngoscopy for many clinicians. As with indirect laryngoscopy, the posterior pharynx must be adequately anesthetized to perform this procedure. In addition, the nasal pharynx also must be anesthetized if this approach is to be used to introduce the nasopharyngoscope.

Posterior pharyngeal anesthesia may be performed in the same manner as for indirect laryngoscopy. If a nebulization technique with a mask is used, the nasal mucosa also will be adequately anesthetized. Even with nebulized lidocaine, adequate anesthesia of the anterior nasal area may be suboptimal. An alternative technique to nasal mucosal anesthesia may be obtained by placing an anesthetic-soaked pledget into the nares and nasal pharynx. The pledget is soaked in a 1 to 2% lidocaine solution, molded into an elongated cigar shape, and passed through the nares along the floor of the nose. The pledget should remain in place for at least 10 minutes to obtain maximum mucosal penetration of the anesthetic solution. An ideal size pledget can be formed from the cotton found in the inner lining of a standard eye patch. The inner and outer edges of the patch are peeled back, leaving a flattened oval piece of cotton. This cotton can be rolled around a single prong of a bayonet forceps to shape the pledget. The pledget must be removed from the single prong, moistened with the anesthetic solution, and placed in the nasal pharynx.

An alternative approach to nasopharyngeal anesthesia uses the expanding Nasopacks (Merocel Corporation, Mystic, CT) employed for epistaxis control. The nasal tampon is trimmed to a size appropriate for the patient, lubricated sparingly with a topical anesthetic jelly, and placed in the normal fashion. Once in place, 1 to 2 mL of lidocaine solution (2%) is applied to the exposed end of the tampon and the tampon is allowed to expand. After approximately 15 minutes, the pack is removed and the endoscopy is performed.

Any solution used to anesthetize the nose should also contain some form of a topical vasoconstrictor to help dilate the nares and facilitate passage of the nasopharyngoscope. Traditionally, cocaine was the topical anesthetic of choice for this purpose because it is the only anesthetic agent with intrinsic vasoconstrictor properties. Although it is still used occasionally in adults, because of the real potential for systemic toxicity from cocaine absorption, its use should be avoided in children. Alternatively, the nose may be pretreated with a vasoconstrictor spray or drops to shrink the nasal mucosa before anesthesia. Use of a topical vasoconstrictor also limits systemic absorption of any anesthetic drug. An alternative nasal topical agent is lidocaine with epinephrine.

SUGGESTED READING

Chuang E, Wenner WJ Jr, Piccoli DA, et al. Intravenous sedation in pediatric upper gastrointestinal endoscopy. Gastrointest Endosc 1995;42:156–160.

Clary B, Skaryak L, Tedder M, et al. Methemoglobinemia complicating topical anesthesia during bronchoscopic procedures. J Thorac Cardiovasc Surg 1997;114:293–295.

Laurito CE, Baughman VL, Becker GL, et al. Effects of aerosolized and/or intravenous lidocaine on hemodynamic response to laryngoscopy and intubation in outpatients. Anesth Analg 1988;67:389–392.

Mallory GB, Stillwell PC. Flexible fiberoptic bronchoscopy. In: Dieckmann RA, Fiser DH, Selbst SM, eds. Pediatric Emergency & Critical Care Procedures. St. Louis: Mosby-Year Book Inc., 1997;240–248.

Manthey DE, Harrison BP. Otolaryngologic procedures. In: Roberts JR, Hedges JR, eds. Clinical Procedures in Emergency Medicine. 3rd ed. Philadelphia: Saunders, 1998; 1120–1149.

Marcus B, Steward DJ, Khan NR, et al. Outpatient transesophageal echocardiography with intravenous propofol anesthesia in children and adolescents. J Am Soc Echocardiogr 1993;6:205–209.

Rodriguez LF, Smolik LM, Zbehlik AJ. Benzocaine-induced methemoglobinemia: report of a severe reaction and review of the literature. Ann Pharmacother 1994;28:643–649.

Sitbon P, Laffon M, Lesage V, et al. Lidocaine plasma concentrations in pediatric patients after providing airway topical anesthesia from a calibrated device. Anesth Analg 1996; 82:1003–1006.

Chapter 28

Procedures of the Ear, Nose, and Throat

Brian Bates

LACERATION REPAIR

Approach and Special Considerations

Because of their prominent anatomic location, the ear and nose are commonly injured in young children. The majority of these injuries are contusions; however, lacerations do occur and pose unique problems for the physician. A relative lack of subcutaneous adipose tissue results in frequent underlying cartilaginous damage when the ear or nose is lacerated. If the area is not adequately cleaned and carefully repaired, unsightly cosmetic deformity can occur.

The decision to use local or topical anesthesia, or both, depends mainly on the location and extent of the injury. Superficial lacerations of the ear and nose that do not disrupt the underlying cartilage or cause notching of the border may be managed using cyanoacrylate tissue adhesive. Although not formally approved by the Food and Drug Administration, it is becoming common practice to use these products for simple lacerations and approval is anticipated to occur soon. For such wounds, local or topical anesthesia is usually not necessary.

Traditionally, the use of local or topical anesthetics containing epinephrine has been reported to be contraindicated for auricular lacerations and lacerations involving the tip of the nose. However, it is generally our practice, and that of our consulting plastic and otorhinolaryngology surgeons, to use either topical LET or injectable lidocaine with epinephrine on the ear or nose when repairing a laceration of the auricle or nose. If LET is used, additional sedation or analgesia usually is not necessary. If, however, local anesthesia or regional blockade is needed, other adjunctive means of analgesia and anxiolysis are often necessary, particularly for younger children. Deep lacerations and those that involve loss of tissue, such as avulsions and amputations, usually require a greater level of sedation and analgesia. Because of the cosmetic importance of the ear and nose, complex lacerations of these areas often require the additional support of a plastic otorhinolaryngology surgeon and are usually managed in the operating suite using general anesthesia. Figure 28.1 illustrates pharmacologic options for lacerations involving the ear and nose.

Factors Influencing the Extent of Pharmacologic Management

Wound Location The sensory innervation of the ear is derived from branches of the fifth, seventh, and tenth cranial nerves. If the laceration is more superficial and infiltration of the wound will not distort the wound edge, then local anesthesia will be adequate. However, if multiple lacerations are present or if local infiltration is not desirable, a regional auricular block should be performed.

One anatomic advantage with ear lacerations is that the child cannot visualize the repair. Having the child positioned so that they can face a parent is often helpful, and various other distractions (toys, books, etc.) can be used to augment the process. In addition, it is important to avoid the inadvertent instillation of irrigation solution into the external auditory canal because this will usually upset the child. This can be avoided by placing a gauze pad into the opening of the external auditory canal.

Repair of nasal lacerations usually requires the use of anxiolytic agents in addition to local anesthesia because the repair occurs in the child's visual field. Although some children prefer to have a drape placed over their eyes during the repair, the majority do not. Most toddlers and young children become more anxious when their eyes are covered.

Wound Dynamics The extent of injury to the skin and underlying cartilage is an important consideration when deciding on the degree of pharmacologic interven-

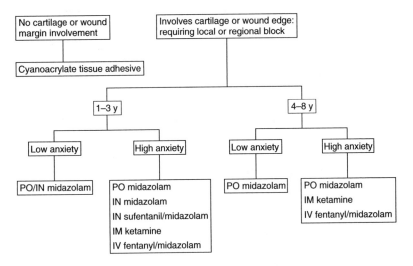

Figure 28.1. Sedation/analgesia options for ear and nasal lacerations.

tion. Superficial injuries that do not, or minimally, involve the underlying cartilage can usually be managed with tissue adhesive or with topical anesthesia and single-layer suturing. Wounds that require significant realignment of tissue margins (edge of the pinna or nasal alae) or involve the underlying cartilage usually require local or regional anesthesia.

Agitation Control The ability to calm the child is important when cosmetically repairing the ear and nose. One should consider this before attempting any repair because it is often difficult to calm a child once they have been frightened.

Age The younger the child, the more important adjunctive pharmacologic measures become. Toddlers (ages 1 to 3) do not understand that they are not supposed to reach into the sterile field; therefore, some degree of restraint is usually indicated. However, they do not usually tolerate restraint well without prior pharmacologic anxiety control.

Anxiety Level More important than age is how much anxiety is displayed by the child. Although most children over the age of 4 years can be calmed and distracted by parents and other care givers, some may not, and early administration of medications can render the repair process less stressful for all involved.

FOREIGN-BODY REMOVAL (FIG. 28.2)

Approach and Special Consideration

Children frequently come to the emergency department for removal of foreign bodies from the ear or nose. This problem most often occurs in the toddler age group, because they begin to explore their own bodies and discover that they can manipulate small objects to the point of placing them where they do not belong. Most of these objects are discovered early by the parents. Unfortunately, it is not uncommon for children to come to the emergency department for the seemingly unrelated complaint of ear pain or a foul-smelling nasal discharge, and only after examination is the foreign object discovered.

Factors Influencing the Extent of Pharmacologic Management

The degree of analgesia and/or sedation required for removing a foreign body from the ear or the nose depends on several factors: 1) the type of foreign body—round and smooth like a bead, irregular like a rock or small toy, soft and pliable like foam or paper, or alive like a small insect; 2) the depth of the foreign body—deep in the ear lying against the tympanic membrane, or superiorly located in the nose dangerously close to the cribriform plate; 3) the duration of the foreign body's existence in the orifice; and 4) the age and anxiety level of the child.

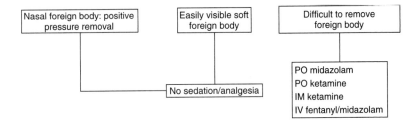

Figure 28.2. Sedation/analgesia options for foreign body removal of the ear and nose.

Type of Foreign Body Smooth objects are often more difficult to grasp and, therefore, require special devices such as right-angle hooks or suction catheters for removal. The wall of the external auditory canal is sensitive and it is difficult to pass an instrument past a foreign object without touching this area. Therefore, providing sedation and analgesia is usually necessary before attempting to remove these types of objects. Any attempt to remove a potentially difficult to grasp object before sedation will usually cause the child to become fearful and virtually impossible to restrain without deep sedation or general anesthesia. Local infiltration of the external auditory canal is often more painful than the actual extraction procedures.

Soft foreign objects such as foam, rubber erasers, and paper are usually easier to remove and can often be grasped using forceps. If the object is not too deep, it can often be removed without touching the wall of the external auditory canal and sedation/analgesia may not be required.

Insects are often alive when they gain access to the child's ear canal and the experience is usually painful. The first intervention should be to asphyxiate the insect using mineral oil (more effective than Auralgan), which usually will significantly reduce the pain associated with the insects presence. After this procedure, irrigation or forceps can be used to remove the insect (irrigation may be less painful and a more successful means of removal because insects often break apart when grasped).

When objects are lodged in the nose, it is often possible to use the positive pressure technique of removal using a bag-valve-mask while occluding the opposite nostril. This method of removal usually does not require any sedation or analgesia. If the technique is not successful or is deemed inappropriate, then the options discussed for removing objects from the ear usually apply.

Depth of Foreign Body The deeper the object is in the ear, the more difficult it is to retrieve. Efforts at blind removal should be avoided because of potential damage to the tympanic membrane. If after adequate sedation/analgesia removal of the object is not successful, one should consider having the otorhinolaryngology surgeon remove the foreign body with the patient under general anesthesia. Otolaryngology consultation is also recommended for objects located deep in the nasopharynx or superiorly located next to the cribriform plate.

Duration of Foreign Body's Presence   The longer the object is in the ear or nose, the more difficult it is to remove. This is particularly the case for objects composed of food, plant material, foam, or paper. These objects tend to swell over time and also may induce an inflammatory response of the surrounding tissue. Harder objects like beads or rocks usually are less problematic. It is important to note that small objects in the ear may be surrounded by cerumen and are often not recognized unless the cerumen is removed.

Age and Anxiety Level of Child   Most children that present with foreign bodies are approximately 1 to 3 years old and are by nature usually more anxious when approached by medical personnel. It is important to anticipate that the child will not tolerate removal of an object from the ear or nose if any direct instrumentation is going to be used. Prior sedation/analgesia and immobilization is usually required.

ABSCESS/HEMATOMA INCISION AND DRAINAGE (FIGS 28.3 AND 28.4)

Approach and Special Consideration

Purulent abscess formation of the ear or nose is unusual. However, when it does occur, it is usually the result of an infected hematoma. Blunt trauma can easily disrupt the perichondrial-cartilage junction shearing the nutrient perichondrial blood vessels, resulting in a localized hematoma. Identifying these hematomas is extremely important. If left untreated, they are likely to become abscessed, causing avascular necrosis of the underlying cartilage and subsequent unsightly cosmetic deformity. The so-called "wrestler's ear" or "cauliflower ear" is the result of avascular necrosis of the cartilage of the pinna. An analogous problem develops with

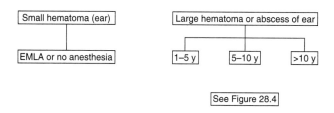

Figure 28.3. Sedation/analgesia options for incision and drainage of abscess/hematomas of the ear.

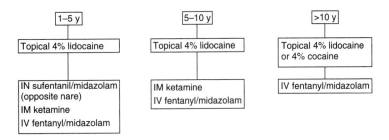

Figure 28.4. Sedation/analgesia options for incision and drainage of abscess/hematomas of the nose.

injury to the nasal septum. If the hematoma/abscess is not identified and drained, avascular necrosis causes a "saddle nose" deformity.

Small hematomas of the ear may be removed by simple sterile needle aspiration and pressure dressing application. This procedure can usually be done without topical anesthesia; however, one option is to apply EMLA cream over the site. Septal hematomas/abscesses of the nose and larger hematomas/ abscesses of the ear require incision and drainage, and systemic sedation and analgesia are usually required. In addition, for nasal hematomas/abscesses, 4% lidocaine (or 4% cocaine in older children) should be applied before incision and drainage.

TYMPANOCENTESIS (FIG. 28.5)

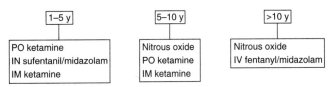

Figure 28.5. Sedation/analgesia options for tympanocentesis.

Approach and Special Considerations

Tympanocentesis is rarely performed in an emergency department setting. However, potential indications for this procedure include otitis media in an immunocompromised or obviously septic child; otitis media with a concomitant brain abscess or mastoiditis; otitis media in an ill neonate; or extreme pain associated with the existing ear infection.

The most important aspect of tympanocentesis is ensuring that the child remains still during the procedure. In most young children, this will require systemic sedation and analgesia. Although instilling local anesthesia in the external auditory canal is possible, the procedure is more painful than tympanocentesis and is generally not recommended.

SUGGESTED READING

Backlin SA. Positive-pressure technique for nasal foreign body removal in children. Ann Emerg Med 1995;25:554–555.

Bruns TB, Simon HK, McLario DJ, et al. Laceration repair using a tissue adhesive in a children's emergency department. Pediatrics 1996;98:673–675.

Canty PA, Berkowitz RG. Hematoma and abscess of the nasal septum in children. Arch Otolaryngol Head Neck Surg 1996;122:1373–1376.

Finkelstein JA. Oral ambu-bag insufflation to remove unilateral nasal foreign bodies. Am J Emerg Med 1996;14:57–58.

Kakish HA, Corneli HM. Removal of nasal foreign bodies in the pediatric population. Am J Emerg Med 1997;15:54–56.

Smith GA, Strausbaugh SD, Harbeck-Weber C, et al. New non-cocaine-containing topical anesthetics compared with tetracaine-adrenaline-cocaine during repair of lacerations. Pediatrics 1997;100:825–830.

Chapter 29
Procedures of the Eye

Mark Joffe

EYE EXAMINATION (FIG. 29.1)

Approach and Special Considerations

Examination of the eye when injury or ocular disease is suspected is often difficult, especially in younger children. Examining the eye carefully is impossible from outside of the visual field. Attempted manipulation in the region of the eye is usually met with extremely vigorous attempts at self-protection from the younger child. Even older children who want to cooperate often cannot overcome the involuntary, protective responses that occur when the eyes are involved. Additionally, children with corneal injuries usually experience severe pain and are especially reluctant to open the affected eye. Physical restraint and forced eye opening are often necessary, but not always easily accomplished. Inadvertent pressure on the globe of a thrashing toddler may be injurious if an open injury is present. Consultation with an ophthalmologist must be prompt if serious ocular disease or injury is present.

The slit lamp is a large, imposing piece of equipment that most young children find frightening. Slit-lamp examination requires a compliant patient. Children under 5 years are seldom relaxed and cooperative enough. In older children, nonpharmacologic measures, such as describing the machine and allowing the child to sit on the parent's lap, are beneficial. Experienced clinicians are sometimes able to actively engage children ("Put your chin here and look into the television") in the slit-lamp examination. Anxiolytics may be helpful, but higher degrees of sedation, which impair the child's ability to cooperate with the examiner, will prove counterproductive.

Most brief examinations can be done with a cooperative patient. Restraint with forced eye opening is used for brief examinations in uncooperative children. When a thorough examination is necessary, and no open globe injury is suspected, and the child has significant anxiety and/or pain, then pharmacologic measures are helpful. Proparacaine can be instilled to relieve corneal pain, and mild sedation may be helpful to complete the examination. When a thorough eye examination is necessary and an open globe injury is suspected, a higher degree of sedation is ap-

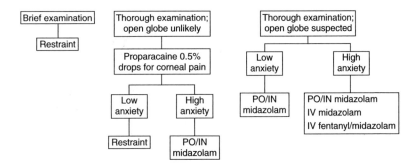

Figure 29.1. Sedation/analgesia options for eye examination.

propriate. Agitation must be controlled. Topical medications to the eye should be avoided until open globe injury is ruled out.

Factors Influencing the Extent of Pharmacologic Management

Risk of Open Globe Injury Opening the eyelids when an open globe injury is possible must be accomplished without pressure on the globe, which can cause extrusion of intraocular contents. Agitation, therefore, must be controlled. Medications that may increase intraocular pressure (e.g., ketamine) are contraindicated in this setting.

Level of Cooperation Required Assessment of visual acuity, extraocular motility, and slit-lamp examination require participation by the patient for accurate evaluation. A significant degree of sedation impairs the patient's ability to cooperate with the examiner.

Age Use of the slit lamp is not possible with most young children even with sedation. Eye examination may be accomplished with restraint. Extremely anxious older children who need a thorough eye examination may benefit from mild sedation/anxiolysis.

Instrument Use The use of instruments in the child's visual field may increase anxiety levels. Although nonpharmacologic measures and topical anesthetic drops are usually sufficient to complete the eye examination, the use of instruments provoke greater anxiety and may require additional pharmacologic management.

FOREIGN-BODY REMOVAL (FIG. 29.2)

Approach and Special Considerations

Patients with suspected ocular foreign bodies require eye examination including eversion of the lids. Lid eversion is more noxious than examination alone and

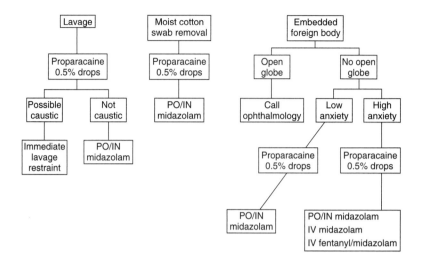

Figure 29.2. Sedation/analgesia options for ocular foreign-body removal.

may increase the need for pharmacologic measures. Optimal examination of the fornices requires cooperation of the patient to look in various directions. Oversedation will preclude this cooperative interaction.

Many foreign bodies can be removed with ocular lavage. Proparacaine anesthetic drops may be instilled after the possibility of a ruptured globe is excluded. Foreign bodies on the underside of the lids can be removed with a premoistened cotton swab. Approaching the eye with the swab from within the child's visual field is frightening for the child and should be avoided.

Embedded foreign bodies can be particularly difficult to remove in young children. If a metal instrument or hypodermic needle is used, a high degree of agitation control is necessary. Even the most cooperative and stoic adult may have a problem when he or she sees a 27-gauge needle approaching the eye. Moderate sedation/anxiolysis and restraint may be helpful in this situation.

OCULAR IRRIGATION

Ocular irrigation for possible caustic exposure to the eye is an emergency procedure that should not wait for sedative administration. If ocular exposure to a caustic substance is suspected, irrigation of the eye should start *immediately*. If immediately available, proparacaine drops can be instilled as the saline is being prepared. If the child is uncooperative, physical restraint and forced eye opening are necessary.

LACERATION REPAIR OF THE EYELID (FIG. 29.3)

Approach and Special Considerations

Lacerations involving the eyelid are common. Repair of an eyelid laceration involves pain and significant anxiety. Manipulation of the eyelids and the unavoidable use of instruments in the field of vision make this repair particularly anxiety provoking. Like other lacerations of the face (see Chapter 30), the cooperation necessary for optimal repair is only achieved in many cases with pharmacologic assistance, especially in younger children.

Sedation requirements are determined by the anticipated time and complexity of repair, need for agitation control, and anxiety level of the patient. Ketamine should not be given to patients at risk for ruptured globe. Ophthalmologic consultation is indicated if injury is suspected to underlying structures.

The prominence of the eyes in one's visual appearance makes optimizing cosmetic results particularly important for lacerations of the eyelids. Small notches or irregularities of the lid margin are especially noticeable. Exact reapproximation of lacerations through the lid margin is necessary. The delicate tissues of the lid require great precision during the repair. The clinician must be certain that movement by the patient will not cause inadvertent injury. Therefore, control of agitation is essential for a successful repair.

If a laceration of the eyelid is associated with injury to underlying structures, ophthalmologic consultation should be sought. These patients will require a greater depth of sedation and more prolonged sedation. General anesthesia is fre-

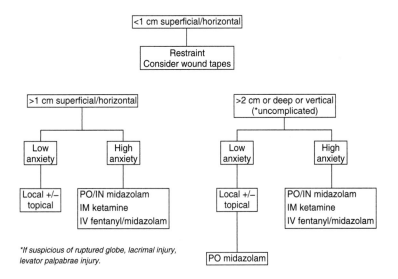

Figure 29.3. Sedation/analgesia options for eyelid lacerations.

quently necessary for optimal repair of complicated lacerations of the eyelid in young children.

Factors Influencing the Extent of Pharmacologic Management

Wound Location   Lacerations close to, or involving the lid margin are more difficult to repair without agitation control. Precise placement of sutures in the recessed area near the medial canthus may be difficult if the patient is not completely still. A greater depth of sedation may be necessary for these wounds.

Wound Dynamics   Vertical lacerations oriented perpendicular to the folds of the eyelid have greater potential for a poor cosmetic result. Deep lacerations of the eyelid need to be explored to assess for associated injuries, which may require a greater degree of sedation. Superficial lacerations along the folds of the eyelid can sometimes be closed with gentle restraint and wound tapes.

SUGGESTED READING

Anderson CTM, Zeltzer LK, Fanurik D. Procedural pain. In: Schechter NL, Berde CB, Yaster M, eds. Pain in Infants, Children and Adolescents. Baltimore, MD: Williams & Wilkins, 1993.

Cheney JP. Ocular foreign body removal. In: Henretig FM, King C, eds. Textbook of Pediatric Emergency Procedures. Baltimore, MD: Williams & Wilkins, 1997.

Gobeaux D, Sardnal F, Cohn H, et al. Intranasal midazolam in pediatric ophthalmology. Cahiers d'Anesthesilogie 1991. 39(1):34–36.

Levin, AV. General pediatric ophthalmic procedures. In: Henretig FM, King C, eds. Textbook of Pediatric Emergency Procedures. Baltimore, MD: Williams & Wilkins, 1997.

Chapter 30
Procedures of the Face and Scalp

Baruch Krauss

LACERATION REPAIR

Approach and Special Considerations

Lacerations of the face and scalp are the most common lacerations in the toddlers. The combination of newly acquired ambulating skills and the larger proportional head size contribute to the high incidence of these types of lacerations. Repair poses unique challenges for clinicians. Toddlers are extremely active and rarely lie in the supine position on a stretcher without assistance for more than a brief period. Furthermore, facial lacerations often require intricate closure techniques to achieve optimal cosmetic results.

Facial and scalp lacerations can be repaired primarily with topical and local anesthesia. Anxiolytic and sedative agents can also be used to increase cooperation, enhance distractibility, and decrease mobility. Facial and scalp lacerations usually take 5 to 45 minutes to repair, and sedation agents should be selected that approximate this time frame.

For those lacerations that can be repaired without sedation, it is important to distinguish those that require only topical anesthesia from those that require both topical and local anesthesia. Superficial lacerations of the face, especially in the orbital and periorbital area where there is only a thin layer of skin overlying the bone, may only need topical anesthesia. Lacerations in deeper tissue usually require both topical and local anesthesia.

Special consideration is necessary for animal bites to the face in toddlers and early school-aged children. These wounds may require debridement and extensive irrigation, which often necessitates a high level of sedation.

Figures 30.1 and 30.2 divide facial and scalp lacerations by location into those involving the forehead/scalp and cheek/chin. Intraoral, perioral, auricular, nasal, and periorbital lacerations are discussed in chapters 28, 29, and 31.

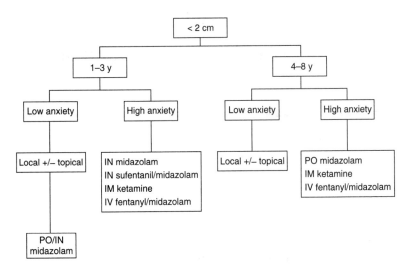

Figure 30.1. Sedation/analgesia options for facial and scalp lacerations.

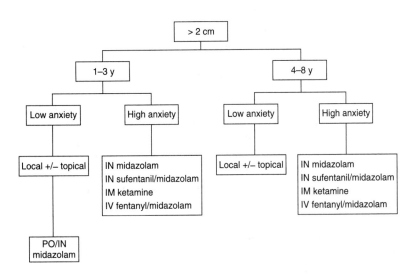

Figure 30.2. Sedation/analgesia options for facial and scalp lacerations.

Factors Influencing the Extent of Pharmacologic Management

Wound Location Wounds located within the child's visual field (chin and cheek lacerations) can be especially challenging in toddlers. However, wounds located outside of the child's visual field (forehead and scalp lacerations) can be managed, in many cases, with topical/local anesthesia augmented by nonpharmacologic strategies.

Wound Dynamics The length and depth of the wound are key determinants of the need for pharmacologic management because the majority of small (less than 2 cm), superficial wounds, especially in children older than 5 years old, can be managed solely with topical/local anesthesia.

Agitation Control Immobility during laceration repair is particularly important for lacerations involving the face. The degree of immobility required for proper cosmetic closure determines the need for and extent of pharmacologic management.

Age Early toddlers (ages 1 to 3) are the most difficult age group to manage. These children are constantly in motion and are apprehensive of strange people and places. A large (more than 2 cm), deep wound of the face in this age group requires some form of pharmacologic management and a high degree of agitation control.

Anxiety Level When children of any age are calm, trusting, and playful much can be accomplished with only the use of topical and local anesthesia. Just as important is when the parents are calm, trusting, and able to assist the clinician in minimizing anxiety and maximizing cooperation through engaging the child in an activity of interest, thereby moving the child's attention away from the procedure itself.

ABSCESS INCISION AND DRAINAGE

Approach and Special Considerations

Despite liberal use of local anesthesia, abscess incision and drainage is often a painful procedure, especially during the expression of pus and wound packing. Therefore, it is important to provide sufficient systemic analgesia and sedation because local anesthesia alone is usually not sufficient (except in the case of small abscesses) to control the pain and anxiety associated with this procedure. Numerous analgesia and sedation options exist (Fig. 30.3).

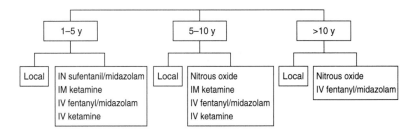

Figure 30.3. Sedation/analgesia options for facial and scalp abscess incision and drainage.

SUGGESTED READING

Bilmire DA, Neale HW, Gregory RO. Use of IV fentanyl in the outpatient treatment of pediatric facial trauma. J Trauma 1985;25:1079–1080.

Green SM, Nakamura R, Johnson NE. Ketamine sedation for pediatric procedures: part 1, a prospective series. Ann Emerg Med 1990;19:1024–1032.

Hennes HM, Wagner V, Bonadio WA, et al. The effect of oral midazolam on anxiety of preschool children during laceration repair. Ann Emerg Med 1990;19:1006–1009.

McNamara R, Loiselle. Laceration repair. In: Henretig FM, King C, eds. Textbook of Pediatric Emergency Procedures. Baltimore: Williams & Wilkins, 1997:1141–1168.

Qureshi FA, Mellis PT, McFadden MA. Efficacy of oral ketamine for providing sedation and analgesia to children requiring laceration repair. Pediatr Emerg Care 1995;11:33–37.

Schilling CG, Bank DE, Borchert BA, et al. Tetracaine, epinephrine (adrenalin), and cocaine (TAC) versus lidocaine, epinephrine, and tetracaine (LET) for anesthesia of lacerations in children. Ann Emerg Med 1995;25:203–208.

Theroux MC, West DW, Corddry DH, et al. Efficacy of intranasal midazolam in facilitating the suturing of lacerations in preschool children in the emergency room. Pediatrics 1993; 91:624–627.

Young GM. Incision and drainage of a cutaneous abscess. In: Henretig FM, King C, eds. Textbook of Pediatric Emergency Procedures. Baltimore: Williams & Wilkins, 1997: 1199–1204.

Chapter 31
Oral Procedures

Edward Walkley

LACERATION REPAIR OF THE ORAL CAVITY AND DENTAL REPAIR AFTER TRAUMA

Lacerations of the oral cavity and fractured teeth present a set of special considerations for the clinician that affect the choice of analgesia and sedation (Figs. 31.1 through 31.5). Most intraoral lacerations will not require repair. Those that do, although not technically difficult, are in an awkward location such as the tongue or mucosa. Lip lacerations, particularly those that involve the vermilion border, must be repaired with accurate approximation to achieve optimal cosmetic results. Many lacerations may require layered closure. Therefore, these repairs require a particularly high level of patient cooperation. Because of age or associated injuries, the level of cooperation may be difficult for most toddlers and some adolescents. The clinician must first determine if the lesion requires repair, select the proper local anesthesia, and carefully weigh the risks and benefits of sedation.

APPROACH AND SPECIAL CONSIDERATIONS

Age

Oral lesions predominantly occur in two age groups: toddlers and adolescents. Toddlers most commonly present with isolated oral injuries associated with falls. Lip lacerations are somewhat less common than the other facial lacerations. The vermilion border may, however, be particularly difficult to see and accurately approximate. Tongue lacerations are more common, usually associated with a fall to the chin and biting with teeth. All oral lacerations may be associated with fractured or dislodged primary teeth. The toddler's level of activity that caused the injury now makes management of these wounds more difficult. Few children will hold their tongue out for suturing after local injection. Few toddlers are capable of lying still long enough for a layered closure of the lip.

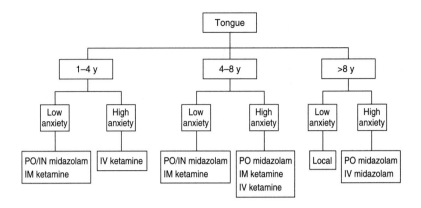

Figure 31.1. Sedation/analgesia options for intra-oral lesions requiring suturing. (This implies lesions in the anterior half of the mouth with easily controlled bleeding and adequate suction. Lesions in the posterior half may require intubation and general anesthesia for optimal safe repair.)

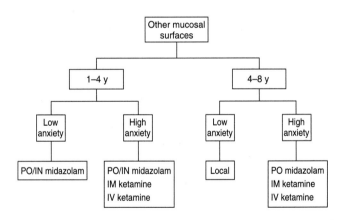

Figure 31.2. Sedation/analgesia options for intra-oral lesions requiring suturing. (This implies lesions in the anterior half of the mouth with easily controlled bleeding and adequate suction. Lesions in the posterior half may require intubation and general anesthesia for optimal safe repair.)

Oral injuries in adolescents are more frequently associated with other traumatic injuries. Although bicycle helmets reduce severe head injuries, they do not reduce oral injuries. Mouth guards are rarely used outside of organized sports. Bicycle, skateboard, and motor vehicle crashes may be associated with either closed head injury or facial or systemic injuries. Although cooperation is generally much easier in adolescents, the associated injuries add special considerations for oral lesions.

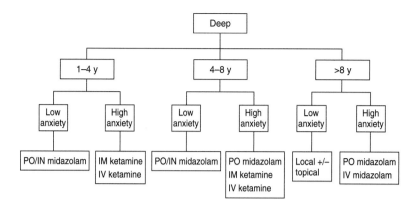

Figure 31.3. Sedation/analgesia options for lacerations of the lip involving the vermillion border.

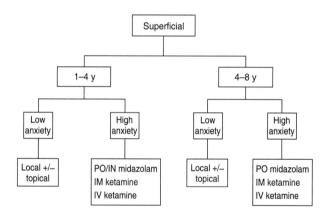

Figure 31.4. Sedation/analgesia options for lacerations of the lip involving the vermillion border.

Local Analgesia

Local injection of buffered lidocaine will produce adequate local anesthesia for all but the most difficult intraoral repair (see chapters 8 and 9). The wound itself may be infiltrated, or the clinician may use one of the mental or dental blocks. Unfortunately, the pain of injection may heighten the anxiety and decrease the ability of toddlers to cooperate. Topical anesthetics have been shown to work extremely well on facial lacerations not involving mucous membranes. Topical anesthetics cause significant blanching of the wound and can make approximation of the vermilion border difficult.

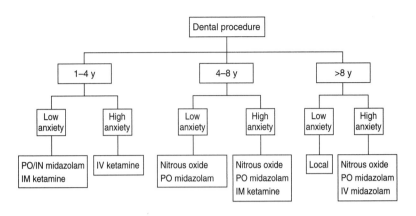

Figure 31.5. Sedation/analgesia options for dental extraction or reimplantation after trauma.

Blood and Oral Secretions

Most oral lesions bleed copiously and most children swallow a lot of that blood. Blood is extremely irritating to the stomach and emesis is frequent. This increases the risk of aspiration during the procedure even if the child has been NPO (has had nothing by mouth) for an appropriate time. The increased risk of emesis must be considered when sedating these patients.

Parental Anxiety

Oral lesions with the presence of blood, broken teeth, and the potential for permanent scarring are particularly anxiety producing for families. Tongue lacerations may require the use of bite blocks or sutures through the tongue, which can be terrifying to the uninitiated lay person as well as the child. Many oral lesions can be easily repaired using a local anesthetic and carefully immobilizing the child, producing minimal trauma to the child; however, this may cause significant anxiety to the parent. Parents should be prepared ahead of time by the nurse and/or physician to minimize their anxiety and maximize their ability to help their child be calm and cooperative during the procedure.

Choice of Agents

Although all of these lesions are relatively simple technically, they tend to take longer than a similar size laceration outside of the oral cavity. Sedation and total immobilization are frequently required. Certain agents should be used with extreme caution for oral procedures. Because of the potential for laryngospasm, ketamine is relatively contraindicated for oral procedures associated with in-

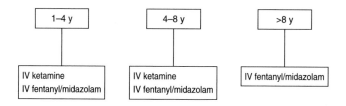

Figure 31.6. Sedation/analgesia options for reduction of mandibular dislocation.

creased secretions or bleeding and particularly those involving the posterior pharynx. The ability of ketamine to produce complete dissociation while the patient maintains a patent airway makes it particularly attractive for oral lesions. The duration of action of ketamine is also suited to most oral repairs. Because sedation is rarely required in youths, emergence reactions are less of a problem (see Chapter 7).

MANDIBULAR DISLOCATION (FIG. 31.6)

This is a relatively uncommon injury in children. In adults, it can occur spontaneously, whereas in children it is frequently traumatic. The procedure is like other dislocation reductions and is briefly and intensely painful after which the patient generally experiences a significant decrease in pain. In addition to the issue of anxiolysis and cooperation associated with intraoral injuries, this procedure requires sedation, analgesia, and muscle relaxation. The optimal sedation regimen would be titratable with a wide safety margin, rapid onset, and short duration and would combine both analgesia and sedative properties. Because mandibular dislocation is most likely to occur in patients over 8 years old, and may involve some increase in secretions, ketamine may be a less desirable agent.

SUGGESTED READING

Bonadio WA. Safe effective method for application of tetracaine, adrenaline, and cocaine to oral lacerations. Ann Emerg Med 1996;28:396–398.

Dionne RA, Gordon SM, et al. Assessing the need for anesthesia and sedation in the general population. J Am Dent Assoc 1998;129:167–173

Delfino J. Public attitudes toward oral surgery; results of a Gallup poll. J Oral Maxillofac Surg 1997;55:564–567.

Green SM, et al. Safety of ketamine for emergency department pediatric sedation. J Oral Maxillofac Surg 1995;53:13–17.

Nelson LP. Emergency management of oral trauma in children. Curr Opin Pediatr 1997;9: 242–245.

Parworth LP, Frost DE, et al. Propofol and fentanyl compared with midazolam and fentanyl during third molar surgery. Parworth LP, Frost DE. J Oral Maxillofac Surg 1998;56:447–453.

Pruitt JW, Goldwasser MS. Intramuscular ketamine, midazolam and glycopyrrolate for pediatric sedation in the emergency department. J Oral Maxillofac Surg 1995;53:13–17.

Roelofse JA, et al. A double-blind randomized comparison of midazolam alone and midazolam combined with ketamine for sedation of pediatric dental patients. J Oral Maxillofac Surg 1996;54:838–844.

Yamamoto LG, et al. Informed consent and parental choice of anesthesia and sedation for repair of small lacerations in children. Am J Emerg Med 1997;15:285–289.

Section III: Chest

Chapter 32
Chest Procedures

David Greenes

ELECTRIC COUNTERSHOCK THERAPY

Approach and Special Considerations

Cardiac dysrhythmias are relatively rare in pediatrics, and dysrhythmias requiring electrical cardioversion or defibrillation are even more uncommon. Nonetheless, the emergency clinician will on occasion be presented with patients with ventricular fibrillation, ventricular tachycardia, or supraventricular tachycardias requiring electric countershock therapy.

Electric countershock therapy is an uncomfortable and frightening experience. Whenever possible, patients undergoing the procedure should be sedated. Because the procedure takes only a few moments, short-acting agents are preferred. Regimens involving sedation alone or sedation and analgesia have both been used with good success.

Factors Influencing the Extent of Pharmacologic Management

Urgency Ventricular fibrillation and pulseless ventricular tachycardia are premorbid rhythms that should be treated immediately with asynchronous defibrillation. When treating these rhythms, absolutely no delay for the administration of sedating medications should be tolerated.

Some patients with ventricular tachycardia with a pulse or with supraventricular tachycardias may be unstable and may be deteriorating rapidly in the emergency department. These patients should also be treated immediately with synchronized electrical cardioversion, and no delay for the preparation and administration of sedating medications should occur.

On the other hand, many patients with ventricular tachycardia or supraventricular tachycardia are stable and are treated with electrical cardioversion only after medical therapies have been unsuccessful. For these stable patients, sedation is indicated.

Underlying Medical Conditions Patients undergoing cardioversion may have multiple medical problems and they may be on several medications. The clinician should think carefully about the potential for drug interactions or other adverse effects before choosing a sedation regimen.

Cardiovascular Depression Much reported experience is in the medical literature using a variety of agents for cardioversion, including midazolam, midazolam/fentanyl, diazepam, thiopental, methohexital, etomidate, and propofol. With the exception of etomidate, all of these agents typically produce some decrease in systolic blood pressure when given for cardioversion. However, these decreases in blood pressure tend to be mild and well tolerated by patients. If potential cardiovascular depression is a concern, the drugs should be given initially in low doses and carefully titrated.

Ketamine may appear to be an attractive agent for patients undergoing cardioversion because it tends to maintain cardiac output and vascular tone. The use of ketamine has generally been avoided, however, probably because of the theoretical risk of a proarrhythmic effect, or of injuring an already compromised heart through increases in myocardial oxygen demand, preload, and afterload.

Efficacy of Cardioversion Concern has been raised in the medical literature that different sedating agents might affect the automaticity of the heart in such a way as to decrease the success rate of cardioversion. In fact, no differences in the rates of successful cardioversion have been noted among the various agents evaluated.

Available Routes of Administration All patients undergoing elective or semielective cardioversion should have an IV placed before the procedure because of the serious risk for decompensation as a result of the electrical therapy. Because IV sedation offers the advantages of titratability and reliability, it is the preferred route of sedation for cardioversion.

If patients require cardioversion urgently before IV access can be obtained, one should perform the procedure immediately, without any sedation. A flow diagram showing the options for sedation is presented in Figure 32.1.

TUBE THORACOSTOMY

Approach and Special Considerations

Tube thoracostomy is performed emergently as a life-saving procedure for trauma patients with tension pneumothorax or rapidly progressing hemothorax. Because tension pneumothorax is a life-threatening condition, relief of the tension needs to be pursued immediately. In this setting, sedation/analgesia is a luxury to be pursued only if the clinician is certain that the patient is stable enough to tolerate the delay. Tube thoracostomy is also frequently performed semielectively for

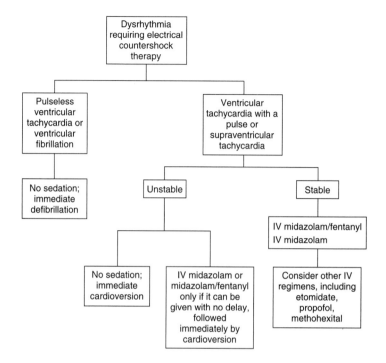

Figure 32.1. Electrical countershock therapy.

patients who have simple pneumothorax and for patients with empyema or other effusions requiring continuous drainage.

Tube thoracostomy is a painful, unpleasant, frightening, and potentially dangerous procedure. A combination of local anesthesia, systemic analgesia, anxiolysis, and sedation will be indicated for most patients undergoing tube thoracostomy. The effects should generally last approximately 10 to 15 minutes, which will allow enough time for the tube to be placed and secured in most instances.

Factors Influencing the Extent of Pharmacologic Management

Need for Immediate Decompression   A tube thoracostomy may be required emergently as in patients with a tension pneumothorax or rapidly accumulating hemothorax. Some of these patients can be stabilized briefly with a needle decompression procedure to allow a few extra moments for premedication before the tube thoracostomy is performed. If patients cannot be stabilized, the tube thoracostomy should be performed immediately, even if no local or systemic sedation/analgesia has been provided. This approach is especially prudent for those critically ill patients who have a depressed level of consciousness.

Degree of Respiratory or Cardiovascular Compromise In choosing a treatment regimen, clinicians should be cognizant of the potential adverse effects, especially given that the patient's underlying condition (e.g., trauma with internal bleeding or pneumonia with significant lung disease) may already be compromising the cardiovascular or respiratory status (see chapter 24).

Therefore, clinicians ideally will start with lower doses and titrate to effect. Agents that are reversible are preferred for these tenuous patients as well. Agents with minimal cardiovascular or respiratory depressing effects (such as ketamine) may be preferred, if no contraindications exist for their use.

Finally, the clinician should remember that performing the procedure without sedation is always an option if the potential risks of sedation outweigh the benefits. The clinician should also consider the option of endotracheal intubation and controlled ventilation for those patients in whom sedation appears necessary but cannot be given safely otherwise.

Type of Tube Being Placed

Conventional Tube Thoracostomy Whenever possible, patients undergoing a conventional tube thoracostomy (Fig. 32.2) should be medicated liberally with local anesthesia. If time permits, topical pretreatment with EMLA cream will make the initial stages of lidocaine administration more comfortable. Typically, as much as 10 to 20 mL of 1% lidocaine are used (remembering the maximum dose of 3 to 5 mg/kg) to anesthetize a large area of skin, subcutaneous tissue, the periosteum, the chest wall, and the pleural lining. Careful attention to local anesthesia will significantly decrease the need for systemic analgesia.

A tube thoracostomy involves vigorous blunt dissection of the chest wall, and local anesthesia is often insufficient. Furthermore, a tube thoracostomy is an invasive procedure that is frightening and unpleasant for many patients, even when pain is controlled. For these reasons, most patients undergoing a conventional tube thoracostomy require moderate systemic levels of analgesia, anxiolysis, and sedation.

Pigtail Catheter As an alternative to a tube thoracostomy, some simple pneumothoraces and effusions may be drained via a smaller pigtail catheter, which is placed using a Seldinger technique. Because the placement of a pigtail catheter involves no blunt dissection, this procedure is less painful and unpleasant for patients. Significantly lower levels of sedation, anxiolysis, and analgesia are required.

The experience of having a pigtail catheter placed is similar to that of diagnostic thoracentesis. For this reason, the sedation of patients undergoing a pigtail catheter thoracostomy is discussed in the section on thoracentesis.

Routes of Administration Available Except in some emergent situations, all patients undergoing tube thoracostomy should have an IV placed before beginning the procedure because of the real possibility of serious cardiovascular or respira-

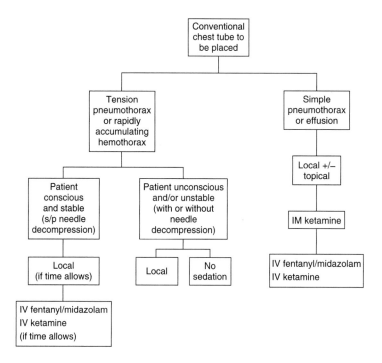

Figure 32.2. Tube thoracostomy.

tory compromise. Because IV sedation offers the advantages of titratability and reliability, it is the preferred route of sedation for a tube thoracostomy.

Patient Age   Regardless of patient age, most patients undergoing a tube thoracostomy will benefit from some degree of systemic sedation and analgesia. Younger patients may need higher degrees of sedation to allow appropriate immobilization so that the procedure can be performed safely and expediently.

Anxiety Level   Even among patients at a given age, anxiety levels may vary widely depending on the patient's temperament, prior medical experiences, intrinsic disease state (respiratory distress or chest pain may contribute significantly to anxiety), and available support systems (anxious parents often contribute to their child's anxiety). Attention should be given to optimizing nonpharmacologic sedation through the use of calming words, distraction, the avoidance of loud noises or harsh lighting, and reassurance to anxious family members.

Unique Adverse Effects in This Setting   As a special note, nitrous oxide should be avoided in any patient with suspected or documented pneumothorax, because the insoluble gas will diffuse from the blood into the pneumothorax, thereby increasing the size of the pneumothorax. For this same reason, nitrous oxide should be avoided during the placement of chest tubes for effusion or hemothorax, where the potential for an iatrogenic pneumothorax exists.

THORACENTESIS/PIGTAIL CATHETER PLACEMENT (FIG. 32.3)

Approach and Special Considerations

Thoracentesis usually is performed semielectively in an inpatient setting or in the emergency department. Most commonly, thoracentesis is performed as a diagnostic procedure to obtain pleural fluid for analysis. When larger volumes of fluid are drained, thoracentesis may be therapeutic as well. The clinical condition of patients undergoing thoracentesis will vary, depending on the size of the effusion and the degree of underlying lung disease, from essentially no symptoms to severe respiratory distress.

Pigtail catheters are placed instead of a tube thoracostomy where a smaller bore catheter will suffice. Pigtail catheters have become increasingly popular for the drainage of simple pneumothoraces and for some pleural effusions. These catheters usually are placed semielectively in the emergency department or in an inpatient setting.

Thoracentesis and pigtail catheter placement are performed in a similar man-

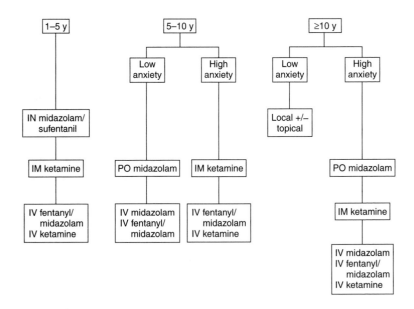

Figure 32.3. Thoracentesis or pigtail catheter thoracostomy.

ner, thus will be discussed together. These procedures cause pain as the needle contacts nerve endings in the skin, subcutaneous tissue, the periosteum of the rib, and the parietal pleura itself. Pigtail catheter placement may be a bit more uncomfortable because of the use of a dilator to enlarge the entry site in the skin and because the procedure requires 1 or 2 extra minutes to complete.

Thoracentesis is performed with the patient sitting upright, leaning over a table or the back of a chair. This position makes management of the airway somewhat more difficult, because the patient's head and neck are unsupported and may flop over, causing airway obstruction when sedation is achieved. The clinician should designate an assistant who will attend to the patient's airway during the procedure, helping to position the airway appropriately, providing supplemental oxygen, and being prepared to suction if necessary. The clinician should remember as well that thoracentesis is generally a semielective procedure. Therefore, if complications arise during sedation, the procedure should be aborted, and the patient should be placed supine on a bed so that optimal airway management and resuscitation efforts can be undertaken.

Because these procedures involve a fairly small and accessible area of body tissue, local anesthesia can be effective in eliminating pain. When time permits, EMLA may be applied to the skin area where the procedure is to be performed. Because the needle will penetrate deeply into the chest wall, however, injected lidocaine should be used as well. When infiltrating lidocaine, care should be taken to anesthetize the entire path of the thoracentesis needle, from the skin and subcutaneous tissue down to the level of the periosteum, and then "walking" along the periosteum over the rib until the pleura itself is reached.

For some patients, even the pain of this local anesthesia may be difficult to bear. In addition, patients undergoing thoracentesis or pigtail catheter placement may be anxious as a result of the respiratory distress they are experiencing or from their fear of the procedure itself. Finally, thoracentesis and pigtail catheter placements are potentially dangerous procedures, with the risk of pneumothorax, hemothorax, injury to intercostal arteries or nerves, or injury to the liver or spleen. It is essential that the patient be fairly immobile during the procedure.

For these reasons, some combination of systemic analgesia, anxiolysis, and sedation may be necessary for a large number of patients undergoing these procedures. The ideal agents should be short-acting, because the entire procedure in most cases will take only 5 to 10 minutes.

Factors Influencing the Extent of Pharmacologic Management

Cardiovascular and Respiratory Stability In all cases, sedation and analgesia should be given only if the benefits of the therapy outweigh the risks. If patients are significantly hypoxic, in respiratory distress, or hemodynamically unstable, it may be more appropriate to perform these procedures without sedation or to defer the procedure until the patient is stabilized. Consideration should also be given to endotracheal intubation and controlled ventilation if sedation is deemed necessary and cannot be given safely otherwise.

Because most patients undergoing these procedures will have at least some potential for respiratory or hemodynamic compromise, the agents that are used should cause a minimum of respiratory or cardiovascular depression. Ideally, therapy should begin at the low end of the dose range with the drug titrated to effect. Reversible agents are particularly advantageous in this setting.

Patient Age If a patient can tolerate the administration of local anesthesia, the remainder of the procedure should be essentially painless. A calm, older patient who understands the reason for the procedure and the need to remain still may require no further medication.

Younger children will frequently require some additional pharmacologic interventions to make the procedure easier for them to tolerate and to achieve the necessary degree of immobilization. In general, the need is probably more for sedation and anxiolysis than for systemic analgesia. Even the local administration of lidocaine may be difficult for some patients, and the discomfort associated with this process may contribute to the patient's level of anxiety. For many younger patients, at least some degree of systemic analgesia and sedation will be needed before the administration of lidocaine.

Anxiety Level More anxious older patients may require significant pharmacologic anxiolysis, sedation, and analgesia, as described for the younger patients. In all cases, attention should be given to maximizing nonpharmacologic sedation by making every effort to keep the patient as relaxed, comfortable, and distracted as possible.

Available Routes of Administration Because of the potential for serious adverse events, all patients undergoing thoracentesis should have an IV placed before beginning the procedure. IV sedation will be preferred in the great majority of cases because it offers the advantages of reliability and titratability. Other routes of administration are acceptable, especially for older or calmer patients who require lighter levels of sedation and/or analgesia. In cases in which only anxiolysis is desired, the oral route might be chosen because of its excellent safety profile.

Unique Adverse Effects in This Setting As discussed for tube thoracostomy, nitrous oxide should be avoided in settings where pneumothorax exists or may be created iatrogenically, because of the potential for the poorly soluble gas to diffuse from the blood stream into the pleural air space, thereby expanding the pneumothorax.

SUGGESTED READING

Canessa R, Lema G, Urzua J, et al. Anesthesia for elective cardioversion: a comparison of four anesthetic agents. J Cardiothorac Vasc Anesth 1991;5:566–568.

Connors KM, Terndrup TE. Tube thoracostomy and needle decompression of the chest. In:

Henrettig FM, King C, eds. Textbook of Pediatric Emergency Procedures. Baltimore: Williams & Wilkins, 1997:389–407.

DiGuilio GA. Thoracentesis. In: Henrettig FM, King C, eds. Textbook of Pediatric Emergency Procedures. Baltimore: Williams & Wilkins, 1997:879–887.

Fennelly ME, Powell H, Galletly DC, et al. Midazolam sedation reversed with flumazenil for cardioversion. Brit J Anaesth 1992;68:303–305.

Gale DW, Grissom TE, Mirenda JV. Titration of intravenous anesthetics for cardioversion: a comparison of propofol, methohexital, and midazolam. Crit Care Med 1993;21:1509–1513.

Gill RM, Sweeney RJ, Reid PR. The defibrillation threshold: a comparison of anesthetics and measurement methods. Pacing Clin Electrophysiol 1993;16:708–714.

Gupta A, Lennmarken C, Vegfors M, et al. Anaesthesia for cardioversion. A comparison between propofol, thiopentone, and midazolam. Anaesthesia 1990;45:872–875.

Khan AH, Malhotra R. Midazolam as intravenous sedative for electrocardioversion. Chest 1989;95:1068–1071.

Scarfone RJ. Cardioversion and defibrillation. In: Henrettig FM, King C, eds. Textbook of Pediatric Emergency Procedures. Baltimore: Williams & Wilkins, 1997:313–326.

Chapter 33
Abdomen and Genitalia

Stephen Teach

HERNIA REDUCTION

Approach and Special Considerations

A hernia is defined as a bulging or protrusion of a structure across a wall designed to contain it. Although there are numerous hernias of the abdominal wall (umbilical, femoral, and direct and indirect inguinal), by far the most common are indirect inguinal hernias. These hernias involve passage of intra-abdominal contents through the inguinal ring, down the inguinal canal along a patent processus vaginalis into the scrotum or labia. Incarceration occurs when the contents cannot be easily reduced. Strangulation occurs when vascular compromise ensues. More common in premature infants and in males, indirect inguinal hernias occur in up to 5% of the general pediatric population, usually in the first year of life.

Rapid reduction of indirect inguinal hernia is essential. Once incarceration occurs, increased swelling and strangulation follow, making reduction increasingly difficult and putting the herniated bowel at risk of ischemia.

Attempts to reduce incarcerated hernias are painful and causes crying, which raises the intra-abdominal pressure and tenses the abdominal wall. Both of these effects make reduction even more difficult. Sedation and analgesia must therefore be sufficient to minimize crying, making successful reduction more likely.

Reduction without sedation and analgesia may be possible with minimal distress and should be attempted before the use of pharmacologic agents. Because the time for reduction may vary from a few seconds of gentle pressure to several minutes of firm pressure, the method employed should ideally be titratable, with options to extend it as long as necessary. Useful nonpharmacologic adjuncts to a proper reduction technique include Trendelenburg positioning, an ice pack to the groin, warm hands, dim light, soft voices, verbal reassurance, and parental touch. Specific approaches to sedation and analgesia are presented in Figure 33.1.

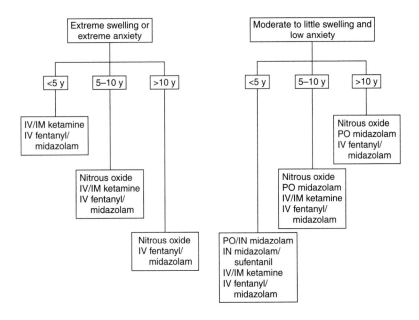

Figure 33.1. Sedation/analgesia options for incarcerated hernia reduction.

Gynecological Evaluation

Approach and Special Considerations A nonelective gynecological examination (a "pelvic exam") may be done as part of an evaluation for trauma, for sex-
ually transmitted diseases, for abdominal pain, or for alleged sexual abuse. In
any case, these examinations may be especially stressful for the school-aged or
adolescent patient. Issues of modesty in a busy, unfamiliar emergency department or clinic setting combined with inadequate time for self-preparation leave
many patients feeling anxious and vulnerable. Adequate sedation and anxiolysis
should therefore be the focus of the practitioner's approach. Constant reassurance and a slow, quiet, gentle approach are essential adjuncts. Unless the examination is performed to repair a laceration or to drain an abscess (see "Incision
and Drainage of Bartholin Cyst" and "Laceration Repair of the External Genitalia and Perineal Area"), then issues of local and systemic analgesia are usually
less important.

In certain cases (e.g., alleged episodes of sexual assault), the practitioner must
acknowledge that no amount of sedation, anxiolysis, and analgesia can prevent retraumatizing the victim. Under such circumstances, the forensic examination may
be best performed under general anesthesia in the operating room. Specific approaches to sedation and analgesia are presented in Figure 33.2.

Incision and Drainage of Bartholin Cyst

Approach and Special Considerations   Incision and drainage of a Bartholin cyst involves a gynecological examination (see "Gynecological Evaluation"). Issues of local and systemic analgesia are covered here.

Unless the abscess is small, effective local analgesia is difficult to obtain. This painful procedure involves an incision into inflamed and swollen tissue, drainage of purulent material, and often packing. Often, slowly infiltrating the skin around the abscess with buffered and warmed 1% lidocaine without epinephrine is the only way to anesthetize the inflamed tissue. Topical analgesia has no role. Systemic analgesia may be necessary in certain cases.

The procedure itself is short. Most can be completed within 10 minutes. The sedation and analgesia used should be titratable with a rapid onset and short duration of action. Specific approaches to sedation and analgesia are presented in Figure 33.3.

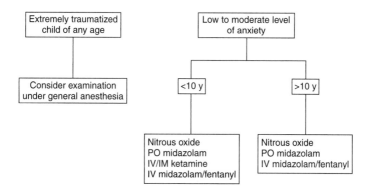

Figure 33.2. Sedation/analgesia options for a gynecological examination.

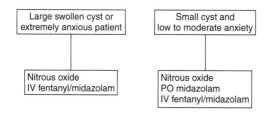

Figure 33.3. Sedation/analgesia options for incision and drainage of a Bartholin cyst. Note: 1) All options assume liberal use of buffered, warmed local anesthetic. 2) Because the majority of these patients are adolescents, use of ketamine should be discouraged.

Laceration Repair of the External Genitalia and Perineal Area

Approach and Special Considerations

Repair of a laceration of the external genitalia or perineal area involves a gynecological examination in a female, or a similar examination in a male (see "Gynecological Evaluation"). Issues of local and systemic analgesia are covered here.

In general, topical anesthesia plays no role. Available topical preparations contain epinephrine to induce vasoconstriction and are therefore contraindicated in lacerations of the penis and clitoris. Similarly, extreme caution must be used with injectable local anesthetics containing epinephrine, which are again contraindicated in lacerations of the penis and clitoris. Certain penile lacerations may be amenable to repair with a dorsal penile nerve block (see "Paraphimosis Reduction").

Special consideration must be given to the child with genital or perineal lacerations incurred during an alleged sexual or physical assault. To avoid retraumatizing the victim of such an assault, strong consideration should be given to completing the forensic examination and laceration repair under general anesthesia in the operating room. Specific approaches to sedation and analgesia are presented in Figure 33.4 and 33.5.

Paraphimosis Reduction

Approach and Special Considerations Paraphimosis results when a tight foreskin cannot be reduced once retracted over the glans penis. As the duration of retraction lengthens, venous congestion and increased swelling results, making reduction increasingly difficult. The condition is most common in young patients whose foreskin is not yet fully retractable. A number of techniques have been described to facilitate reduction. If the swelling and anxiety level are not great, then manual reduction without sedation or analgesia should be attempted.

For more complicated cases, a dorsal penile nerve block to achieve penile analgesia may be effective. This procedure involves infiltration of local anesthetic (usually 1% lidocaine) at the base of the penis on the dorsal aspect. Use of preparations of local anesthetic with epinephrine are contraindicated. After sterile preparation, 1 mL (for a neonate) to 5 mL (for an adolescent) of local anesthetic is injected on both sides of the dorsal penile neurovascular bundle (at the 10-o'clock and 2-o'clock positions). Injection is best made with as small a needle as possible, just inside Buck's Fascia. A palpable "pop" is usually felt when the fascia is crossed. Aspiration should always precede injection. Complications, although rare, include bleeding, hematoma formation, and the possibility of infection.

Whether or not a dorsal penile nerve block is used, additional sedation, anxiolysis, and analgesia may be necessary. If the foreskin is badly swollen, prolonged manual compression to decrease the edema may be necessary. The regimen chosen for sedation and analgesia should therefore be sufficiently flexible and titrat-

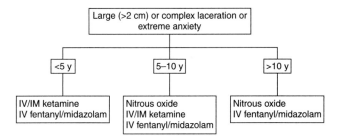

Figure 33.4. Sedation/analgesia options for laceration repair of the external genitalia and perineal region. Note: All options assume liberal use of buffered, warmed local anesthetic.

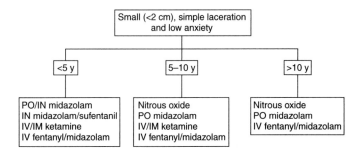

Figure 33.5. Sedation/analgesia options for laceration repair of the external genitalia and perineal region.

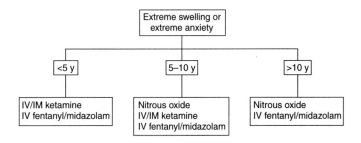

Figure 33.6. Sedation/analgesia options for paraphimosis reduction. Note: All options assume that a dorsal penile nerve block has been considered.

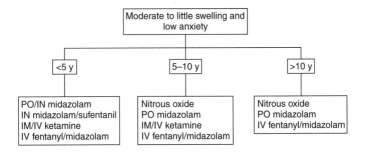

Figure 33.7. Sedation/analgesia options for paraphimosis reduction.

able so it can be prolonged if necessary. Specific approaches to sedation and analgesia are presented in Figure 33.6 and 33.7.

SUGGESTED READING

Hernia Reduction

Bronsther B, Abrams MW, Elboim C. Inguinal hernias in children— a study of 1000 cases and a review of the literature. JAMA 1972;27:522–584.

Clark MC. Hernia reduction. In: Henretig FM, King C, eds. Textbook of Pediatric Emergency Procedures. Baltimore: Williams & Wilkins, 1997:927–933.

Gynecological Evaluation

Giardino AP, Christian CW. Adolescent pelvic examination. In: Henretig FM, King C, eds. Textbook of Pediatric Emergency Procedures. Baltimore: Williams & Wilkins, 1997: 975–981.

Ludwig S. Child abuse. In: Fleisher GR, Ludwig S, eds. Textbook of Pediatric Emergency Medicine. 3rd ed. Baltimore: Williams & Wilkins, 1994:1429–1463.

Millstein SG, Adler NE, Irwin CE. Sources of anxiety about pelvic examinations among adolescent females. J Adolesc Health Care 1984;5:105–111.

Primrose RB. Taking the tension out of pelvic exams. Am J Nurs 1984;84:72–74.

Incision and Drainage of a Bartholin Cyst

Young GM. Incision and drainage of a cutaneous abscess. In: Henretig FM, King C, eds. Textbook of Pediatric Emergency Procedures. Baltimore: Williams & Wilkins, 1997: 1199–1204.

Laceration Repair of the External Genitalia and Perineal Area

Bartfield JM, Gennis P, Barbera J, et al. Buffered versus plain lidocaine as a local anesthetic for simple laceration repair. Ann Emerg Med 1990;19:1387–1389.

Lewis L, Stephan M. Local and regional anesthesia. In: Henretig FM, King C, eds. Textbook of Pediatric Emergency Procedures. Baltimore: Williams & Wilkins, 1997:465–496.

Mader TJ, Playe SJ, Garb JL. Reducing the pain of local anesthetic infiltration: warming and buffering have a synergistic effect. Ann Emerg Med 1994;23:550–554.

McNamara R, Loiselle. Laceration repair. In: Henretig FM, King C, eds. Textbook of Pediatric Emergency Procedures. Baltimore: Williams & Wilkins, 1997:1141–1168.

Paraphimosis Reduction

Green M, Strange GR. Paraphimosis reduction. In: Henretig FM, King C, eds. Textbook of Pediatric Emergency Procedures. Baltimore: Williams & Wilkins, 1997:1007–1010.

Lewis L, Stephan M. Penile nerve blocks. In: Henretig FM, King C, eds. Textbook of Pediatric Emergency Procedures. Baltimore: Williams & Wilkins, 1997:487–489.

Chapter 34
Musculoskeletal Procedures

Robert Kennedy, David Jaffe

FRACTURE REDUCTION

Approach and Special Considerations

Fractures and joint dislocations are among the most painful pediatric emergencies. Successful management in the emergency department requires effective relief of pain and anxiety. Many regimens have been shown to provide analgesia and anxiolysis during fracture care, yet no consensus exists on which are safest and most effective because few direct comparisons of techniques have been reported. No single regimen provides the best means of fracture pain and anxiety management for all patients.

Most children benefit from balanced sedation with anxiolytic and analgesic agents. Parental presence during sedation also may lessen patient and parental anxiety and decrease the amount of sedative medication required. The addition of amnestic agents such as midazolam can prevent patient recall of residual procedural pain, but these agents often potentiate respiratory depression and lessen the amount of analgesic that can be administered safely. Combination of techniques (e.g., nitrous oxide plus hematoma block) may increase effectiveness, lessen adverse effects, and hasten recovery from sedation by decreasing the amount of individual medications required. Intensely painful or difficult fracture reductions may be managed with deep levels of sedation during the reduction, injection of lidocaine into the fracture hematoma (hematoma block), and placement of a local nerve block (e.g., axillary) or intravenous regional anesthesia (Bier block). Fractures requiring little or no manipulation may need little or no sedation if effective analgesia is provided.

Published medication dosages estimate amounts likely to be safe and reasonably effective for most patients, yet individual patient responses may determine that greater or lesser amounts of medication than recommended are needed to provide the desired effect. "Titration to effect" with repeated fractional dosing enables use of the least amount of medication to achieve the desired effect. Repeated administration of fractional doses lessens adverse effects when compared with administration of a larger single dose and allows use of the smallest effective dose of a medication, thus hastening recovery. This approach minimizes adverse effects but requires use of methods that enable rapid medication absorption such as intravenous or inhalational administration.

Adverse effects of medications, such as respiratory depression, nausea, and blunting of protective airway reflexes, limit the amount of medication that can safely be administered and thus prevent complete procedural anesthesia. Patients should be considered to have "full stomachs" because of the ileus that many fractures induce. If these patients then become more deeply sedated than expected, they will and be at increased risk for hypoxia and aspiration.

Strategies of effective fracture pain management are determined by patient responses and may include balancing analgesic and anxiolytic medications, using short-acting potent analgesics with longer-lasting "baseline" analgesics, employing local anesthetics, monitoring carefully for adverse effects, and paying attention to nonpharmacologic methods of anxiety reduction.

Oral Agents

Oral analgesics have the major benefit of painless administration but are difficult to titrate to effect. They are best used to provide a baseline of analgesia for mildly painful fractures. The following oral medications can be augmented during fracture reduction by hematoma block.

Codeine with or without acetaminophen, 1 to 2 mg/kg of codeine orally 30 to 60 minutes before casting (e.g., before obtaining radiographs) provides pain relief for mildly painful fractures.

Oxycodone with or without acetaminophen, 0.15 to 0.3 mg/kg of oxycodone orally 30 to 60 minutes before casting (e.g., before obtaining radiographs) may cause less nausea and vomiting than codeine.

Ketamine 6 to 10 mg/kg orally 30 minutes before casting provides mild analgesia, sedation, anxiolysis and amnesia but may require 1 to 2 hours for recovery.

Midazolam 0.5 to 0.75 mg/kg orally 20 to 30 minutes before casting provides anxiolysis with mild sedation and amnesia.

Inhalational Agent

Nitrous oxide 50% inhaled, blended with oxygen, painlessly and safely provides rapid anxiolysis, moderate analgesia, and amnesia in 90% of patients. Recovery occurs within 5 minutes of cessation of administration. Nitrous oxide can be used as a single agent for reduction and casting, or, for moderately to severely painful fractures, can be combined with a fracture hematoma block. The commonly available apparatus for nitrous oxide administration uses a demand valve and is limited in use to children older than 4 to 8 years of age; however, if a continuous circuit apparatus is available, nitrous oxide may be effectively administered to younger children.

Local Anesthetics

Lidocaine is the preferred anesthetic for local blocks because its short half-life enables neurologic reexamination before discharge and because systemic toxicity is less than longer-acting agents such as bupivacaine. Provision of analgesia with local infiltration of lidocaine may significantly lessen the need for or extent of sedation for painful procedures.

Fracture Hematoma Block This technique has been shown to manage forearm and ankle fracture pain effectively. Using sterile technique, the fracture hematoma is first partially aspirated to confirm correct needle position. The hematoma is then slowly injected with 1 to 4 mg/kg of 1 to 2% lidocaine. Although sufficient analgesia may be provided within 15 minutes with this technique, many children benefit from sedation with nitrous oxide or midazolam. Use of oral analgesics may aid in controlling prereduction and postreduction pain. Although complications associated with hematoma blocks are rare, they include infection, temporary interosseous nerve paralysis, and compartment syndrome. A comparison in adults of hematoma block without sedation to regional intravenous anesthesia found greater pain with the hematoma block.

Axillary Block Transarterial axillary nerve block using 5 mg/kg of 1% lidocaine has been shown to provide analgesia and muscle relaxation for reduction of forearm fractures. Although it is likely children would benefit from adjunctive sedation, the benefits of this practice have not been reported. While this technique requires careful placement of lidocaine in the axillary nerve sheath, its advantages include lack of need for intravenous access and provision of analgesia for the entire forearm. Rapid recovery allows neurovascular reexamination before discharge. Contraindications include coagulopathy, infection of overlying skin or lymph nodes and, neurologic abnormality of the extremity.

Intravenous Regional Anesthesia (Bier Block) This technique has been successful in the management of forearm fractures. After venous access has been obtained in the dorsum of the hand or the antecubital fossa of the fractured arm, the fractured forearm is exsanguinated by elevation or by gentle wrapping with an elastic bandage. A single or double tourniquet (often a blood pressure cuff) is then applied on the upper arm and inflated to 225 to 250 mm Hg. Lidocaine (1 to 5 mg/kg, 0.125 to 0.5%) is next infused over 1 minute into the fractured arm. After 10 to 15 minutes, the arm is anesthetized and the fracture reduction can be performed. After satisfactory reduction, the cuff is deflated either in a single release or multiple releases, and the patient is observed for 15 to 60 minutes. Use of 1 to 1.5 mg/kg lidocaine diluted to 0.125% (mini-dose Bier block) has been shown to be effective, enabling rapid release of the tourniquet without systemic toxicity and requiring only brief postrelease observation. A comparison in adults of regional intravenous anesthesia to hematoma block without sedation found greater pain with the hematoma block.

This technique may be less effective for elbow and hand fractures. Patients may benefit from adjunctive sedation and hematoma block. Disadvantages include the need for vascular access in the fractured arm and, by some protocols, the need for a second "safety" IV in other than the injured arm, and the potential toxicity from excess lidocaine release. An experienced health care provider must be dedicated to assuring the tourniquet remains inflated. This technique is contraindicated in patients with seizure disorders, underlying heart block, or sickle cell disease.

Intramuscular Agents

Demerol, Phenergan, and Thorazine   The combination of meperidine (Demerol), promethazine (Phenergan), and chlorpromazine (Thorazine) (DTP) for fracture reduction is discouraged because of its high rate of therapeutic failure, serious adverse reactions, and protracted sedation. Other agents provide better analgesia and sedation profiles.

Ketamine   Intramuscular ketamine, 4 mg/kg, has been shown to produce effective dissociation and analgesia to enable fracture reduction. Onset to dissociation is usually within 5 to 10 minutes and recovery by 120 to 180 minutes.

Intravenous Agents

Morphine   Morphine administered intravenously, 0.1 to 0.2 mg/kg, titrated to the effect of pain relief, is the "standard" for analgesia. Its rapid onset and long effect enable early and ongoing pain relief. However, when additional administration of a benzodiazepine is required for anxiolysis, prolonged respiratory depression may occur.

Fentanyl/Midazolam or Ketamine/Midazolam   Comparison of intravenous fentanyl/midazolam with ketamine/midazolam administered for emergency orthopedic fracture reduction and joint relocations found that ketamine/midazolam was more effective than fentanyl/midazolam for relief of pain and anxiety in children. Respiratory depression occurred less frequently with ketamine/midazolam than with fentanyl/midazolam (6% vs. 25% transiently had oxygen saturations less than 90% while breathing room air), but respiratory support may be needed with either regimen. Both regimens were effective in facilitating fracture reduction (> 98%) and producing amnesia in nearly all children. Vomiting occurred more frequently with ketamine/midazolam than with fentanyl/midazolam, and emergence dysphoria occurred in small and statistically equivalent numbers with both regimens.

Nondisplaced Fractures (Fig. 34.1)

For fractures to be casted in place, oral pain medications are frequently effective. Because absorption takes 30 to 60 minutes, early administration, e.g., before radiographic evaluation, enhances efficacy and efficiency. Painful nondisplaced fractures such as tibial fractures may require parenteral medication such as morphine or fentanyl during casting. Anxious children may also benefit from oral anxiolytics such as midazolam or ketamine 20 to 30 minutes before casting.

Angulated Fractures (Fig. 34.2)

Simple Reductions Fractures that require straightening with a single maneuver may be effectively managed by several regimens. Effective regimens include use of nitrous oxide with hematoma blocks, intravenous regional blocks, axillary blocks, intramuscular ketamine, intravenous ketamine/midazolam, or intravenous fentanyl/midazolam.

Displaced Fractures and Difficult Reductions (Fig. 34.3)

Displaced fractures of the distal radius and/or ulna frequently require painful manipulation during reduction. These patients require deeper levels of sedation or effective local or regional anesthesia along with anxiolysis. Use of intravenous regional anesthesia (Bier block), intramuscular ketamine, or intravenous fentanyl/midazolam or ketamine/midazolam have all been shown to provide effective pain management for reduction of these fractures. Hematoma blocks may augment these methods of sedation by lessening the need for sedation and its related respi-

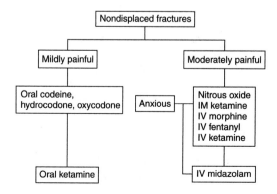

Figure 34.1. Sedation/analgesia options for nondisplaced fraction reduction.

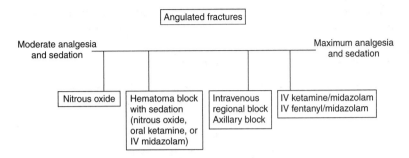

Figure 34.2. Sedation/analgesia options for angulated fracture reduction.

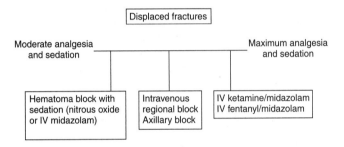

Figure 34.3. Sedation/analgesia options for displaced fracture reduction.

ratory depression. Nitrous oxide with a hematoma block may enable reduction of some of these fractures; however, more failures with this technique have been reported compared with the techniques above.

JOINT RELOCATION

Approach and special considerations

Joint dislocations and reductions are painful and frightening. Radial head (nursemaid's elbow), phalangeal, and patellar dislocations can optimally be managed with nitrous oxide alone, especially in younger patients if a continuous circuit apparatus is available. Alternatives include use of oral agents or digital blocks for anxious patients. Management of shoulder, elbow (e.g., ulna fracture with radial head dislocation [Monteggia's fracture]), hip, knee, and ankle dislocations usually requires deeper levels of sedation with intramuscular or intravenous agents. Regional intravenous anesthesia and axillary or hematoma blocks tend to be less effective because of the anatomic locations of these injuries.

ARTHROCENTESIS

Approach and Special Considerations

Aspiration of septic joints or those distended by blood can be frightening and painful. Use of local anesthesia usually provides adequate analgesia, but many patients benefit from additional judicious use of an anxiolytic agent such as nitrous oxide, midazolam, or low-dose ketamine. Patients should be monitored according to the level of sedation achieved, particularly in darkened fluoroscopy rooms. Parental presence during the procedure can also lessen anxiety.

SUGGESTED READING

General

Christoph RA, Buchanan L, Begalia K, et al. Pain reduction in local anesthetic administration through pH buffering. Ann Emerg Med 1988;17:117–120.

Committee on Drugs. Guidelines for monitoring and management of pediatric patients during and after sedation for diagnostic and therapeutic procedures. Pediatrics 1992;89: 1110–1115.

Graff KJ, Kennedy RM, Jaffe DM. Conscious sedation for pediatric orthopaedic emergencies. Pediatr Emerg Care 1996;12:31–35.

Kennedy RM, Porter FL, Miller JP, et al. Comparison of fentanyl/midazolam to ketamine/midazolam for pediatric orthopedic emergencies. Pediatrics (in press).

Maxwell LG, Yaster M. The myth of conscious sedation. Arch Pediatr Adolesc Med 1996;150:665–667.

Varela CD, Lorfing KC, Schmidt TL. Intravenous sedation for the closed reduction of fractures in children. J Bone and Joint Surg 1995;77–A:340–345.

Weisman SJ, Bernstein B, Schechter NL. Consequences of inadequate analgesia during painful procedures in children. Arch Pediatr Adolesc Med. 1998;152:147–149.

Hematoma Block

Alioto RJ, Furia JP, Marquardt JD. Hematoma block for ankle fractures: a safe and efficacious technique for manipulations. J Ortho Trauma 1995;9:113–116..

Hennrikus WL, Shin AY, Klingelberger CE, et al. Self-administered nitrous oxide analgesia combined with hematoma block for outpatient reductions of fractures in children. J Bone Joint Surg 1995;77:335–339.

Johnson PQ, Noffsinger MA. Hematoma Block of distal forearm fractures. Is it safe? Ortho Rev 1991;20(11):977–979.

Meining RP, Quick A, Lobmeyer L. Plasma lidocaine levels following hematoma block for distal radius fractures. J Ortho Trauma 1989;3(3):187–191.

Intravenous (Bier) Block

Abbaszadegan H, Jonsson U. Regional anesthesia preferable for Colles' fracture: controlled comparison with local anesthesia. Acta Ortho Scand 1990;61(4):348–349.

Blasier RD, White R. Intravenous regional anesthesia for management of children's extremity fractures in the emergency department. Pediatr Emerg Care 1996;12(6):404–406.

Blyth MJG, Kinninmonth AWG, Asante DK. Bier's block: a change of injection site. J Trauma 1995;39:726–728.

Bolte P, Stevens S, Scott J, et al. Mini-dose Bier block intravenous regional anesthesia in the emergency department treatment of pediatric upper-extremity injuries. J Pediatr Ortho 1994;14:534–537.

Colizza WA, Said E. Intravenous regional anesthesia in the treatmnent of forearm and wrist fractures and dislocations in children. Can J Surg 1993;36:225–228.

Juliano J, Mazur R, Cummings W, et al. Low-dose lidocaine intravenous regional anesthesia for forearm fractures in children. J Pediatr Ortho 1992;12:633–635.

Axillary Block

Cramer KE, Glasson S, Mencio G, et al. Reduction of forearm fractures in children using axillary block anesthesia. J Ortho Trauma 1995;9:407–410.

Chapter 35
Skin and Soft Tissue Procedures

Michael Gerardi

Soft tissue procedures are painful and sometimes frightening for a child. Local anesthetics and field blocks usually provide adequate analgesia. However, to optimally manage these procedures, procedural sedation is often required to 1) alleviate a patient's fear and enhance cooperation, 2) improve the overall degree of analgesia, and 3) facilitate the administration of local anesthetic agents. The decision whether to use procedural sedation is predicated on the response to specific considerations (Table 35.1).

FOREIGN-BODY REMOVAL

Removal of a foreign body often becomes more difficult than one initially expects. It is probably better to assume that foreign-body identification and removal will be difficult and therefore provide more than adequate anesthesia from the onset. Local anesthetic should be infiltrated in large enough of an area to allow extension of wound margins if necessary to search for and retrieve the foreign matter. This is especially important with wounds involving the hands in which one not only has to explore for debris but also directly visualize tendons and ligaments to evaluate for lacerations.

When possible, an anesthetic with epinephrine should be used because it will cause local vasospasm and help decrease blood flow into the wound and, thus, enhance visibility. When a foreign body is located in a particularly sensitive area (eyelids, face, soles of feet, etc.), sedation before local anesthesia may be necessary. Sedation should also be strongly considered for procedures that are more likely to provoke anxiety, such as repairs and wound explorations about the eyes, nose, face, and genital area.

INGROWN TOENAIL REMOVAL

Special attention should be paid to guaranteeing adequate digital block because anything less than 100% local anesthesia will lead to patient pain and resistance. Unfortunately, it is sometimes difficult to apply adequate local nerve blocks to the

Table 35.1.   Decision Analysis for Pharmacologic Management

1. Why is sedation needed in the first place? Is the procedure painful and frightening or does it require extreme cooperation?
2. Are the risks of sedation appropriate for the procedure involved?
3. Do the parents consent to the use of sedation?
4. How long will the procedure take? If it is a short procedure, is it worth the added risk and expense to the patient? If it is a long procedure, is there an appropriate agent that can be titrated to allow adequate sedation throughout the entire length of the procedure?
5. Are there significant side effects that limit the usefulness of a particular drug?
6. Are there enough nurses and support personnel present to safely allow the use of sedation?
7. What is the recovery period for a given agent? Are there enough treatment areas and staff in the emergency department to allow adequate observation during recovery?
8. When had the child last eaten? Is a delay in waiting for a sufficient fasting time worth the time lost in caring for the wound?

digits. The situation is often complicated by induration and sometimes concomitant infection. These cause the digit to be swollen and extremely tender. If a delay has occurred in seeking medical attention, the pain is exacerbated by recruitment of neuronal c-fibers that amplify the pain from the wound. Inadequate digital block will make it impossible to perform the procedure.

The local anesthetic applied as a digital block should be used in generous amounts to ensure adequate anesthesia. The more distal the wound, the more critical it is to be certain to get the inferior digital nerves to assure distal anesthesia of the digit. Many times, initial infiltration of local anesthetic is unsuccessful in providing adequate anesthesia. In this case, repeat infiltration of anesthetic should proceed until the patient has nothing but mild pressure sensations without pain sensations.

Ingrown toenails, contused digits, and subungual hematomas continue to cause pain after the nail removal and drainage. Therefore, longer-acting agents such as bupivacaine should be considered in these situations. Longer-acting agents last longer (in hours) but take a longer time to infiltrate into the nerves; therefore, one should allow adequate time (10 to 15 minutes) for adequate anesthesia after the injection.

BURN DEBRIDEMENT

Using local anesthetics to provide adequate analgesia over large surface areas is nearly impossible. Therefore, systemic analgesia is required to provide adequate analgesia. Because of the severe emotional stress often accompanying the pain in acute burns, sedation may also be needed.

Morphine sulfate is the analgesic that is most easily titrated and administered in acute situations. Morphine sulfate 0.1 to 0.2 mg/kg should be administered intravenously or intramuscularly as soon as possible to alleviate the severe pain associated with burns. In the absence of intravenous access, intramuscular morphine is remarkably effective, although not as easy to titrate as via the intravenous route.

Sometimes, the pain is so severe in these situations that parenteral opioids alone in traditional doses do not relieve the pain. Burn patients are also frequently terrified, which makes pain control more difficult. Therefore, adjunctive medications can be of great assistance. Hydromorphone has more of an anxiolytic effect than other opioids; therefore, it is effective in situations in which emotional distress is contributing significantly to the pain.

Benzodiazepines are effective anxiolytics and can be used as adjunctive synergistic agents to alleviate anxiety and decrease the total amount of opioids required for adequate pain relief. Midazolam has amnestic as well as anxiolytic effects, which make it an ideal adjunctive drug in painful crises.

Ketamine is particularly effective and useful in burn patients. It provides the ideal qualities of sedation, analgesia, and amnesia with an excellent cardiorespiratory profile for the painful burn debridement and dressing process.

ABSCESS INCISION AND DRAINAGE

Abscesses are wounds that need special attention because of the extreme sensitivity and pain directly over the wound as well as in the deep and surrounding tissues. Because of the induration accompanying abscesses, pain is exaggerated with manipulation of the abscess, removal of loculated fluid collection, and packing. In addition, abscesses tend to occur in areas that are more sensitive to manipulation such as the axilla, perineum, and perirectal tissues. Application of local anesthetic to these abscesses is extremely painful and, therefore, precautions should be taken to minimize the discomfort associated with application of the local anesthetic.

Furthermore, if an abscess is larger or deeper than a superficial follicular abscess, parenteral sedation and analgesia should be considered. Options include oral or parenteral analgesia with an opioid, benzodiazepine sedation, a combination of both (especially with a perirectal abscess), or nitrous oxide. Once a patient has been adequately sedated or given enough opioid to diminish sensitivity to manipulation, local anesthetic techniques can be employed.

Before infiltrating local anesthetic into the site of drainage, ice or a local vapocoolant spray may be used to desensitize the area. The pain from the local injection of an abscess can be so severe that it cannot be tolerated, which is the reason systemic analgesia and sedation are indicated.

Rather than injecting directly into the pointing area of an abscess, the local anesthesia can be given as a field block. The advantage of this technique is that this avoids injecting anesthetic into the most sensitive area of the wound. A field block has the added advantages of allowing the extension of the incision site to facilitate lysis of loculations, giving the option of wider exploration, and decreasing the pain with packing.

Iontophoresis can also be used proximal to the abscess or over it as an adjunctive anesthetic before local anesthesia and during the procedure.

SUGGESTED READING

Abramowicz M, ed. Drugs for pain. Medical Letter Jan 1993;35:887.

Algren JT, Algren C. Sedation and analgesia for minor pediatric procedures. Ped Emerg Care 1996;12(6):435–441.

Baraff LJ. Conscious sedation of children (editorial). Ann Emerg Med 1994;24:1170–1172.

Baxter JK. Stewart smiled (letter). Pediatrics 1993;91(5):1018.

Coté CJ. Pediatric anesthesia. In: Miller RD, ed. Anesthesia, 4th ed. New York: Churchill Livingstone, 1994;2:2097–2124.

Coté CJ. Sedation for the pediatric patient: a review. Pediatr Clin North Am 1994;41(1):31–58.

Holzman RS, Cullen DJ, Eichhorn JH, et al. Guidelines for sedation by nonanesthesiologists during diagnostic and therapeutic procedures. J Clin Anesth 1994;6:265–276.

Ilkanipour K, Juels CR, Langdorf MI. Pediatric pain control and conscious sedation: a survey of emergency medicine residencies. Acad Emerg Med 1994;1:368–372.

Proudfoot J, Roberts M. Providing safe and effective sedation and analgesia for pediatric patients. Emerg Med Rep 1993;14(24).

Proudfoot J, Petrack E. The six skills of highly effective pediatric sedation. Ped Emerg Med Reports Aug 1997;2(8):79–90.

Sacchetti A, Schafermeyer R , Gerardi MJ, et al. Pediatric analgesia and sedation. Ann Emerg Med 1994;23:237–250.

Woolard DJ, Terndrup TE. Sedative-analgesic agent administration in children: analysis of use and complications in the emergency department. J Emerg Med 1994;12:453–461.

Yaster M. Pain relief (editorial). Pediatrics 1995;95(3):427–428.

Yealy DM. Acute pain management. Acad Emerg Med 1994;1(2):186–189.

Chapter 36
Lumbar Puncture and Bone Marrow Aspiration

Richard Bachur

LUMBAR PUNCTURE

Approach and Special Considerations

Despite the simplicity of the procedure, discussion of a lumbar puncture (LP) is anxiety provoking for parents and older children. Lumbar punctures have traditionally been performed with only local anesthesia in children and without any anesthesia in infants and toddlers. As with other procedures in infants, clinicians often convinced themselves that the injection of local anesthesia is no less painful than the actual spinal needle without anesthesia; therefore, the use of anesthesia would only prolong the procedure. In the older child as with an adult, local anesthesia alone can make the procedure painless; however, the success of the procedure depends on the voluntary maintenance of the patient's position or the experience and muscle of the "holder" to maintain the patient's position. Unfortunately, this dependence on cooperation or on the strength of the holder can often lead to unsuccessful or "traumatic" taps and certainly raises the risk of complications (e.g., dural tears, backache, radicular symptoms). Additionally, manometry during the procedure cannot be performed accurately in a struggling child.

Special consideration must be given to the proper positioning of the patient. The best position, either lateral decubitus or sitting, requires flexion of the spine. This flexion negatively impacts breathing by potentially causing upper airway obstruction, chest wall compression, and increased abdominal pressure. These effects may be exaggerated with any form of sedation. The negative physiologic effects are further magnified if the patient has any concurrent respiratory distress and is being forcefully restrained (held in *extreme* flexion or having the weight of an adult on the child's chest). Air hunger (secondary to positioning) with associated combativeness must be recognized, and alternatives to physical restraint must be considered. Additionally, the necessary positioning obviates the need for careful monitoring: the physician does not face the patient to observe the level of consciousness or color, and often sterile drapes blind the physician from chest wall motion, especially in young infants. Holders should be warned of the dangers of over-restraint, and proper monitoring should be employed, especially if any sedatives are given.

General Considerations

1. The use of sedation must always be weighed against any risk of the medications. The procedure should be performed with the least amount of pharmacologic intervention possible.
2. Experienced holders are necessary. Proper positioning of the patient, the physician, and the assistant is paramount for maintaining sterility, minimizing time to completion, and performing the LP successfully.
3. Topical/local anesthesia should be used in all cases except in the youngest infants in which it is optional.
4. Sedation should never be used in the absence of local anesthesia.
5. The ability to maintain proper positioning without excessive force should be the major determinant for use of sedation. The patient's response to injection of local anesthesia should *not* determine the need for using sedation or administering more sedation.

Factors Influencing the Extent of Pharmacologic Management (Fig. 36.1)

Age

Neonates and Young Infants LPS can usually be successfully and quickly performed without any local anesthesia. Topical anesthesia (EMLA) can be safely used in this age group. Local anesthesia (lidocaine 1%) may transiently make the spinous processes harder to palpate, especially if excessive amounts are given intradermally.

Toddlers and Older Children Except in extreme circumstances, local anesthesia is necessary. Topical anesthesia (EMLA) can be used, but it should always be followed by local anesthesia.

Anxiety Level The success of the procedure depends on the ability of the patient to be maintained in proper position. Anxiety after administration of local anesthesia is inversely related to the patient's understanding of its value. In the older child, anxiety diminishes, and in the young child, anxiety increases. If the child cannot cooperate or be held correctly by a trained assistant, pharmacologic sedation is indicated.

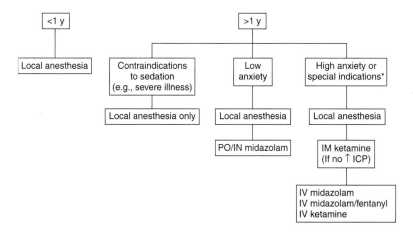

Figure 36.1. Sedation/analgesia options for lumbar puncture. Topical/local anesthesia should be used except in the youngest infants where it is optional. (*See text for special indications for lumbar puncture.)

Indication for the Procedure When cerebrospinal fluid pressure must be measured, the patient must be relaxed (ideally in only mild spinal flexion once the needle is properly positioned). Additionally, if medication is to be infused through a needle or catheter, the patient must be relatively motionless during the infusion to avoid extravasation. Finally, in cases in which diagnosis depends on a "clean" tap, the ability to maintain the patient's position is critical.

Severity of Illness This may dictate the urgency of the procedure, alter the level of consciousness, or influence the risk of pharmacologic intervention.

BONE MARROW ASPIRATION

Approach and Special Considerations

Bone marrow aspiration (BMA), with or without biopsy, is another relatively simple procedure that can be anxiety provoking for parents and older children. The procedure is potentially painful, never delicate, and, to the lay observer, can appear barbaric. Additionally, the need for the procedure already draws emotion from the parents because of the diagnostic possibilities. And because BMA is often the first of many procedures for a newly diagnosed patient with cancer, avoiding/treating unnecessary pain and anxiety is paramount.

The duration of the procedure is relatively short and does not require the patient to stay motionless. Because most BMAs are performed with the patient prone, the head cannot be maintained in a perfect neutral position; therefore, if an airway emergency occurs, the procedure should be aborted and the patient rolled supine.

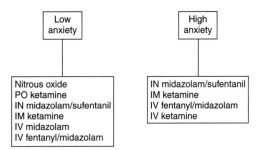

Figure 36.2. Sedation/analgesia options for bone marrow aspiration. Adequate local anesthesia is absolutely necessary.

The procedure requires excellent local anesthesia to the skin, soft tissues, and periosteum. Because multiple aspirations/biopsies are often done at a particular site, a wide area of local anesthesia must be given. Because BMAs are often done semielectively, topical anesthesia with EMLA should be used whenever possible.

Factors Influencing the Extent of Pharmacologic Management (Fig. 36.2)

Prior Experience with Other Procedures   For many patients, BMA is done repeatedly and, therefore, experience with prior sedation regimens may prove useful.

Physiologic Derangements   Patients who require BMA often have multisystem problems that may alter the response to sedation. Special consideration must be given to patients with the following:

- Tumors that affect the airway (including mediastinal masses)
- Severe anemia (with resulting congestive heart failure)
- Coagulopathies (avoid intramuscular administration)
- Increased intracranial pressure
- Renal and hepatic function, which affect metabolism/excretion of medications

SUGGESTED READING

Cote CJ. Sedation for the pediatric patient: a review. Pediatr Clin North Am 1994; 41:31–58.

Ferrari L, Barst S, Pratila M, et al. Anesthesia for diagnostic and therapeutic procedures in pediatric outpatients. Am J Pediatr Hematol-Oncol 1990;12(3):310–313.

Green SM, Nakamura R, Johnson NE. Ketamine sedation for pediatric procedures: Part 1, A prospective series. Ann Emerg Med 1990;19:1024–1032.

Green SM, Johnson NE. Ketamine sedation for pediatric procedures: part 2, review and implications. Ann Emerg Med 1990;19:1033–1046.

Henry DW, Burwinkle JW, Klutman NE. Determination of sedative and amnestic doses of lorazepam in children. Clin Pharmacol 1991;10(8):625–629.

Marx CM, Stein J, Tyler MK, et al. Ketamine-midazolam versus meperidine-midazolam for painful procedures in pediatric oncology patients. J Clin Oncol 1997;15(1):94–102.

Petrack EM, Marx CM, Wright MS. Intramuscular ketamine is superior to meperidine, promethazine, and chlorpromazine for pediatric emergency department sedation. Arch Pediatr Adolesc Med 1996;150(7):767–781.

Pinheiro JM, Furdon S, Ochoa LF. Role of local anesthesia during lumbar puncture in neonates. Pediatrics 1993;91(2):379–82.

Schecter NL, Weisman SJ, Rosenblum M, et al. The use of transmucosyl fentanyl citrate for painful procedures in children. Pediatrics 1995;95(3):335–339.

Chapter 37
Central Venous Catheter Placement

Richard Saladino

APPROACH AND SPECIAL CONSIDERATIONS

Indications for central venous catheter placement in the pediatric patient are many and include an urgent need for venous access in life-threatening illnesses and injuries, failure to gain peripheral access, central venous pressure monitoring, and administration of inotropic medicines (such as epinephrine and dopamine) and venoirritants (such as calcium chloride).

As a general approach, placement of a central venous catheter will be in one of two contexts. The very ill or multiply injured child will require local analgesia at the site of placement, but will likely not require a significant degree of sedation. Sedative medications may complicate management and be contraindicated in patients with shock. However, children who are more alert and aware of their surroundings will certainly benefit from both a local anesthetic and systemic sedation.

Sites of Catheterization

The three common sites used for central venous catheter placement in the pediatric patient are the femoral, subclavian, and internal jugular veins. By far, the preferred and most often used access site in the child is the femoral vein. Regardless, local anesthesia is indicated and easily applied.

For femoral vein catheter placement, the use of a local anesthetic may preclude the need for sedation, especially in the older child (Fig. 37.1). Conversely, because of the proximity to the face, an approach to the neck or subclavian veins will more likely require anxiolysis and sedation, regardless of age.

Urgency

In the very ill or injured child, response to pain may not be readily apparent; however, local anesthesia should always be used. Local infiltration of lidocaine (0.5 to 1%)

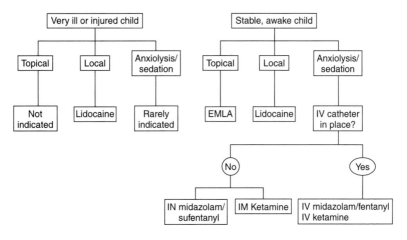

Figure 37.1. Sedation/analgesia options for central venous catheterization.

is sufficient in these cases and rarely requires more than 15 to 45 seconds to apply. The duration of action of lidocaine will outlast the time required for the procedure.

In the less significantly ill or injured child, an anxiolytic or sedative agent or both preceding local anesthesia and the actual procedure will reduce anxiety and provide a more cooperative patient. This will enhance the success rate and therefore reduce the time to complete the procedure. A short-acting agent such as midazolam may provide sufficient calming to proceed with the procedure. The addition of fentanyl is rarely necessary, but in combination with midazolam will provide anxiolysis and sedation in the uncooperative patient, especially those requiring subclavian or internal jugular venous catheterization. If a peripheral venous catheter has not been or cannot be placed, anxiolysis and sedation may be accomplished via the intranasal route of administration. Midazolam and sufentanil can be used in combination and titrated to effect. Alternatively, in appropriate clinical situations, ketamine can be administered intramuscularly for sedation. If time permits, a topical anesthetic such as EMLA during the preparation time may reduce the need for both local and systemic analgesia and sedation.

Underlying Circulatory and Respiratory Function

The very ill or injured child may have compromise of both circulatory and respiratory functions. In addition, such patients may have a degree of obtundation. Local anesthesia is indicated, but anxiolytics and sedative agents may further embarrass respiratory effort or blood pressure or both, and should be avoided. Somewhat less ill patients may in fact be agitated and will benefit from systemic sedation and/or analgesia. Small doses should be titrated to effect, and the patient should be carefully monitored throughout the procedure.

SUGGESTED READING

Harrison N, Langham BT, Bogod DG. Appropriate use of local anaesthetic for venous cannulation. Anaesthesia 1992;47:210–212.

Langham BT, Harrison DA. Local anaesthetic: does it reduce the pain of insertion of all sizes of venous cannula? Anaesthesia 1992;47:890–891.

Selby IR, Bowles BJM. Analgesia for venous cannulation: a comparison of EMLA (5 minutes application), lignocaine, ethyl chloride, and nothing. J Royal Soc Med 1995;88:264–267.

Selby IR, Bowles BJM. Analgesia for venous cannulation (letter). J Royal Soc Med 1996; 89:237.

Van Wijk MGF, Smalhout B. A post-operative analysis of the patient's view of anaesthesia in a Netherlands' teaching hospital. Anaesthesia 1990;45:679–682.

Chapter 38
Radiologic Imaging

Kathleen Brown

Children who present to outpatient medical settings will frequently need non-elective radiologic imaging as part of their evaluation or treatment. These procedures will often require a degree of patient cooperation that even a well child would find difficult. Children who are in pain, frightened, anxious, or confused secondary to their illness or injury will have an even greater difficulty cooperating for these procedures. In addition, the radiographic procedure itself may be uncomfortable or painful and therefore require sedation or analgesia (e.g., aspiration of a hip joint under fluoroscopy).

FACTORS INFLUENCING THE EXTENT OF PHARMACOLOGIC MANAGEMENT

The Study Being Performed

The degree of sedation and/or analgesia required for radiographic imaging studies will vary greatly depending on the specific imaging study being performed and the length of time it takes to perform the study. A child without a painful injury who requires a plain radiographic will almost never need sedation or analgesia. However a child who requires fluoroscopy-guided aspiration of the hip joint will most likely require both sedation and systemic and local analgesia. Young children, even if they are cooperative, will rarely be able to hold still long enough to obtain an abdominal computed tomography (CT). Studies that last longer than a few minutes, such as magnetic resonance imaging (MRI), will require sedation even in older children or adults.

The Patient's Acute Illness or Injury

A patient with a severe head injury who is unconscious will normally not require any sedation to obtain a head CT. However, a patient with a head injury who is combative may require considerable sedation. A patient with a painful injury such as an extremity fracture may require sedation and/or analgesia to obtain even plain radiographs.

The Patient's Age

Infants and toddlers will often require sedation for nonpainful procedures such as a head CT because they are developmentally unable to cooperate sufficiently to remain motionless for even brief periods of time. School-aged children will usually be able to cooperate for painless radiographic procedures without any sedation.

The Patient's Anxiety Level

An infant who is sleeping because it is nap time will often be able to undergo a CT scan without any sedation. One who is awake and frightened will most likely require sedation to cooperate for the same study.

COMPUTED TOMOGRAPHY

Computed Tomography of the Head

A CT scan of the brain is a painless procedure that requires the patient to remain motionless for a relatively brief period. The most common reason for obtaining a noncontrast head CT scan in the outpatient setting is to rule out intracranial hemorrhage secondary to trauma. Spiral CT scanners can obtain a study of the head in less than 3 minutes, whereas older generation scanners may take 10 to 15 minutes to obtain the same scan. If a contrast scan is required, then the study will take significantly longer. Cooperative older (more than 3 years) children are often able to perform this task without difficulty and no sedation is needed. The commonly encountered reasons why a child may be uncooperative for a CT of the head are listed in Table 38.1 and the sedation/analgesia options are outlined in Figure 38.1.

Abdominal Computed Tomography

Abdominal CT is a painless procedure that requires the patient to remain motionless for a longer period than for a CT of the head. Nonelective abdominal CT is used for the evaluation of trauma, abdominal masses, and as part of the diagnostic evaluation for other medical or surgical conditions. An optimal abdominal CT scan will also require that the patient receive oral and/or intravenous contrast. Oral medications should be avoided in patients with suspected abdominal injuries or disorders. Trauma patients will often need a CT of the head in addition to the

Table 38.1.   Factors Affecting a Child's Ability to Remain Motionless for a Head CT

1. Developmentally incapable
     Young age
     Developmental delay
2. Anxiety
     Strange environment
     Nature of their injury or illness
     Parental/staff anxiety
3. Pain
     Acute injury or illness
     The presence of immobilization devices
     Coexisting painful procedures
4. Altered level of consciousness
     Head Injury
     Intoxication
     CNS infection
     Seizure activity

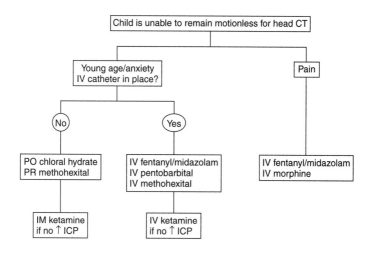

Figure 38.1. Sedation/analgesia options for head computed tomography. *ICP,* intracranial pressure.

abdominal CT. In this case, the flow diagram for sedation of the child who requires a CT of the head should be used.

ULTRASOUND

Outpatient nonelective ultrasound may be done as part of the diagnostic evaluation for appendicitis, pyloric stenosis, renal abnormalities, or pregnancy. The performance of a diagnostic ultrasound is usually not painful and does not require the patient to remain motionless. Therefore, this study is generally well tolerated. Most children are able to cooperate sufficiently to produce an adequate study without pharmacologic management. However, children who are extremely anxious, or in pain, especially if the pain involves the area to be imaged, may require some sedation or analgesia in order to cooperate (Fig. 38.2).

BARIUM ENEMA

A barium enema is performed as part of the diagnostic evaluation of appendicitis, intussusception, malrotation with volvulus, inflammatory bowel disease, or other lower gastrointestinal disease processes. A barium enema is also the definitive treatment for the patient with an intussusception. Infants and toddlers with intussusception are often lethargic secondary to their disease process and will rarely

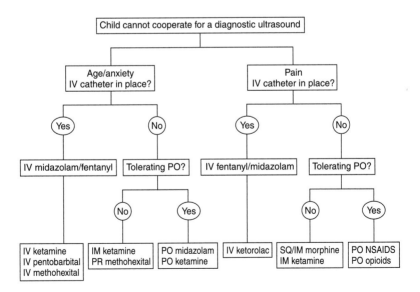

Figure 38.2. Sedation/analgesia options for diagnostic ultrasound. *NSAIDs,* nonsteroidal anti-inflammatory drugs; *SQ,* subcutaneous.

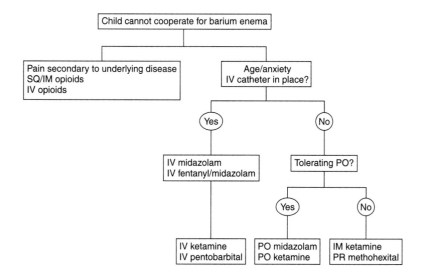

Figure 38.3. Sedation/analgesia options for barium enema. *SQ,* subcutaneous.

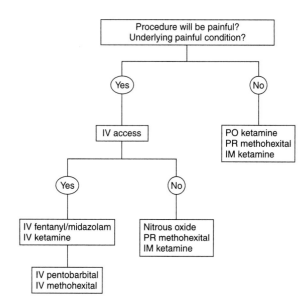

Figure 38.4. Sedation/analgesia options for fluoroscopy-guided procedures. Local anesthesia should be used in all cases.

need sedation to perform a barium enema. Patients with other suspected gastrointestinal disease processes who need a barium enema will often be in pain. Coupled with the discomfort produced by the procedure, sedation and analgesia are often needed to perform the barium enema (Fig. 38.3). These patients will almost always have suspected gastrointestinal disorders and often will have vomiting as a symptom, thus the oral route for medication should be avoided.

FLUOROSCOPY-GUIDED PROCEDURES

Children who need a fluoroscopy-guided procedure will almost always require sedation and/or analgesia (Fig. 38.4). The most common reason for fluoroscopy is aspiration of a septic joint, which is most commonly the hip. These patients will be in pain, and the procedure itself is painful. Intravenous agents are preferred in this setting.

SUGGESTED READING

Sedation/Analgesia for Radiographic Imaging

Egelhoff JC, Ball WS, Koch BL, et al. Safety and efficacy of sedation in children using a structured sedation program. AJR 1997;168:1259–1262.

Frush DP, Bisset GS. Sedation of children for emergency imaging. Rad Clin North Am 1997;35:789– 797.

Kucera ED, Karmazyn B, Cohen MD, et al. Imaging modalities in pediatric oncology. Rad Clin North Am 1997;35:1281–1300.

Louon A, Reddy VG. Nasal midazolam and ketamine for paediatric sedation during computerized tomography. Acta Anesth Scand 1994;38:259–261.

Murphy MS. Sedation for invasive procedures in pediatrics. Arch Dis Child 1997;77:281–284.

Sacchetti A, Schafermeyer R, Gerardi M, et al. Pediatric analgesia and sedation. Ann Emerg Med 1994;23:237–250.

Specific Sedation/Analgesia Agents

AAP Committee on Drugs and Committee on Environmental Health. Use of chloral hydrate for sedation in children. Pediatrics 1993;92:471–473.

Chudnofsky CR, Wright SW, Dronen SC, et al. The safety of IV fentanyl use in the emergency department. Ann Emerg Med 1989;18:635–639.

Connors KM, Terndrup TE. Nasal versus oral midazolam for sedation of anxious children undergoing laceration repair. Ann Emerg Med 1994;24:1074–1079.

Dachs RJ, Innes GM. Intravenous Ketamine sedation of pediatric patients in the emergency department. Ann Emerg Med 1997;29:146–150.

Gamis AS, Knapp JF, Glenski JL. Nitrous oxide analgesia in the pediatric ED. Ann Emerg Med 1989;18:177–181.

Greenberg SB, Faerber EN, Aspinall CL, et al. High-dose chloral hydrate sedation for children undergoing MR imaging: safety and efficacy in relation to age. AJR 1993;161:639–41.

Hennes HM, Wagner V, Bonadio WA, et al. The effect of oral midazolam on anxiety of preschool children during laceration repair. Ann Emerg Med 1990;19:1006–1009.

Malis DJ, Burton DM. Safe pediatric outpatient sedation: The chloral hydrate debate revisited. Otolaryngol Head Neck Surg 1997;116:53–57.

Parker RI, Mahan RA, Gugliano D. Efficacy and safety of intravenous midazolam and ketamine as sedation for therapeutic and diagnostic procedures in children. Pediatrics 1997;99:427–431.

Quereshi FA, Mellis PT, McFadden MA. Efficacy of oral ketamine for providing sedation and analgesia to children requiring laceration repair. Pediatr Emerg Care 1995;11:33–37.

Stewart RD. Nitrous oxide sedation/analgesia in emergency medicine. Ann Emerg Med 1985; 14:139–148.

White PF, Way WL, Trevor A. Ketamine its pharmacology and therapeutic uses. Anesth 1982;56:119–136.

Wright SW, Chudnofsky CR, Dronen SC et al. Midazolam use in the emergency department. Am J Emerg Med 1990;8:97–100.

Index